Review of Radiologic Physics

Review of Radiologic Physics

Walter Huda, Ph.D.
Associate Professor of Radiology
  and Director of Medical Physics
University of Florida College of Medicine
Gainesville, Florida

Richard M. Slone, M.D.
Assistant Professor of Radiology
Mallinckrodt Institute of Radiology
Washington University School of Medicine
St. Louis, Missouri

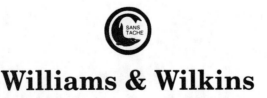

Williams & Wilkins

BALTIMORE • PHILADELPHIA • HONG KONG
LONDON • MUNICH • SYDNEY • TOKYO
A WAVERLY COMPANY

Acquisitions Editor: Elizabeth A. Nieginski
Project Editor: Amy G. Dinkel
Production Coordinator: Marette D. Magargle

Copyright © 1995
Williams & Wilkins
Suite 5025
Rose Tree Corporate Center
Building Two
Media, PA 19063 USA

Printed in the United States of America.

Library of Congress Cataloging-in-Publication Data

Huda, Walter.
    Review of radiologic physics / by Walter Huda, Richard M. Slone.
      p. cm.
    Includes bibliographical references and index.
    ISBN 0-683-04230-0
    1. Radiology, Medical—Outlines, syllabi, etc. 2. Medical
physics—Outlines, syllabi, etc. I. Slone, Richard M. II. Title.
    [DNLM: 1. Health Physics—examination questions. WN 18 H883r
1994]
R896.5.H83   1994
616.07'54'076—dc20
DNLM/DLC
for Library of Congress

           94-25711
           CIP

    95 96 97 98
1 2 3 4 5 6 7 8 9 10

Dedication

To my parents,
Stefan and Paraskevia Huda, for their
resolute support and encouragement

Walter Huda

To my son, Logan, who loves books, and to my wife, April,
for her support

Richard Slone

Ordinary language is totally unsuited for expressing what physics really asserts, since the words of everyday life are not sufficiently abstract. Only mathematics and mathematical logic can say as little as the physicist means to say.

—Bertrand Russell

X-rays: their moral is this—that a right way of looking at things will see through almost anything.

—Samuel Butler

Contents

Acknowledgments

Radiology residents taking the review course on which this book is based supplied valuable information about the written exams and comments on the appropriateness of the text and accompanying questions. Grateful thanks go to all these ex-residents including David Bulley, Cathy Carruthers, Maria Chiechi, Timothy Daniels, Cheryl DeBose, Kelly Diamond, Deborah Dipersio, Eugene Erquiaga, Catherine Johnson, Glen Jung, Stephen Kennedy, Jong Kim, Barry Kraus, Sylvester Lee, Allen Powell, Robert Quarles, Chuck Scheil, Nanette Schuerer, Kevin Shamlou, Hilda Sambuk, Richard Steinman, Brett Storm, Roger Tart, Margaret Weeks, Karl Weingarten, and Carol Younathan.

The creation of examination questions that test comprehension without introducing ambiguity is non-trivial. All of the questions in this book were tested on experienced imaging physicists. Those that they could not immediately answer were presumed to be unclear or ambiguous, and removed. Our special thanks go to the following physicists who willingly took on the onerous task of reviewing most of the text and questions contained in this book: Jim Atherton, Jeff Bews, John Schreiner, and Wil van der Putten. Appreciation is also offered to the following individuals who conscientiously reviewed the specialty chapters: Pat Abbitt, Kyongtae Bae, Ray Ballinger, Cliff Belden, Richard Briggs, Raymond Carrier, Patrick Datoc, Geoff Dean, Larry Filipow, Jeff Fitzsimmons, Janice Honeyman, Terry James, Stephen Kennedy, Tom Pilgram, Dan Rickey, Shailendra Shukla, Barbara Steinbach, and Martin Yaffe. Valuable input pertaining to the technologist's perspective on radiologic physics was supplied by Dean Ann Brake, Gary Brink, Ed Dice, Karen Dodge, Johnnie Moore, and Carole Palmer. Guoying Qu and Zhenxue Jing are credited for their conscientious review of the penultimate version of this text. All remaining ambiguities, errors, and omissions clearly remain the responsibility of the authors.

A large vote of thanks is due to Christine Hoppock for expert manuscript preparation, editorial support, and diligent project management through countless manuscript revisions. Thanks are also due to Evelyn Cairns for pioneering the initial draft.

Introduction

I. What Is Radiologic Physics?

Radiology is arguably the most technology dependent specialty in medicine, and it has seen monumental changes over the past decade. Computer integration with constant technical innovations has changed the workplace and influenced the role radiology plays in the diagnosis and treatment of disease. Radiologists and technologists need to understand the technology and the physical principles that constitute the advantages, govern the limitations, and determine the risks of the equipment they use.

Radiologic physics is not an esoteric subject of abstract equations and memorized definitions, but rather the total process of creating and viewing a diagnostic image. This process is influenced by a range of physical principles that need to be comprehended to better understand their clinical applications. Radiologic physics covers the important medical imaging modalities of radiographic and fluoroscopic imaging, mammography, computed tomography (CT), magnetic resonance imaging (MRI), nuclear medicine, and ultrasound.

All imaging modalities have a "cost" associated with their use. MRI and ultrasound do not have any specific risks, and the cost is generally the time required to perform the study. For modalities that employ ionizing radiation, one of the costs is the radiation dose to the patient and staff working with these systems. Accordingly, radiation protection principles are important. Radiologists and technologists should understand the quantitative magnitude of the radiation dose to the patient and personnel exposed and be able to ensure that radiation levels are kept *as low as reasonably achievable* (ALARA principle) and within regulatory limits.

II. Why Study Radiologic Physics?

Both residents and technologists need to acquire an understanding of the underlying imaging science for each diagnostic modality and be able to pass their respective radiologic physics exams. However, it is important to appreciate that neither will actually practice physics, and there is no need to learn how to measure modulation transfer function curves in screen/film radiography, write programs to perform filtered back projection algorithms in CT, or design radio frequency pulses for fat suppression in MRI.

It is important, however, for well-rounded radiologists and technologists to have a basic understanding of (1) image quality parameters, such as noise, spatial resolution, and contrast; (2) how image quality is affected by radiographic techniques; (3) how to evaluate commercial imaging equipment in terms of its ability to perform the required patient examinations; (4) the radiation dose and risks associated with radiographic exposure; and (5) how to communicate with medical physicists and service personnel regarding imaging problems.

The focus of the text and allied questions is on the physics underlying the creation of clinical images, with particular emphasis on the factors impacting image quality, notably image contrast, spatial resolution, and noise. Residents and technologists need to understand the achievable performance of imaging systems and how this equipment should best be used to solve specific patient imaging problems.

III. Review Book Structure

This review book is designed to help prepare residents and technologists for the radiologic physics portion of their board and registry exams. It provides a source for comprehensive self-study in the area of diagnostic radiologic physics. The text assumes a background of instruction in radiologic physics and is *not* intended to replace a standard radiologic physics text. This book is designed, rather, to provide a concise yet complete source of review to refresh and reinforce the concepts of radiologic physics expected of residents and technologists.

The text is divided into 13 chapters, with subsections covering everything from basic physics to image quality. Each chapter begins with a summary of the "key" information in point form pertaining to the area under review. This is followed by questions designed to provide a self-test of the reader's knowledge and comprehension in each area. The questions include multiple choice, true–false, and matching format. The philosophy adopted by the authors is that material comprehension, rather than rote memorization, will guarantee success in the exam. The book also contains two practice examinations with questions that cover all of the topics in the book. Finally, the book contains a glossary of key terms commonly used in radiologic physics and an appendix with a summary of units used in radiology.

Radiation measurements are generally given in SI units, with non-SI units provided in brackets. An exception to this rule is the use of Roentgen to specify radiation exposure because conversion into Coulombs per kilogram would likely result in unnecessary confusion. In general, practical choices were preferred over semantic purity.

IV. Radiology Residents and the ABR Exam

The written portion of the radiology boards is taken by board eligible residents in the fall of their senior year. It is administered by the American Board of Radiology (ABR) over a two-day period in late September or October of each year. The physics portion of the exam is taken on the first day, and the diagnostic radiology section is taken the following day. Four hours are allowed for the physics section, and most residents comfortably finish the exam in the allowed time. A non-programmable calculator is allowed. The test has contained an average of 300 questions in recent years. Approximately one half of the questions are true–false, and the remaining questions are matching and multiple choice. Residents failing only the physics portion of the exam can take a make-up exam in the winter, enabling them to take the oral exam in June of their senior year.

Approximately two thirds of the questions cover diagnostic physics and equipment including basic physics, x-ray tubes, image intensifiers, recording systems, ultrasound, CT, MRI, contrast media, image quality, radiation exposure, and safety. The remaining questions cover the physics of nuclear medicine (basic physics, equipment, dosimetry, measurements, and statistics) and radiation biology (cell and tissue kinetics; subcellular, cellular, tissue, and whole body effects and response).

V. Radiology Technologists and the ARRT Exam

The American Registry of Radiologic Technologists (ARRT) is the credentialing board for radiology technologists. The ARRT written exam is offered three times a year to technologists who have completed formal training in an accredited radiology technologists program. The written exam includes about 200 questions in five general areas including (1) radiation protection, (2) equipment operation and maintenance, (3) image production and evaluation, (4) radiographic procedures, and (5) patient care. The first three sections comprise approximately 55% of the total exam and are the focus of this book.

Topics that all radiologic technologists need to cover include the biological effects of radiation, techniques to minimize radiation exposure, sources of radiation exposure, methods of protection, basic properties of radiation, units of radiation measurement, dosimeters, personnel monitoring, components of radiographic equipment including x-ray generators, tubes and transformers, fluoroscopic units, beam restriction, screens and cassettes, shielding, image contrast, density and the effects of kVp and mAs, grids, filtration, and screen/film combinations. Technologists planning to specialize in the imaging modalities of nuclear medicine, ultrasound, MRI, and CT should find the more advanced chapters devoted to these topics useful. Radiographic procedures and patient care issues are *not* addressed in this book.

1

Basic Physics

I. Introduction

A. Motion

–The **mass** of a body is a measure of its inertia, or resistance to acceleration, measured in **kilograms** (kg).

–**Velocity** is the constant speed of a body moving in a given direction and is measured in **meters per second** (m/s).

–**Acceleration** is the rate of change of velocity and is measured in **meters per second per second** (m/s²).

–**Force** causes a body to deviate from a state of rest or constant velocity (push or pull). **Force = mass × acceleration** and is measured in newtons (N).

–The **weight** of a body is the force of gravitational attraction on its mass.

–**Work** is the product of the force and distance moved and is measured in **joules** (J).

B. Energy and power

–**Energy** is the ability to perform work and is measured in **joules**.

–Energy takes on various forms including electrical, nuclear, mechanical, chemical, and thermal.

–Energy may be **kinetic,** caused by motion (e.g., a speeding bullet), or **potential**, which is the ability to perform work when a mass is moved from a higher to a lower potential (e.g., energy produced at a hydroelectric station).

–Einstein showed that mass and energy are interconvertible as expressed by $E = m \times c^2$, where E is energy, m is mass, and c is velocity of light.

–Based on this interconversion of mass and energy, **rest mass energy** is the energy equivalent of a particle.

–In diagnostic radiology, the **electron volt** (eV) is a convenient unit of energy, where $1 \text{ eV} = 1.6 \times 10^{-19}$ J.

–**Power** is the rate of performing work. The average value of power is the energy used divided by time and is measured in **watts** (W), where 1 W = 1 J/s.

–Table 1-1 lists the power and energies of a range of sources.

Table 1-1. Power and Energy Associated with a Range of Sources

Energy Source	Power Rating (W or kW)	Energy Used in 1 Second (Joules)
Flashlight	2 W	2 J
Domestic light bulb	50 W	50 J
Microwave	500 W	500 J
Stove burner	2 kW	2,000 J
X-ray generator	80 kW	80,000 J
Major power plant	1,000,000 kW (1 GW)	1,000,000,000 J
[One horse power]	*[750 W]*	*[750 J]*

C. Electricity

–The **electric charge** of electrons and protons is 1.6×10^{-19} **coulomb** (C). **Electrons** are negatively charged; **protons** are positively charged.

–**Electric current,** measured in **amperes** (A), is the flow of electrons through a circuit. An ampere is the amount of charge that flows divided by time (1 A = 1 C/s).

–Electrons accelerated through V volts gain a kinetic energy of V electron volts. See Figure 1-1.

–In electric circuits, the power (P) dissipated is the product of electric current (I) and voltage (V) or $P = I \times V$ watts.

D. Physical forces

–The four physical forces in the universe are **gravitational, electrostatic, strong,** and **weak**. These are measured by relative strength. See Table 1-2.

–**Gravity** pulls objects to the Earth. In radiologic physics, the effects of gravity are small and are ignored.

–The **electrostatic force** causes protons and electrons to attract and holds atoms together.

–**Strong forces** hold the nucleus of an atom together.

–**Weak forces** are involved in beta decay.

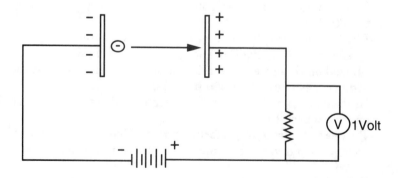

Figure 1-1. One electron volt (1 eV) is the kinetic energy gained when a single electron is accelerated between two plates that differ in potential by 1 V. Before leaving the negatively charged plate, the electron has potential energy of 1 eV.

Table 1-2. Relative Strength of Physical Forces

Type of Force	Relative Strength	Range of Interaction	Force Function
Gravitational	1	Infinite	Binds earth to the sun
Weak	$\sim 10^{24}$	$< 10^{-18}$ m	Involved in beta decay
Electrostatic	$\sim 10^{35}$	Infinite	Binds electrons in atoms
Strong	$\sim 10^{38}$	$< 10^{-15}$ m	Binds protons and neutrons in the nucleus

II. Matter

A. Atoms

–**Matter** is made up of atoms, which are composed of **protons, neutrons,** and **electrons**.

–**Protons** have a positive charge and are found in the nucleus of atoms.

–**Neutrons** are electrically neutral and are always found in the nucleus.

–The relative number of neutrons in an atom affects the stability of the nucleus.

–**Electrons** are much lighter than protons and neutrons and are found outside the nucleus.

–Isolated protons and electrons are **stable,** whereas an isolated neutron is **unstable** and has a half-life of approximately 11 minutes.

–The **atomic number (Z)** is the number of protons in the nucleus of an atom and is unique for each element.

–The **mass number (A)** is the total number of protons and neutrons in the nucleus.

–In the notation $_Z^A X$ or $^A X$, X is the unique letter or letters designating the element, A is the mass number, and Z is the atomic number.

–Electrically neutral atoms have Z electrons and Z protons.

–One gram-mole of a substance contains 6×10^{23} atoms, normally expressed as N_o, the **Avogadro number**.

–Mass on the atomic scale is measured in **atomic mass units** (amu).

–One atomic mass unit is one twelfth the mass of a carbon atom (^{12}C), or 1.6×10^{-27} kg.

–Protons and neutrons have a mass of approximately 1 amu.

–Electrons have a much smaller mass of 9.1×10^{-31} kg, or 0.00055 amu.

–The **electron density** of a substance is $\rho \times N_o \times (Z/A)$ electrons/cm^3, where ρ is the density measured in **grams per cubic centimeter (g/cm^3)**.

–For most atoms making up humans (e.g., oxygen, carbon, nitrogen, calcium), Z/A is approximately constant (0.5). Thus, electron density is generally proportional to the physical density ρ.

B. Atomic structure

–The nucleus of an atom is made up of tightly bound protons and neutrons, which are called **nucleons,** and contains most of the atomic mass.

–In the **Bohr model** of an atom, **electrons surround the nucleus in shells** (e.g., K-shell, L-shell) as shown for tungsten in Figure 1-2.

–Each shell is assigned a principal quantum number (n) beginning with 1 for the K-shell, 2 for the L-shell, and so on.

TUNGSTEN ¹⁸⁴ W

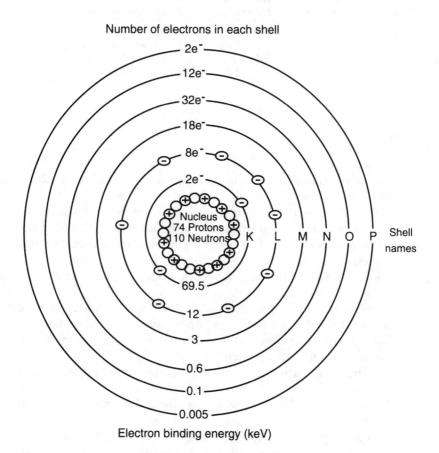

Figure 1-2. Bohr model of the atom showing Tungsten with a total of 74 protons, 74 electrons, and 110 neutrons. The electron binding energy decreases rapidly with electron distance from the nucleus.

–The number of electrons each shell can contain is $2n^2$.
–The K-shell in tungsten ($n = 1$) has 2 electrons, the L-shell ($n = 2$) has 8 electrons, the M-shell ($n = 3$) has 18 electrons, and so on.
–No more than **8 electrons** can be in the outer shell of an atom.
    –The number of electrons in the outer shell (valence electrons) determines the atom's chemical properties.

C. Electron binding energy
    –Atomic electrons are held in place by the **electrostatic pull** of the positively charged nucleus.
    –The work that is required to remove an electron from an atom is called the **electron binding energy**.
        –The binding energy of **outer shell electrons** is small, that is, **several electron volts (eV)**.
        –The binding energy of **inner shell electrons** is large, that is, **thousands of electron volts (keV)**.

Table 1-3. Atomic Number, K-shell Binding Energy, and Approximate Density of Selected Elements

Element	Atomic Number (Z)	K-shell Binding Energy (keV)	Physical Density (g/cm^3)
Hydrogen	1	0.01	< 0.001
Carbon	6	0.3	1.8–2.3
Nitrogen	7	0.4	0.001
Oxygen	8	0.5	0.001
Calcium	20	4.0	1.6
Copper	29	9.0	8.9
Selenium	34	12.7	4.3–4.8
Molybdenum	42	20.0	10.2
Silver	47	25.5	10.5
Iodine	53	33.2	4.9
Barium	56	37.4	3.5
Tungsten	74	69.5	19.3
Lead	82	88.0	11.3

–K-shell binding energies increase with atomic number (Z) as listed in Table 1-3.

–Electrons moving from a high to a low atomic energy may emit excess energy as **electromagnetic radiation**.

D. Nuclear binding energy

–The particles in an atomic nucleus are held together by **strong forces**.

–The **total binding energy** of the entire nucleus is the energy required to separate all of the nucleons.

–The binding energy of a single nucleon (i.e., neutron or proton) is the energy required to remove it from the nucleus.

–The **average binding energy** per nucleon is the total binding energy divided by the number of nucleons.

–The average binding energy per nucleon increases from approximately 1 million electron volts (MeV) for deuterium with a mass number of 2, to between 7 and 9 MeV for nuclei with mass numbers greater than 20.

–A high binding energy indicates stability.

–The average binding energy per nucleon increases after radioactive decay, because the daughter is more stable than the parent.

III. Radiation

A. Electromagnetic waves

–Radiation is the transport of energy through space.

–**Wavelength (λ)** is the distance between successive crests of waves.

–**Amplitude** is the intensity defined by the height of the wave.

–**Frequency (*f*)** is the number of wave oscillations per unit of time expressed in cycles per second, or **hertz** (Hz).

–The **period** is the time required for one wavelength to pass (1/*f*).

–For any type of wave motion, velocity (*c*) = *f* × λ m/s, where *f* is measured in hertz and λ in meters.

–Electromagnetic radiation travels in a straight line at the speed of light (3×10^8 m/s in a vacuum).

–X-rays are an example of electromagnetic radiation.

–The product of the wavelength (λ) and frequency (f) of electromagnetic radiation is equal to the speed of light.

–Electromagnetic radiation represents a **transverse wave,** in which the electric and magnetic fields oscillate perpendicular to the direction of the wave motion.

–Figure 1-3 shows the electromagnetic spectrum from long wavelength radio waves to short wavelength x-rays and gamma rays.

B. Photons

–Electromagnetic radiation is **quantized,** meaning that it exists in **discrete** quantities called photons.

–**Photons** may behave as waves or particles, but **have no mass.**

–**Photon energy** (E) is **directly proportional** to **frequency** and **inversely proportional** to **wavelength**.

–X-ray wavelengths may be measured in angstroms (Å), where 1 Å is 10^{-8} cm, or 10^{-10} m, or 0.1 nm.

–Photon energy is $E = h \times f = h \times (c/\lambda) = \mathbf{12.4/\lambda}$, where E is in keV, h is Planck's constant, and λ is wavelength in angstroms.

–A 10-keV photon has a wavelength of 1.24 Å, which is equal to the diameter of a typical atom.

–A 100-keV photon has a wavelength of 0.124 Å.

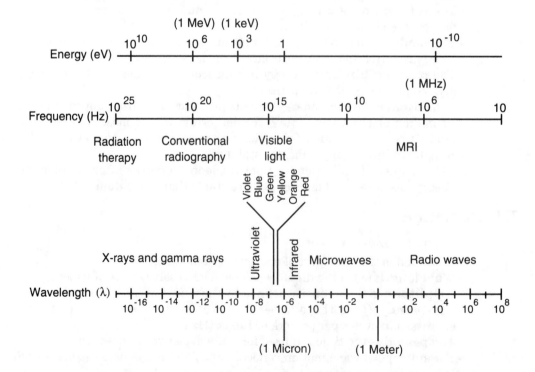

Figure 1-3. Electromagnetic spectra ranging from radio waves to x-rays and gamma rays.

–By convention, photons are called **x-rays** if produced by electron interactions and **gamma rays** if produced in nuclear processes.

C. Particulate radiation

–**Particulate radiation** involves electrons, positrons, protons, neutrons, and alpha particles, whose properties are listed in Table 1-4.

–**Charged particles lose energy** when passing through matter by interacting with atomic electrons.

   –Energy lost from energetic particles can eject electrons from atoms or raise atomic electrons to higher energies.

   –**Electrons and positrons** lose approximately 1 keV when traveling through 1 μm of soft tissue.

   –**Alpha particles** lose approximately 100 keV when traversing 1 μm of soft tissue.

   –**Neutrons** produce recoil protons, which lose energy as they travel through matter.

D. Ionization

–**Ionization** occurs when an electron is ejected from a neutral atom, leaving behind a **positive ion**.

–Electromagnetic radiation with sufficient energy to remove electrons is called ionizing radiation.

–**Ionizing radiation** includes x-rays and gamma rays.

–Radiation may be **directly ionizing** (involving charged particles) or **indirectly ionizing** (involving uncharged particles such as neutrons, x-rays, and gamma rays).

–The average amount of energy needed to generate one electron–ion pair in air is approximately 33 eV.

–Ionizing radiation loses energy in the absorbing medium by exciting atomic electrons from low to high energies.

–The energy deposited in the absorbing medium by ionizing radiation can result in deleterious chemical modifications to molecules such as DNA.

–Energy deposited by radiation is ultimately transformed into increased molecular motion (heat). The heating effect of ionizing radiation is negligible.

–For a computed tomography (CT) scan of the head, the total amount of energy deposited is approximately 0.2 J, whereas a 500-W microwave oven deposits 5000 J in 10 seconds.

Table 1-4. Mass, Charge, and Rest Mass Energy of Selected Elementary Particles

Particle	Relative Mass	Charge	Rest Mass Energy
Electron (e^-)	1	–1	511 keV
Proton (p)	1836	+1	938 MeV
Neutron (N)	1839	0	940 MeV
Alpha particle (α)	7350	+2	3.8 GeV
Positron (e^+)	1	+1	511 keV

IV. Radionuclides

A. Introduction

–Nuclei having different numbers of protons, neutrons, or both are called **nuclides**.

–Unstable nuclides are called **radionuclides,** and atoms with unstable nuclei are called **radioisotopes**.

–The mass number (A) of a nuclide is the sum of the number of protons (Z) and neutrons (N), or $A = Z + N$. ^{131}I has 131 nucleons; $Z = 53$ and $N = 78$.

–Nuclides having the same mass number A are called **isobars**.

–Nuclides having the same atomic number ($protons$) are called **isotopes**.

–Nuclides having the same number of $n$eutrons are called **isotones**.

–Figure 1-4 illustrates these relations and shows that stable high atomic mass atoms have proportionally more neutrons.

–An **isomer** is the *excited* state of a nucleus.

–Table 1-5 lists the three isotopes of hydrogen. Hydrogen and deuterium are stable, but tritium is radioactive with a half-life of 12 years.

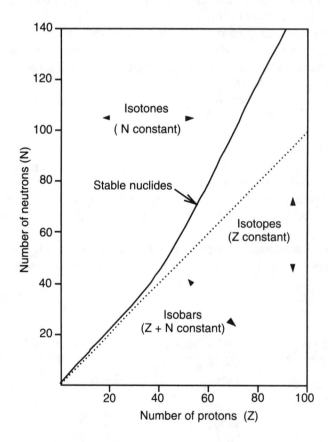

Figure 1-4. Relation between the number of protons, or atomic number (Z), and the number of neutrons in the nucleus of stable nuclides. As the mass number increases, the ratio of neutrons to protons increases from 1:1 to approximately 1:1.5 for stable nuclides.

Table 1-5. Isotopes of Hydrogen

Symbol	Protons (Z)	Neutrons (N)	Mass Number (A)	Name Nucleus	Atom
^{1}H	1	0	1	Proton	Hydrogen
^{2}H	1	1	2	Deuteron	Deuterium
^{3}H	1	2	3	Triton	Tritium

B. Nuclear stability

–For common and stable low mass number nuclides, the number of neutrons (N) is approximately equal to the number of protons (Z). For example, ^{12}C has six protons and six neutrons and ^{16}O has eight protons and eight neutrons.

–For stable high mass number nuclides, the number of neutrons exceeds the number of protons.

–For example, tungsten has 74 protons and 110 neutrons.

–Very heavy nuclei (Z > 82) tend to be unstable.

–The three processes by which an unstable nuclide or radionuclide attains stability are **alpha, beta,** and **gamma decay**.

–The transformation from unstable to stable nuclides is called **radioactive decay**.

–The original nuclide is called the **parent** and the products are **daughter** nuclei.

–In nuclear transformations, energy, mass number, and electric charge are conserved.

C. Radioactivity

–**Half-life ($T_{1/2}$)** is the time required for half of the material to decay.

–**Activity** is the number of transformations per unit of time.

–Activity is expressed mathematically as $dN(t)/dt$, where $N(t)$ is the number of atoms at time (t).

–**Lambda (λ)** is the **decay constant** and $dN(t)/dt = N(t) \times \lambda$.

–Activity is $N \times \lambda$, where N is the number of atoms.

–The relation between λ and the half-life of the radioactivity ($T_{1/2}$) is $\lambda = \log_e(2)/T_{1/2} = 0.693/T_{1/2}$.

–The SI unit of activity is the becquerel (Bq), and the non-SI unit is the curie (Ci). Both units are used to describe a quantity of radioactive material.

–One **becquerel** is 1 transformation per second.

–One **curie** is 3.7×10^{10} transformations per second.

–1 mCi = 37 MBq; 1 μCi = 37 kBq.

V. Decay Modes

A. Isomeric

–**Gamma rays** are high-energy photons (electromagnetic radiation) that result from nuclear processes.

–The **ground state** is the lowest energy state of a nucleus and is, therefore, the **most stable** arrangement of nucleons.

–**Excited states** have increased energies, are **unstable,** and have a transient existence before transforming into a more stable state.

–**M** ctastable **states** (isomeric states) are also **unstable** but have relatively long lifetimes before transforming to another state. To be called metastable, the half-life must exceed 10^{-12} seconds. The metastable state of an atom is denoted by a lower case m following the mass number (e.g., ^{99m}Tc).

–Nuclear transformations to a more stable state (isomeric transitions) release energy in the form of a **gamma ray**.

–After an **isomeric transition,** both parent and daughter nuclei have the same mass number, atomic number, and number of neutrons.

–Rather than emitting gamma rays, energy may be transferred to an orbital electron, which is then emitted from the atom as an **internal conversion electron**.

B. Beta minus decay

–In **beta minus (β^-) decay,** a neutron inside the nucleus is converted into a proton, and the excess energy is released as an energetic electron, called a **beta particle,** and an **antineutrino**.

–The **antineutrino** has no rest mass, no electric charge, and rarely interacts with matter.

–Beta minus decay occurs in nuclei with too many neutrons.

–In beta minus decay, the atomic number increases by 1, but the mass number remains constant.

–The beta particles (electrons) emitted during beta minus decay have a range of energies (spectrum) up to a maximum energy (E_{max}).

–The average energy of beta emitters is approximately one third the maximum.

–^{32}P is a pure beta emitter with a maximum beta particle energy of 1.71 MeV and a mean beta particle energy of approximately 570 keV.

–^{3}H, or tritium, (E_{max} = 18 keV) and ^{14}C (E_{max} = 156 keV) are low energy beta minus emitters that are ubiquitous in biomedical research.

C. Beta plus decay

–In **beta plus (β^+) decay** (sometimes called positron emission), a proton inside the nucleus is converted into a neutron, and the excess energy is emitted as a positively charged electron, called a **positron,** and a **neutrino**.

–A **neutrino** has no electric charge and no rest mass, and is similar to an antineutrino.

–Beta plus decay occurs in nuclei with too few neutrons (too many protons).

–In beta plus decay, the atomic number decreases by 1 and the mass number stays the same.

–A **positron** is an electron with a unit-positive charge instead of a unit-negative charge that interacts with matter like an electron.

–Energetic positrons lose their energy by ionization and excitation of atomic electrons.

–When the positron loses all of its kinetic energy, it annihilates with an electron.

–The mass (energy) of the positron and electron (511 keV each) are converted into two 511 keV photons that are emitted 180 degrees apart.

–Positron emitters generally have short half-lives (^{11}C, 20 minutes; ^{15}O, 2 minutes; ^{18}F, 110 minutes).

D. Electron capture

–In **electron capture,** a proton inside the nucleus is converted into a neutron by capturing an electron from one of the atomic shells (e.g., K, L, M) and a **neutrino** is emitted.

–Electron capture is most likely from the K-shell, followed by electron capture from the L-shell, M-shell, and so on.

–Electron capture occurs in nuclei with too few neutrons (too many protons).

–In electron capture, the atomic number decreases by 1 and the mass number stays the same.

–If the electron is captured from the K-shell (K-shell capture), the resultant K-shell vacancy is filled by an outer shell electron.

–The excess energy is emitted as a characteristic x-ray, or **Auger electron**.

–Electron capture may compete with beta plus decay.

–Important electron capture radionuclides used in nuclear medicine include ^{57}Co, ^{67}Ga, ^{111}In, ^{123}I, ^{125}I, and ^{201}Tl.

E. Alpha decay

–In **alpha decay,** a radionuclide emits an alpha particle consisting of two neutrons and two protons (i.e., helium nucleus).

–Alpha decay is most common in atoms with atomic numbers (Z) greater than 82.

–In alpha decay, the atomic number decreases by 2 and the mass number by 4.

–Alpha particles have an energy between 4 and 7 MeV.

–Alpha particles can travel from 1 to 10 cm in air, but less than 0.1 mm in tissue. For this reason, alpha particles pose little risk as an external radiation source, but pose a high risk if ingested or injected.

–Table 1-6 summarizes the major modes of radioactive decay.

Table 1-6. Radioactive Decay Modes for Unstable Nuclei Containing Protons (Z), Neutrons (N), and Mass Number (A) [= $Z + N$]

Decay Mode	Daughter Nucleus Value			Comments
	Mass No.	Atomic No.	Neutron No.	
Isomeric transition	A	Z	N	Metastable if half-life > 10^{-12} sec
Beta minus (β^-)	A	$Z+1$	$N-1$	Emits electrons and antineutrinos
Beta plus (β^+)	A	$Z-1$	$N+1$	Emits positrons and neutrinos
Electron capture	A	$Z-1$	$N+1$	Emits neutrinos and x-rays*
Alpha decay	$A-4$	$Z-2$	$N-2$	Occurs in heavy nuclei ($Z > 82$)

*Characteristic x-rays are emitted as the inner shell electron vacancies are filled.

Review Test

1. Which of the following is NOT a unit of energy?

(A) Erg
(B) Joule
(C) Watt
(D) British thermal unit (BTU)
(E) Electron volt (eV)

2. True (T) or False (F).

(A) The coulomb (C) is a unit of electric current
(B) The amp is a unit of electric current
(C) 10 coulombs flowing in 2 seconds is equal to 5 amps
(D) One electron has a charge of 3.1×10^{-31} C
(E) One proton has a charge of 1.6×10^{-19} C
(F) The neutron has no charge

3. Match the following.

(A) Electrons flowing through a medium
(B) Attraction or repulsion between two bodies
(C) Mass or electromagnetic radiation
(D) Restricts electric current
(E) Energy expended per unit time

(i) Resistance
(ii) Energy
(iii) Force
(iv) Current
(v) Power

4. Match the following forces and descriptions.

(A) Gravitational
(B) Electrostatic
(C) Weak
(D) Strong

(i) Binds electrons to the nucleus
(ii) Binds nucleons together
(iii) Binds the moon to the earth
(iv) Involved in beta decay

5. Match the following terms with the correct definitions.

(A) Mass number
(B) Atomic number
(C) Avogadro's number
(D) Atomic mass unit

(i) 6×10^{23}
(ii) 1/12 mass of ^{12}C
(iii) Number of electrons in a neutral atom
(iv) Number of nucleons in a nucleus

6. Match the particle to the correct electrical charge.

(A) Alpha particle
(B) Neutron
(C) Electron
(D) Positron

(i) −1
(ii) 0
(iii) +1
(iv) +2

7. What is the maximum number of electrons in the following atomic shells?

(A) K-shell
(B) L-shell
(C) M-shell

8. The electron binding energy is

(A) independent of the electron distance from the nucleus
(B) independent of the nuclear charge
(C) several MeV
(D) overcome for the electron to be ejected from the atom
(E) a result of the strong interaction

9. Match the following materials with the correct K-edge energy.

(A) Hydrogen (Z=1)
(B) Oxygen (Z=8)
(C) Calcium (Z=20)
(D) Iodine (Z=53)
(E) Lead (Z=82)

(i) 4 keV
(ii) 0.01 keV
(iii) 88 keV
(iv) 0.5 keV
(v) 33 keV

10. Iodine-131 and Iodine-125 have different

(A) chemical properties
(B) Z values
(C) numbers of neutrons
(D) numbers of protons

11. True (T) or False (F). A neutral cobalt 60 atom (Z = 27) has

(A) 27 protons in the nucleus
(B) 60 electrons around the nucleus
(C) 33 neutrons in the nucleus
(D) K-shell electron binding energy levels of 60 keV
(E) outer shell binding energy levels of several eV
(F) a weight about 60 times a hydrogen atom

12. All electromagnetic radiation has the same

(A) intensity
(B) frequency
(C) wavelength
(D) velocity
(E) energy

13. Match the following types of radiation with the appropriate frequency.

(A) Radio waves
(B) Microwaves
(C) Visible light
(D) Ultraviolet
(E) X-rays

(i) 10^{14}
(ii) 10^{18}
(iii) 10^{16}
(iv) 10^{7}
(v) 10^{10}

14. Which of the following statements regarding electromagnetic radiation is false?

(A) Travels at the speed of light (3×10^8 m/s)
(B) Exhibits particulate properties
(C) Has a photon energy proportional to frequency
(D) Travels at a speed proportional to frequency
(E) The product of frequency and wavelength is constant

15. Which characteristic increases with increasing *photon energy*?

(A) Wavelength
(B) Frequency
(C) Mass
(D) Charge
(E) All of the above

16. An atom which has lost an outer shell electron is called

(A) unstable
(B) metastable
(C) an ion
(D) a radioisotope
(E) all of the above

17. Which of the following is NOT directly ionizing radiation?

(A) Auger electrons
(B) Positrons
(C) Neutrons
(D) Alpha particles
(E) Internal conversion electrons

18. Match the type of radiation with its description.

(A) Beta rays
(B) RF radiation
(C) Neutrinos
(D) X-rays

(i)   Ionizing particulate radiation
(ii) Nonionizing particulate radiation
(iii) Ionizing electromagnetic radiation
(iv) Nonionizing electromagnetic radiation

19. The addition of what kind of particle to an atom would create a new element?

(A) Neutron
(B) Proton
(C) Electron
(D) None of the above

20. When ^{60}Co (Z = 27) decays to ^{60}Ni (Z = 28), which of the following is emitted?

(A) Positrons
(B) Electrons
(C) Alpha particles
(D) 140 keV x-rays
(E) Neutrinos

21. Match the following modes of decay with the corresponding change in mass number (A) and atomic number (Z).

(A) Beta minus decay
(B) Beta plus decay
(C) Alpha decay
(D) Isomeric transition

(i)   Z and A remain the same
(ii) Z increases by 1; A remains the same
(iii) Z decreases by 1; A remains the same
(iv) A decreases by 4; Z decreases by 2

22. Electron capture can result in emission of

(A) antineutrinos
(B) high LET radiation
(C) characteristic x-rays
(D) positrons
(E) neutrons

23. In alpha decay

(A) A changes by 2
(B) Z changes by 4
(C) nuclei with A < 82 are most likely candidates
(D) an energetic helium nucleus is emitted
(E) charge is not conserved

24. Match the following terms with the appropriate nuclides.

(A) Isotopes
(B) Isotones
(C) Isomers
(D) Isobars
(i) ^{99}Tc/^{99m}Tc
(ii) ^{131}I/^{123}I
(iii) ^{14}N/^{14}C
(iv) ^{3}H/^{4}He

25. An activity of 3.7×10^7 Bq corresponds to

(A) 1 mCi
(B) 10 mCi
(C) 100 mCi
(D) 1 Ci
(E) none of the above

Answers and Explanations

1–C. The watt is a unit of power. It is the rate at which energy is used, expressed in joules per second.

2. A–False; electric current is the rate of flow of charge, or C/s; **B–True; C–True;** current is coulomb divided by seconds [10/2] amps; **D–False;** the electron has a charge of -1.6×10^{-19} C; **E–True; F–True.**

3. A–iv; an electric current is the rate of flow of charge; **B–iii;** gravitation is an example of attraction between two bodies and electrostatic repulsion between charges of the same polarity; **C–ii;** both have energy with the rest mass energy of a particle given by E = mc²; **D–i;** resistance is given by the voltage divided by the current flow so, for a given voltage, increasing the resistance reduces the current; **E–v;** power is the rate at which energy is expended and is given in watts, with 1 watt = 1 J/s.

4. A–iii; B–i; C–iv; D–ii.

5. A–iv; B–iii; C–i; D–ii.

6. A–iv; B–ii; C–i; D–iii.

7. Shell capacity is determined by $2n^2$, where n is the principal quantum number. **A–2 for the K-shell** (n is equal to 1); **B–8 for the L-shell** (n is equal to 2); **C–18 for the M-shell** (n is equal to 3).

8–D. The electron binding energy is the energy that must be supplied to pull the electron away from the atom. It *decreases* with increasing distance from the nucleus, *increases* with Z, is never more than about 100 keV, and is due to electrostatic forces between the positive nucleus and negative electron.

9. A–ii; B–iv; C–i; D–v; E–iii. The K-edge energy increases with the atomic number.

10–C. All isotopes of iodine have 53 protons (Z), but differing numbers of neutrons (Iodine-125 has 72 neutrons and Iodine-131 has 78 neutrons.) The outer shell electrons affect the chemical properties of an element.

11. A–True; the number of protons is equal to Z, which is 27; **B–False;** for a neutral atom, the number of electrons is equal to Z, which is 27; **C–True;** the total number of nucleons is 60, and since there are 27 protons, there must be 33 neutrons; **D–False;** the binding energy depends on the atomic number Z; for cobalt, the K-shell binding energy is only 7.7 keV; **E–True;** all outer shell electrons have binding energies of only a few eV; **F–True;** most of the atomic mass is in the nucleus, and ^{60}Co has 60 times the nucleons of ^{1}H.

12–D. The velocity of light (electromagnetic radiation) is a constant in a vacuum (3×10^8 m/s).

13. A–iv; B–v; C–i; D–iii; E–ii. Radio waves have the lowest frequencies and x-rays the highest.

14–D. The speed of light in a vacuum is always a *constant* and independent of frequency ($c = f \times \lambda$).

15–B. Frequency increases with energy ($E = h \times f$, where h is Plank's constant). Wavelength decreases with increasing photon energy.

16–C. An ion.

17–C. Neutrons, since they have no charge. All charged particles are directly ionizing; neutrons ionize by producing recoil protons, and photons ionize by generating electrons.

18. A–i; B–iv; C–ii; D–iii. Beta rays and neutrinos are particulate; x-rays and beta rays are ionizing.

19–B. The addition of a proton will create a new element with an atomic number of Z + 1.

20–B. The atomic number of the daughter increases by 1. Therefore, this is an example of beta minus decay, where a neutron in the nucleus is converted into a proton, and an energetic electron (beta particle) and antineutrino are emitted.

21. A–ii; B–iii; C–iv; D–i.

22–C. In electron capture, an inner-shell electron is absorbed by the nucleus, leaving a vacancy that is subsequently filled by an outer-shell electron resulting in the emission of characteristic radiation.

23–D. An alpha particle has two protons (Z = 2) and two neutrons (A = 4), which is a helium nucleus. (Alpha decay generally occurs in nuclei with Z > 82 and charge is *always* conserved.)

24. A–ii; both have the same number of protons in the nucleus and are thus isotopes; **B–iv;** ^{3}H (tritium) has two neutrons, as does ^{4}He (the helium nucleus is also known as an alpha particle); **C–i;** ^{99m}Tc is an excited nuclear state of ^{99}Tc with a half-life of 6 hours; **D–iii;** both ^{14}N and ^{14}C have 14 nucleons and are therefore isobars.

25–A. 37 MBq is 1 mCi (1 Ci is 3.7×10^{10} Bq).

2

X-ray Production

I. X-ray Generators

A. Introduction

–In the United States, the electric power supply from utility companies is normally 120 volts (V) **alternating current (AC),** which oscillates at a frequency of 60 cycles per second (Hz).

–A **generator** increases the voltage and **rectifies** the waveform from AC to **direct current (DC).**

–Generators permit x-ray operators to control three key parameters of x-ray operation: **x-ray tube voltage,** measured in kilovolts (kV), **tube current,** measured in milliamperes (mA), and **exposure time,** measured in milliseconds (ms).

–**Voltage** is applied **across** the x-ray tube, and **current** flows **through** the x-ray tube.

–The power dissipated equals the product of tube voltage (V) and current (I), or $V \times I$, and is measured in watts (W).

–**Typical transformer ratings** in x-ray departments are **100 kV** and **800 mA,** which corresponds to a power of 80 kW.

B. Transformers

–**Transformers** are used to change the size of the input voltage.

–**Step-up transformers** increase the voltage, and **step-down transformers** decrease the voltage.

–If two wire coils are wrapped around a common iron core, current in the primary coil produces a current in the secondary coil by electromagnetic induction.

–The voltages in the two circuits (V_p and V_s) are proportional to the number of turns in the two coils (N_p and N_s), expressed mathematically as $N_p/N_s = V_p/V_s$, where p refers to primary and s to secondary.

–The product of the voltage (V) and current (I) in the primary and secondary circuits must be equal (conservation of energy), which can be expressed mathematically as $V_p \times I_p = V_s \times I_s$.

–The step-up transformers used in x-ray generators have a secondary coil with many more turns (1:500) to produce a high voltage accross the tube.

–Generators also have a step-down transformer with fewer turns in the secondary coil for the x-ray tube filament circuit, which only requires about 10 V.

–An **autotransformer** permits adjustment of the output voltage using movable contacts to change the number of coil turns in the circuit.

C. Rectification

–The electric current from an AC power supply flows alternately in both directions, resulting in a voltage waveform shaped like a sine wave.

–**Rectification** changes the AC voltage at the input to the transformer into a DC voltage across the x-ray tube. Rectification is achieved using **diodes,** which only permit current to flow in one direction.

–With **half-wave rectification,** one direction of current is eliminated.

–In **full-wave rectification** (achieved using a minimum of four diodes), two pulses per cycle are produced.

–**Three-phase generators** obtain power from three lines of current, each 120 degrees out of phase with the others.

–Diodes are arranged in combinations of **deltas** and **wye** circuits to produce 6- and 12-pulse outputs.

–Modern high-frequency generators transform input voltage to high frequencies that may be rectified to yield a nearly constant waveform.

–High-frequency generators are smaller and more efficient.

D. Voltage waveform

–The **peak voltage (kVp)** is the **maximum** voltage that crosses the x-ray tube during a complete waveform cycle.

–The voltage **waveform ripple** is the maximum voltage minus the minimum voltage per cycle expressed as a percentage of the maximum voltage.

–Single-phase half- and full-wave rectified systems have 100% ripple.

–Three-phase 6-pulse systems typically have 13% ripple, and 12-pulse systems have approximately 4% ripple.

–High-frequency generators have ripple comparable to 12-pulse systems.

–A low ripple is desirable because a more constant voltage is produced. Modern radiology equipment uses three-phase or high-frequency generators with low ripples.

–Figure 2-1 shows the waveforms for different types of generators and their corresponding ripple values.

II. X-ray Production

A. Introduction

–**Diagnostic x-rays** are produced when electrons with energies of 20 to 150 keV are stopped in matter.

–Electrons accelerated to the positive anode gain a kinetic energy of V eV, determined solely by the value of the applied voltage (V).

–The kinetic energy of the electron is transformed into heat and x-rays when the electrons strike the anode.

–Electrons rapidly lose their energy by ionization and excitation of electrons in the anode material. These electrons penetrate tens of micrometers (μm) into the anode.

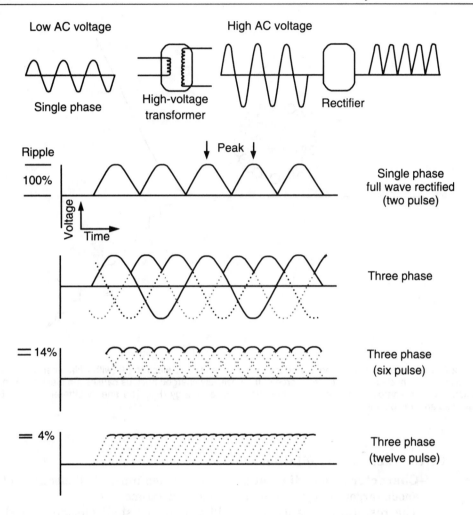

Figure 2-1. A transformer is used to increase the voltage supplied by the power company to the high voltages (20,000 to 150,000 V) needed for x-ray production. Full-wave rectification with single-phase results in 2 pulses per cycle. Three-phase can be rectified to yield either a 6- or 12-pulse waveform, which provides a more constant voltage.

–X-rays are generated by two different processes known as **bremsstrahlung** and **characteristic x-ray** production.

B. Bremsstrahlung radiation

   –**Bremsstrahlung** (breaking or general) x-rays are produced when incident electrons interact with nuclear electric fields, which slow them down and change their direction as shown in Figure 2-2. Some of the electron kinetic energy is emitted as an x-ray photon.

   –Bremsstrahlung x-rays produce a **continuous spectrum** of radiation, up to a maximum energy determined by the maximum kinetic energy of the incident electron. Maximum photon energies correspond to minimum x-ray wavelengths.

   –Bremsstrahlung x-ray production increases with the accelerating voltage (kV) and the atomic number (Z) of the anode.

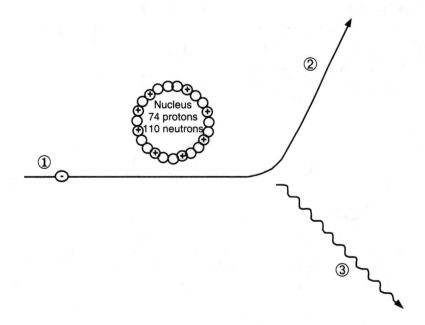

Figure 2-2. Bremsstrahlung radiation is produced when an energetic electron (*1*) (with initial energy E$_1$) passes close to an atomic nucleus. The attractive force of the positively charged nucleus causes the electron to change direction and lose energy. The electron (*2*) now has a lower energy (E$_2$). The energy difference (E$_1$ – E$_2$) is released as an x-ray photon (*3*).

C. Characteristic radiation

–**Characteristic radiation** is produced when inner shell electrons of the anode target are ejected by the incident electrons.

–The resultant vacancies are filled by outer shell electrons, and the energy difference is emitted as characteristic radiation (e.g., K-shell x-rays, L-shell x-rays) as shown in Figure 2-3.

–Excess energy may also be emitted as an **Auger electron**.

–Each anode material emits characteristic x-rays of a given energy as listed in Table 2-1. K-shell characteristic x-ray energies are slightly lower than the K-shell binding energy.

–K-shell electrons are ejected only if incident electrons have energies greater than the K-shell binding energy.

–For tungsten, K-shell characteristic x-rays are only produced when the applied voltage exceeds 70 kV (K-shell binding energy is 69.5 keV).

–For molybdenum, K-shell characteristic x-rays are only produced when the applied voltage exceeds 20 kV.

–L-shell radiation also normally accompanies K-shell radiation. L-shell characteristic x-rays have very low energies and are absorbed by the glass of the x-ray tube. Only K-shell characteristic x-rays are important in diagnostic radiology.

–Most incident electrons interact with outer shell electrons and produce heat but not x-rays.

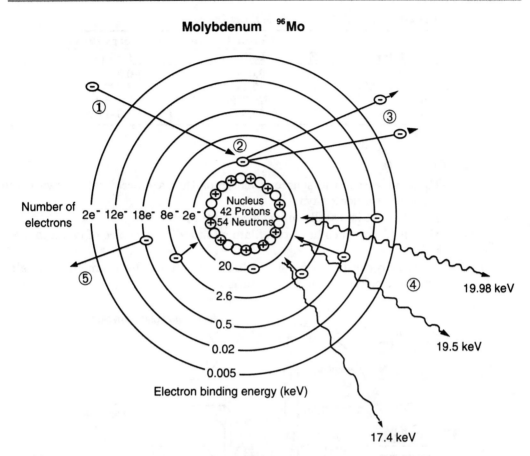

Figure 2-3. Characteristic radiation is produced when an incoming electron (*1*) interacts with an inner shell electron (*2*) and both are ejected (*3*). When one of the outer shell electrons moves to fill the inner shell vacancy, the excess energy is emitted as characteristic radiation (*4*). Sometimes the excess energy is emitted as an Auger electron (*5*) rather than as characteristic radiation.

III. X-ray Tubes

A. Introduction

–Figure 2-4 is a diagram of a radiographic x-ray tube.

–X-ray tubes contain a negatively charged **cathode** containing the **filament** that serves as an electron source.

–The **anode** is positively charged and includes the target where x-rays are produced.

–The anode may be stationary or rotating.

–The anode and cathode are contained in an evacuated envelope to prevent the electrons from colliding with gas molecules.

–The envelope is contained in a **tube housing** that protects the tube and provides shielding to prevent leakage radiation.

–The housing contains an oil bath to provide electrical insulation and help cool the tube.

–The primary x-rays exit through a window in the tube housing.

Table 2-1. Selected Characteristic X-ray Energies

		Characteristic X-ray Energy (keV)	
Anode Material	**Z**	**K-Shell**	**L-Shell**
Copper (Cu)	29	8.0–8.9	0.9
Molybdenum (Mo)	42	17.4–19.6	2.3–2.6
Tin (Sn)	50	25.0–28.5	3.4–4.1
Tungsten (W)	74	58.0–67.2	8.3–11.3

B. Filaments

–The **filament** is the source of electrons that are accelerated toward the anode to produce x-rays.

–The filament is usually made of coiled tungsten wire.

–Most modern tubes have two filaments to allow a choice of two focal spot sizes.

–A **focusing cup** or **cathode block** surrounds the filament and helps direct the electrons toward the target.

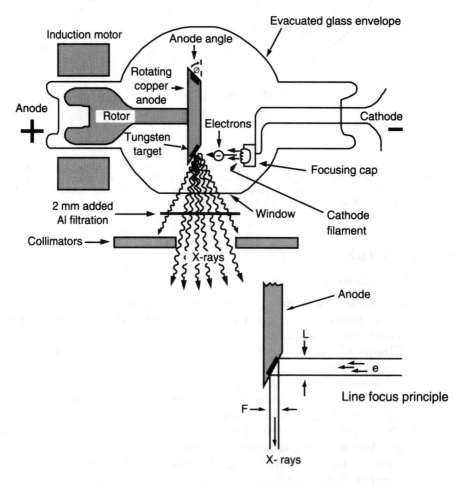

Figure 2-4. Major components of an x-ray tube. The tube is typically surrounded by an oil bath and lead housing. The magnified view of the target illustrates the line focus principle, whereby the focal spot size (*F*) is smaller than the electron beam (*L*) because of the anode angle.

–**Typical voltages across** the x-ray tube filament are **10 V,** and **currents through** the cathode filament are **4 A.**

–The power dissipated from the filament ($I \times V$) is typically 40 W.

–The high resistance in the filament causes temperature to rise (> 2200°C), resulting in the **thermionic emission** of electrons.

C. X-ray tube current

–Electrons emitted from a heated filament form a negative cloud around the filament called a **space charge,** which prevents further emission of electrons.

–The **tube current,** measured in milliamperes, is the flow of electrons from the filament to the anode. This results when a negative potential is applied to the filament, or cathode, and a positive potential is applied to the anode.

–At low peak voltage (< 40 kV), the potential is insufficient to cause all the electrons to be pulled away from the filament, and a residual space charge remains which limits the tube current.

  –Therefore, at low kilovoltage, the tube potential controls the tube current; this is called **space charge limited**.

–At the **saturation voltage,** all electrons are immediately pulled away from the filament, and the tube current is maximized.

  –The tube current cannot be further increased by increasing tube potential (kilovoltage).

–Tube currents range from several milliamperes to hundreds of milliamperes and are selected by the technologist performing the radiographic exposure.

–The x-ray tube output is directly proportional to the x-ray tube current.

–A typical current for radiography is 100 to 1000 mA and up to 5 mA for fluoroscopy.

D. Anode

–The **anode** is the target electrode.

–Electrons striking the anode produce heat and x-rays.

–**Tungsten** is the most common target material because of its high atomic number ($Z = 74$) and melting point.

  –Rhenium is often added to reduce the pitting and cracking caused by overheating.

–Molybdenum ($Z = 42$) and rhodium ($Z = 45$) are used for targets in mammography.

–A **stationary anode** consists of a tungsten target embedded in a copper block.

  –Although copper is a good heat conductor, heat dissipation is limited.

  –Stationary anodes are used in portable x-ray units.

–A **rotating anode** greatly increases the target area and raises the heat capacity.

E. Focal spots

–The **focal spot** is the apparent source of x-rays in the tube and may be characterized by a **length and width,** or by a **diameter** (measured in millimeters).

–Focal spots must be small to produce sharp images, but they also must tolerate a high heat loading without melting the target.

–The **actual focal spot** size is the area of the target struck by the electrons and is determined by the filament size and focus cup.

   –The focal spot size enlarges as the mA increases due to the repulsion of adjacent electrons. This effect is called **blooming**.

–The **effective focal spot** size is the dimension of the x-ray source as viewed from the image.

–The **line focus principle** is used to permit larger heat loading while minimizing the apparent size of the focal spot by orienting the anode at a small angle to the direction of the x-ray beam (see Figure 2-4).

–The anode angle is the angle between the target surface and the central beam.

   –Typical anode angles range from about 7 to 20 degrees.

   –Radiation field coverage increases with target angle.

–**Nominal** (reported) **focal spot** sizes range from about 0.1 mm to approximately 1.2 mm.

   –Manufacturers' specifications state that the **measured focal spot size** may be up to 50% larger as listed in Table 2-2.

   –Focal spot sizes can be measured using pinhole cameras, star test patterns, or slit cameras.

IV. X-ray Tube Heating

A. Energy deposition

–The **efficiency** of x-ray production is approximately $kV \times Z \times 10^{-6}$.

–This efficiency is approximately 1% for materials with high atomic numbers (Z) at 100 kVp.

–The amount of heat energy deposited during an x-ray exposure is known as **the loading**.

–X-ray tube loading depends on the peak kilovoltage, voltage waveform, tube current, exposure time, and number of exposures.

   –For a constant x-ray tube voltage (V) and current (I), the energy deposited during an x-ray exposure is $V \times I \times t$ joules, where t is the exposure time measured in seconds.

   –This energy is temporarily stored in the anode, which has a heat capacity of several hundred thousand joules.

–X-ray tube loading is assessed by using an x-ray tube rating chart and an anode thermal characteristics chart.

Table 2-2. Focal Spot Sizes Used in Diagnostic Radiology

Focal Spot Size (mm)		Clinical Applications
Nominal	**Measured**	
0.1–0.15	0.15–0.2	Magnification mammography
0.3	0.45	Mammography; magnification radiography
0.6–1.2	0.9–1.8	Conventional radiography
0.6	0.9	Fluoroscopy

B. Heat units (HUs)

–If the voltage is not constant, the calculation of energy deposition in joules is more complicated.

–For systems with single-phase power supplies and full-wave rectification, the quantity $kVp \times mA \times time$ is termed **heat units** (HUs). 1 HU = 0.71 J.

C. Tube rating

–The **rating** of an x-ray tube is based on maximum allowable kilowatts (kW) at an exposure time of 0.1 second.

  –For example, a tube with a rating of 80 kW (80,000 W) tolerates a maximum exposure of 80 kVp and 1000 mA at 0.1 second.

–Typical focal power ratings, defined for 0.1-second exposure times, range from 5 to 100 kW depending on focal spot size.

–The loading on the focal spot, anode, and x-ray tube housing must be considered to ensure none of these components overheat.

–**Increasing the exposure time** or **using a larger focal spot size** may be required to achieve the required x-ray tube output.

D. X-ray tube heat dissipation

–X-ray tubes are designed to efficiently dissipate heat.

–Modern anodes are circular and rotated at high speeds (3000 to 10,000 rpm) to spread heat loading over a large area.

–Heat is transferred from the focal spot by **radiation** to the tube housing and **conduction** into the anode. Anodes also lose heat by conduction and radiation.

–X-ray tubes are usually immersed in oil for electrical insulation and to aid heat dissipation by **convection**.

–Air fans are sometimes used to increase the rate of heat loss.

–Cooling of the anode is described by an anode thermal characteristics chart.

V. X-ray Output

A. Quantity

–Most x-ray photons are produced by bremsstrahlung radiation. A graph of x-ray tube output showing the number of photons at each x-ray energy is called a **spectrum**.

–When an x-ray tube with a tungsten target is used, characteristic radiation accounts for between 10% and 30% of the x-ray beam intensity between 80 and 150 kVp.

–X-ray output is directly proportional to both the tube current and exposure time.

–Increasing either or both increases the production of x-rays.

  –Doubling the current at constant exposure time has the same effect as doubling the exposure time at constant tube current.

  –The product of the tube current (mA) and exposure time (s) is expressed in mAs. X-ray tube output is directly proportional to the mAs value.

  –Doubling the mAs doubles the number of x-rays emitted but does not change the energy distribution of the x-ray photon spectrum.

  –Figure 2-5A shows how the number of photons at each energy level increases when the tube current is increased, but the spectrum shape does not change.

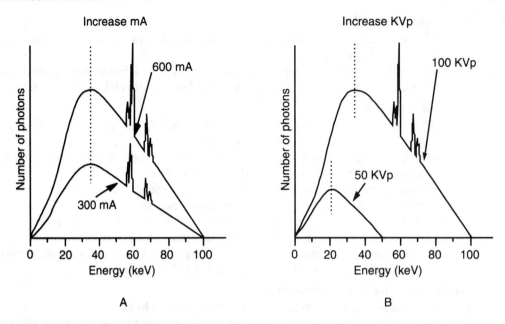

Figure 2-5. Effect of current and voltage on x-ray spectra. **A,** When the mA is increased and the peak voltage and exposure time are constant, the intensity of the x-rays increases but the energy distribution stays the same. **B,** When peak voltage is increased and the milliamperes and exposure time are constant, the intensity, peak, and mean energy of the x-rays increase.

–The **quantity** of x-rays produced can also be increased by increasing the kilovoltage, but this also changes the quality or shape of the x-ray spectrum as shown in Figure 2-5*B*.

B. Quality

–The quality of an x-ray beam is obtained from the **average x-ray energy** of the x-ray spectrum.
  –Increasing the peak kilovoltage (kVp) increases the x-ray tube output, peak energy, and mean energy of the beam.
  –This increases the beam quality as shown in Figure 2-5*B*.
–Increasing beam quality increases the x-ray beam **penetrating power** because the average photon energy is higher.
–Table 2-3 lists typical x-ray outputs as a function of kilovoltage.
–Changing the kVp by a given percentage increases the x-ray tube output more than the same percentage increase in mAs.

Table 2-3. Typical X-ray Outputs for a Three-phase Generator

Peak Voltage (kVp)	X-ray Output (mR/mAs) at 100 cm	
	2.5 mm Al filtration	3.5 mm Al filtration
80	10	8
100	15	12
120	20	17

–A rule of thumb is that increasing the kVp by 15% has the same effect as doubling the mAs.

–For example, changing tube voltage by 10 kVp (from 65 to 75 kVp) normally has the same effect on film density as doubling the mAs.

–The target material, voltage waveform, and tube filtration also affect the beam quality.

C. Unwanted radiation

–**Leakage radiation** is radiation that is transmitted through the x-ray tube housing.

–**Secondary radiation** is characteristic radiation that is produced as a result of the primary x-ray beam interacting with materials other than the target. X-ray tubes are surrounded by lead to absorb unwanted primary and secondary radiation.

–**Scattered radiation** has been deviated in direction after leaving the tube.

–**Stray radiation** is the sum of the leakage and scattered radiation.

–Low-energy radiation in the beam is absorbed by the patient and does not contribute to the image.

    –Filtration, therefore, is routinely used in conventional radiography to remove these low-energy x-rays and thereby reduce patient dose.

    –Filtration does not affect peak energies.

D. Heel effect

–X-rays produced within the target are attenuated as they pass out of the anode material.

–This attenuation is greater in the anode direction than in the cathode direction because of differences in the path length within the target.

–This is known as the **Heel effect** and results in a higher x-ray intensity at the cathode end and a lower x-ray intensity at the anode end.

–The magnitude of the Heel effect depends on the anode angle (see Figure 2-4), source to image detector distance (SID), and field size.

    –To reduce the Heel effect, anode angle should be increased, SID increased, and field size decreased.

–The Heel effect can be taken advantage of by placing denser parts of the body at the cathode side and thinner parts at the anode side.

    –In mammography, for example, the more intense cathode side is used to irradiate the denser chest wall region.

E. Inverse square law

–X-ray beam intensity decreases with distance from the tube because of the divergence of the x-ray beam.

–The decrease in intensity is proportional to the square of the distance from the source and is an expression of energy conservation.

–This nonlinear fall-off in intensity with distance is called the **inverse square law**.

    –For example, doubling the distance from the x-ray source decreases the x-ray beam intensity by a factor of 4; increasing the distance by a factor of 10 decreases the beam intensity by a factor of 100.

–In general, if the distance from the x-ray source is changed from x_1 to x_2, then the x-ray beam intensity changes by $(x_1/x_2)^2$.

Review Test

1. Alternating electric current sources produce

(A) static electric fields
(B) static magnetic fields
(C) unidirectional flow of electrons
(D) oscillatory flows of electrons
(E) all of the above

2. Transformers in an x-ray machine

(A) work on the principle of electromagnetic induction
(B) need a filament as a source of electrons
(C) are used to transform electron energy into x-rays
(D) utilize thermionic emission
(E) cannot be used to generate low voltages

3. Match the device found in an x-ray circuit with its purpose.

(A) Transformer
(B) X-ray tube filament
(C) Diode
(D) Milliammeter

(i) Allows current to flow in one direction only
(ii) Increases or decreases voltage
(iii) Thermionic emission of electrons
(iv) Measures tube current

4. Match the following waveforms with the theoretical percentage ripple.

(A) Constant potential
(B) Single phase
(C) Three phase (6 pulse)
(D) Three phase (12 pulse)

(i) 0%
(ii) 3.5%
(iii) 14%
(iv) 100%

5. Electrons passing through matter lose energy primarily by

(A) production of bremsstrahlung
(B) photoelectric interactions
(C) collision with atomic electrons
(D) Compton interactions
(E) thermionic emission

6. 100 keV electrons incident on a tungsten target can produce

(A) Bremsstrahlung x-rays with a maximum energy of 100 keV
(B) Bremsstrahlung x-rays with average energy of 100 keV
(C) characteristic x-rays of 100 keV
(D) negligible (< 1%) heat in the target
(E) 100 keV photoelectrons

7. The continuous x-ray spectrum obtained from an x-ray tube is due to

(A) transitions of atomic electrons from higher to lower energy levels
(B) deceleration of electrons in the anode
(C) target heating by the electrons
(D) ejection of K-shell electrons
(E) ionization of target atoms

8. The *maximum* photon energy in x-ray beams is determined by the

(A) atomic number (Z) of the target
(B) atomic number (Z) of the filament
(C) voltage across the filament (V)
(D) voltage between anode and cathode (kV)
(E) tube current (mA)

9. Match the following radiations with the production parameters.

(A) Characteristic radiations of 19 keV
(B) Low energy photons have been removed by filtration
(C) Maximum photon energy is 100 keV
(D) Characteristic radiation at about 65 keV

(i) Applied x-ray tube voltage is 100 kV
(ii) X-ray tube has equivalent of 3 mm Al filtration
(iii) Anode is made of molybdenum
(iv) Anode is made of tungsten

10. The number of electrons accelerated across an x-ray tube is determined by

(A) anode speed
(B) focal spot size
(C) filament current
(D) x-ray tube filtration
(E) none of the above

11. X-ray production with a tungsten anode at 100 kVp is primarily

(A) Bremsstrahlung radiation
(B) characteristic radiation
(C) Compton scatter
(D) photoelectric
(E) none of the above

12. Anodes for production of x-rays have

(A) low atomic numbers (Z)
(B) air cooling to help dissipate their heat
(C) beryllium covering to prevent thermionic emission
(D) high-heat capacities to tolerate high temperatures
(E) all of the above

13. The line focus principle may be explained as

(A) apparent focus is smaller than true size
(B) another name for the heel effect
(C) x-ray intensity falls as square of distance
(D) reduction in intensity at anode edge
(E) all of the above

14. The size of an x-ray tube focal spot is

(A) larger than the nominal value by up to 50%
(B) dependent on applied mA ("blooming")
(C) smaller for magnification radiography
(D) measured using pinhole cameras
(E) all of the above

15. Match the focal spot size with the application.

(A) 0.1 mm
(B) 0.3 mm
(C) 0.6 mm
(D) 1.0 mm
(E) 1.5 mm

(i) Radiography focal spot
(ii) Fluoroscopy focal spot
(iii) Magnification neuroradiography
(iv) Magnification mammography
(v) Measured large focal spot

16. The formula mA $\times$ kV $\times$ time for a constant potential x-ray generator is the

(A) maximum safe technique value
(B) total energy deposited
(C) exposure level at 1 meter
(D) focal spot loading (power)
(E) none of the above

17. Calculate the anode heat loading for the following exposures.

(A) 100 seconds of fluoroscopy @ 100 kV and 5 mA
(B) Chest x-ray @ 100 kV, 1,000 mA, and 10 ms
(C) Lateral C-spine @ 100 kV, 500 mA, and 100 ms
(D) 10 s cardiac cine run @ 100 kV, 1,000 mA, 10 ms, and 50 frames per second
(E) 10 s digital run @ 100 kV, 100 mA, 10 ms, and 10 frames per second

18. Heat generated in an anode is primarily dissipated by

(A) convection
(B) conduction
(C) combustion
(D) air cooling
(E) radiation

19. True (T) or False (F). For an x-ray tube rating of 80 kW, the following exposures (0.1 sec) would be allowed.

(A) 100 kV and 800 mA
(B) 100 kV and 1000 mA
(C) 80 kV and 1000 mA
(D) 90 kV and 900 mA

20. True (T) or False (F). The energy of an x-ray tube characteristic x-ray is

(A) proportional to the energy of the projectile electrons
(B) dependent on the shell structure of the target atom
(C) about 65 keV for tungsten anodes
(D) dependent on x-ray filtration
(E) about 19 keV for molybdenum anodes

21. Changing the x-ray tube current (mA) is most likely to modify which of the following x-ray beam parameters?

(A) Maximum energy
(B) Quantity
(C) Quality
(D) Patient penetration (%)
(E) All of the above

22. Increasing the x-ray tube kVp will result in an increase of the average x-ray

(A) velocity
(B) wavelength
(C) energy
(D) mass
(E) none of the above

23. X-ray beam quality is primarily deter-mined by

(A) focal spot size
(B) filament current
(C) x-ray tube current
(D) filament voltage
(E) x-ray tube voltage

24. True (T) or False (F). The heel effect is more pronounced

(A) closer to the focal spot
(B) at high mA
(C) with a small target angle
(D) perpendicular to the anode-cathode-anode axis
(E) at the anode edge of the x-ray field

25. Match the following types of radiation with the appropriate definition.

(A) The useful beam
(B) Secondary radiation
(C) Stray radiation
(D) Leakage radiation
(E) Scattered radiation

(i) Radiation transmitted through the x-ray tube housing
(ii) Primary radiation limited by the collima-tor
(iii) Radiation changed in direction
(iv) Radiation resulting from absorption of other radiation
(v) Sum of the leakage and scattered radia-tion

Answers and Explanations

1–D. In North America, voltage changes direc-tion 60 times per second (60 Hz), resulting in an oscillating flow of electrons in the circuit.

2–A. Transformers are used to generate high (or low) voltages and operate according to the laws of electromagnetic induction.

3. A–ii; B–iii; the filament is the source of electrons for x-ray tube currents, which are generated by thermionic emission when the filament is heated; **C–i; D–iv.**

4. A–i; by definition a constant potential has no ripple; **B–iv;** AC waveforms oscillate to the maximum voltage in both directions; **C–iii; D–ii.**

5–C. Up to 99% of the electron energy is lost by collisions with outer shell atomic electrons (i.e., ionizations and excitations), which will appear as heat in the x-ray tube target.

6–A. About 1% of the energy is converted into x-rays. Most of the x-rays are produced by bremsstrahlung, whose spectrum has a maxi-mum photon energy of 100 keV, and an aver-age energy between 1/3 and 1/2 of the maximum.

7–B. Bremsstrahlung means "braking radia-tion" and occurs when an electron undergoes rapid deceleration in the nuclear electric field.

8–D. Voltage across the x-ray tube. The maxi-mum kinetic energy of electrons incident on the anode is equal to the maximum voltage; and it is possible for electrons to lose all this energy in a bremsstrahlung process.

9. A–iii; molybdenum has a K-shell binding energy of 20 keV; **B–ii;** 3 mm Al is a standard amount of filtration used in most of radiology; **C–i;** 100 keV bremsstrahlung radiation is the maximum that can be produced when the tube voltage is 100 kV; **D–iv;** tungsten has a K-shell binding energy of 69 keV, and the charactersitic x-rays are just below this energy.

10–C. The filament current determines the filament heating and the corresponding rate of release of electrons, which determines the x-ray tube current.

11–A. Bremsstrahlung. Characteristic x-ray production only accounts for about 10% to 20% of a typical x-ray beam produced at 100 kVp.

12–D. Anodes need high-heat capacities to prevent their melting when subjected to high-power loadings.

13–A. The line focus principle results in an apparent focal spot that is smaller than the area of the anode irradiated by the x-ray tube current, and depends on the anode angle (see Figure 2-4).

14–E. All the statements are true regarding focal spot sizes.

15. A–iv; B–iii; C–ii; D–i; E–v.

16–B. This expression for a constant potential generator gives the total energy deposited in the anode (power is the kV × mA).

17. A–50 kJ; B–1 kJ; C–5 kJ; D–500 kJ; E–10 kJ. In each case, the energy deposited in the anode is the product of the voltage (V), current (A), and exposure time (s), and also the total number of frames if applicable.

18–E. Heat dissipation occurs primarily by radiation through the x-ray tube vacuum into the housing (anodes get white hot during prolonged exposures).

19. A–True; power deposition of 80 kW; **B–False;** power deposition of 100 kW exceeds rating value of 80 kW; **C–True;** power deposition of 80 kW; **D–False;** power deposition of 81 kW. Note that in each case the power deposition is kV × mA.

20. A–False; characteristic x-ray production only requires that incident electrons have energy levels greater than the electron shell–binding energy; **B–True;** each element has a definite structure and emits well-defined energy x-rays which are, therefore, termed characteristic; **C–True; D–False;** filters primarily serve to attenuate low-energy x-rays; **E–True**.

21–B. The x-ray beam intensity is directly proportional to the x-ray tube current.

22–C. Increasing the kVp results in an increase in the average photon energy.

23–E. The x-ray tube voltage determines the x-ray beam quality; the higher the voltage, the higher the average x-ray energy, and the more penetrating the x-ray beam.

24. A–True; for a fixed-field size, the closer to the focus, the more pronounced the heel effect due to geometrical factors; **B–False;** heel effect is independent of mA; **C–True;** the smaller the angle, the greater the heel effect; **D–False;** the heel effect occurs *along* the cathode-anode axis, not *perpendicular* to it; **E–True;** the x-ray beam intensity is lowest at the anode side.

25. A–ii; B–iv; C–v; D–i; E–iii.

3

Interaction of Radiation and Matter

I. X-ray Interactions

A. Introduction

–When passing through matter, **photons** may **pass through** unaffected (i.e., penetrate), **be absorbed** (and transfer their energy to the absorbing medium), or **be scattered** (i.e., change direction and possibly lose energy).

–Important factors affecting these photon interactions include the **incident photon energy** and the **density, thickness,** and **atomic number** (Z) of the medium.

–The arrangement of atoms in the molecule (i.e., molecular structure) has a negligible effect on photon interactions.

–X-ray photons transfer energy to electrons, normally in substantial amounts that are measured in kiloelectron volts (keV).

–These energetic electrons, in turn, lose energy by interacting with the orbital electrons from other atoms and producing additional ionizations.

–An energetic electron may produce several hundred additional ion pairs.

–The approximate maximum distances, or ranges, traveled by energetic electrons are listed in Table 3-1.

–**Compton scatter** and the **photoelectric effect** (PE effect) are the two most important x-ray interactions in diagnostic radiology. Other interactions include **coherent scatter, pair production,** and **photodisintegration**.

B. Coherent scatter

–**Coherent scatter** occurs when an **incident photon changes direction without losing energy**.

–Coherent scatter does not result in any energy deposition in the patient (i.e., dose) but contributes to undesirable scatter.

–Because no energy is transferred to the atom, ionization does not occur.

Table 3-1. Distances Traveled by Energetic Electrons in Media of Different Effective Atomic Number ($\bar{Z}$) and Physical Density (ρ)

Electron energy (keV)	Air $\bar{Z} = 7.8$ $\rho = 0.0012$ g/cm³	Water $\bar{Z} = 7.5$ $\rho = 1.0$ g/cm³	Bone $\bar{Z} = 12.3$ $\rho = 1.7$ g/cm³
10	0.25 cm	3 μm	2 μm
30	1.7 cm	18 μm	12 μm
50	4.1 cm	43 μm	28 μm
100	13.5 cm	140 μm	94 μm
150	26.5 cm	280 μm	180 μm

–Coherent scatter is usually present in diagnostic radiology but is a relatively minor concern.

–Coherent scatter accounts for less than 10% of all photon interactions occurring in tissue at diagnostic energies.

C. Pair production

–**Pair production** occurs when a high-energy photon interacts with the nucleus of an atom. The photon disappears, and the energy is converted into an **electron** and a **positron**.

–Pair production has a photon energy threshold of 1.022 MeV, which is the energy required to produce an electron (511 keV) and positron (511 keV) pair.

–Because of the high threshold energy (1.022 MeV), pair production is not encountered in diagnostic radiology but is important in megavoltage radiotherapy.

D. Photodisintegration

–**Photodisintegration** occurs when a high-energy photon is absorbed by a nucleus, resulting in **immediate disintegration** of the nucleus.

–The **energy threshold** for photodisintegration is appoximately **15 MeV**.

–Photodisintegration is, therefore, only important at the high photon energies encountered in megavoltage radiotherapy and high-energy accelerator physics.

II. Photoelectric and Compton Effects

A. Photoelectric effect

–The **PE effect** occurs between tightly bound (inner shell) electrons and incident x-ray photons.

–The PE effect occurs when a photon is totally absorbed by an inner shell electron and a **photoelectron is emitted**.

–In addition to the photoelectron emission, a positive atomic ion is formed.

–The photoelectron loses energy by ionizing other atoms in the tissue and contributes to patient dose.

–The photoelectron energy equals the difference between the incident photon energy and the electron binding energy.

–The inner shell electron vacancies are filled by outer shell electrons, and the excess energy is emitted as **characteristic radiation**.

Calcium ^{40}Ca

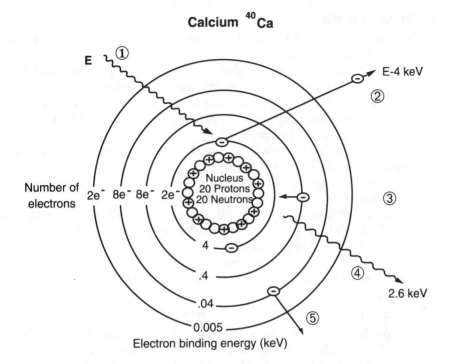

Figure 3-1. The photoelectric effect occurs when an incident x-ray (*1*) is totally absorbed by an inner shell electron, which is ejected as a photoelectron (*2*). The vacancy (*3*) is filled by an outer shell electron, and the energy difference is emitted as characteristic radiation (*4*) or as an Auger electron (*5*).

–An alternative to the emission of a characteristic x-ray is for the energy to be used to eject an **Auger electron** from the shell.

–Figure 3-1 shows a photoelectric interaction.

B. Probability of photoelectric effect

–For the PE effect to occur, the incident x-ray must have energy greater than the binding energy of the inner shell electron.

  –The binding energy of the K-shell electrons (K-edge) in iodine is 33 keV, and a sharp increase in the interaction of photons occurs when the x-ray photon energy exceeds 33 keV.

–The absorption of photons increases markedly as the x-ray photon energy is increased from below to above the binding energy of the K-shell electrons (K-edge).

  –Above the K-edge energy, the PE effect declines rapidly in proportion to photon energy (*E*), that is, the PE effect is **proportional to $1/E^3$**.

–The PE effect is also **proportional to Z^3**. The more tightly bound an electron is, the greater is the probability of the PE effect, if *E* is greater than the binding energy.

–The PE effect is important if the atomic number (*Z*) is high and the photon energy is just above the K-edge.

–Important K-shell binding energies are oxygen (*Z* = 8) 0.5 keV, calcium (*Z* = 20) 4 keV, iodine (*Z* = 53) 33 keV, barium (*Z* = 56) 37 keV, and lead (*Z* = 82) 88 keV.

C. Compton scatter

–In **Compton scatter,** incident photons interact with loosely bound (**outer shell**) electrons.

–A Compton interaction results in a **scattered photon** that has less energy than the incident photon and travels in a new direction.

–A **scattered electron** carries the energy lost by the incident photon.

–This electron loses energy by ionizing other atoms in the tissue, thereby contributing to the patient dose.

–As a result of the Compton interaction, a positive atomic ion, which has lost an outer shell electron, remains.

–Compton interactions occur most commonly with electrons with a low binding energy.

–Outer shell electrons have binding energies of only a few electron volts, which is negligible compared to the high energy (30 keV) of a typical diagnostic energy x-ray photon.

–Figure 3-2 shows a Compton interaction.

–Compton interactions account for most scattered radiation encountered in diagnostic radiology.

D. Probability of a Compton interaction

–The **probability** of a Compton interaction is **proportional to the number of outer shell electrons** available in the medium (electron density) and **inversely proportional to the photon energy ($1/E$).**

–Scattered photons may move in any direction, including 180 degrees to the direction of the incident photon (**backscattered**).

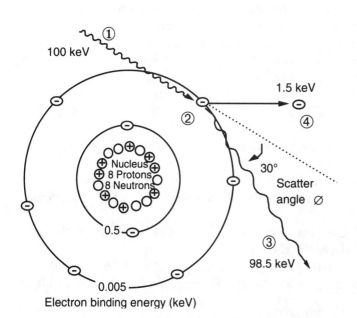

Oxygen ^{16}O

100 keV
①
1.5 keV
②
④
⊕ Nucleus
⊕ 8 Protons
○ 8 Neutrons
30°
Scatter angle ∅
0.5
③
98.5 keV
0.005
Electron binding energy (keV)

Figure 3-2. Compton scattering occurs when an incoming x-ray photon (*1*) interacts with an outer shell electron (*2*). The x-ray photon loses energy and changes direction (*3*). The Compton electron carries away the energy lost by the scattered photon (*4*).

Table 3-2. Energies of Compton-scattered Photons Deflected Through 90 and 180 Degrees

	Photon Energy (keV)	
Incident	**Scattered 90°**	**Scattered 180°**
60	54	49
80	69	61
100	84	72
120	97	82

Note. Energy difference between incident and scattered photons is transferred to the Compton-scattered electron.

–As the angle of deflection decreases, the energy retained by the scattered x-ray increases.
  –Energy transfer to the electron is maximum when the photon is backscattered.
  –The incident and Compton scattered x-ray energies at different scatter angles are listed in Table 3-2.
  –For soft tissue, the PE and Compton effects are equal in magnitude at a photon energy of about 25 keV.

III. Attenuation of Radiation

A. Linear attenuation coefficient

  –The **linear attenuation coefficient (μ)** is the fraction of incident photons "lost" from the beam when traveling a unit distance.
  –The attenuation coefficient accounts for all possible x-ray interactions, including the PE effect and Compton scatter.
    –The attenuation coefficient generally decreases with increasing photon energy and increases with atomic number and density.
    –An attenuation coefficient of 0.1/cm (0.1 cm^{-1}) means that 10% of the incident photons are lost (absorbed or scattered) in traveling 1 cm, with the remaining 90% being transmitted.
  –**Monochromatic** (monoenergetic) x-rays are absorbed according to the **exponential formula $N = N_0\,e^{-\mu t}$,** where N_0 is the initial number of photons incident on an absorbing medium of thickness t (cm), N is the number of photons transmitted, and μ (cm^{-1}) is the attenuation coefficient.

B. Mass attenuation coefficient

  –The linear attenuation coefficient normally depends on the density of the absorbing material. For any absorbing medium, however, the attenuation is the same with only half the thickness but double the density.
    –For example, compression of lung has no effect on photon transmission because the amount of absorbing material (i.e., total number of atoms) remains the same. However, the values of both the attenuation coefficient (μ) and density (ρ) change as the lungs are expanded or compressed.
  –The **mass attenuation coefficient** is the linear attenuation coefficient (μ) divided by the density (ρ).
    –This allows attenuation to be described as a function of the mass of the material traversed rather than the distance traveled by photons.

–The mass attenuation coefficient is independent of the density of the material.

–The thickness of the absorbing medium must be specified using the **mass thickness g/cm²,** or $\rho \times t$, when the mass attenuation coefficient (μ/ρ) is used to specify attenuation.

–X-ray attenuation is determined by the product of the mass thickness and mass attenuation coefficient, that is, $(\rho \times t) \times (\mu/\rho)$.

–This product equals $\mu \times t$, giving the attenuation factor $e^{-\mu t}$ because the densities (ρ) cancel out.

–Figure 3-3 shows the mass attenuation coefficient for different materials as a function of x-ray energy.

C. Half-value layer

–The thickness of material that attenuates an x-ray beam by 50% is the **half-value layer (HVL).**

–The thickness of material that attenuates an x-ray beam by 90% is called the **tenth value layer (TVL)** because it transmits only one tenth of the incident intensity.

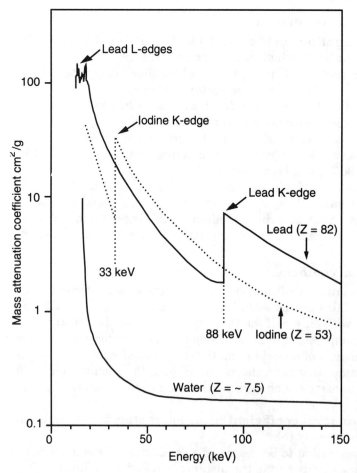

Figure 3-3. Mass attenuation coefficient as a function of photon energy. Notice the sharp increase at the K-edge of lead and iodine due to the PE effect at the K-edge of these materials.

Table 3-3. Selected Half-Value Layer/Tenth-Value Layer Data for Monoenergetic Photons

Energy (keV)	Muscle (cm)		Bone (cm)		Lead (mm)	
	HVL	**TVL**	**HVL**	**TVL**	**HVL**	**TVL**
30	1.8	6.1	0.4	1.5	0.02	0.07
50	3.0	9.9	1.2	4.0	0.08	0.26
100	3.9	13.0	2.3	7.7	0.11	0.37
150	4.5	14.8	2.8	9.3	0.31	1.0

   –At average diagnostic x-ray beam energies, the HVL for soft tissue typically ranges from 2.5 to 3.0 cm.
     –For a 20-cm thick patient, the primary transmission for an abdominal
     radiograph is approximately 1%. (Intensity is reduced to 50% after 3
     cm, 25% after 6 cm, 12% after 9 cm, and so on.)
   –Approximate values for transmission of the primary beam through a
   patient is 10% for chest radiographs, 5% for mammograms, 1% for skull
   radiographs, and 0.5% for abdominal radiographs.
   –At the low energies (28 kVp spectra) used in mammography, the HVL for
   soft tissue is about 1 cm.
   –The relation between the linear attenuation coefficient (μ) and HVL is
   $HVL = \log_e(2)/\mu = 0.693/\mu$.
   –Table 3-3 shows typical HVLs and TVLs for a range of monoenergetic x-
   ray beams.

IV. Diagnostic X-ray Beams

A. Introduction

   –X-ray beams in diagnostic radiology consist of a range of photon energies
   (spectrum) and are known as **polychromatic**.
   –To measure the reduction in the intensity of polychromatic x-ray beams,
   the attenuation coefficient for the absorbing medium at the **effective
   photon energy** must be known.
     –The effective photon energy is taken to be between one third and one
     half of the maximum photon energy.

B. Filters

   –The x-ray beam emerging from the x-ray tube may contain a high number of low-energy photons.
     –Low-energy photons have a negligible chance of getting through the
     patient, thereby contributing to patient dose but adding nothing to the
     image.
   –Some of the very low-energy x-rays are stopped as they exit the tube by
   the glass window, which acts as an inherent x-ray beam filter.
     –Beryllium provides almost no filtration and is sometimes used as a win-
     dow in mammography x-ray tubes.
   –Filters are also added to the x-ray tube window to increase the filtration
   effect as listed in Table 3-4.
   –Filters preferentially absorb low-energy photons.
   –Filtration does not affect the maximum energy of the x-ray beam spec-
   trum.

Table 3-4. Representative Filtration Values

Technique	kVp	Typical Added Filtration
Screen/film mammography	26–30	30 μm Molybdenum
Radiography	< 50	> 0.5 mm Aluminum
Radiography	50–70	> 1.5 mm Aluminum
Radiography	> 70	> 2.5 mm Aluminum
High-voltage studies (chest)	> 100	Copper/aluminum
High-energy imaging	> 200	Tin/copper/aluminum*

*Thoraeus filter.

  –Figure 3-4 shows the effect of filtration on an x-ray spectrum. Low-energy photons are preferentially lost when passing through a filter or any other absorbing medium.

C. Beam hardening

  –**Beam hardening** refers to the **preferential loss** of lower energy photons with filtration.

  –The x-ray beam output is decreased with increased filtration (see Table 2-3), but the average x-ray energy is increased.

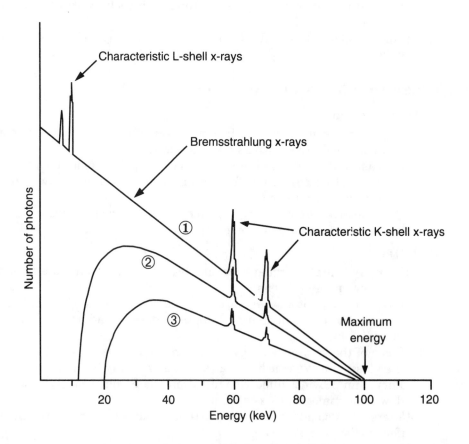

Figure 3-4. X-ray emission spectra from a tungsten target produced at 100 kV. Curve *1* is the theoretical spectrum without any filtration. Curve *2* is the typical spectrum with the inherent filtration of the x-ray tube and added filtration. Curve *3* shows the effect of additional filtration.

–The x-ray beam becomes **more penetrating** as the mean photon energy increases. Filtered beams with higher mean photon energies are called **harder** x-ray beams.

  –After filtration by one HVL, a greater thickness of material is required to further reduce the more penetrating beam intensity by an additional 50%.

  –This means that the **second HVL** is always **greater than** the **first HVL** for polychromatic x-ray beams.

–Beam hardening does not occur with monochromatic x-ray beams because the HVL remains constant.

–**Hard beams** are produced at high peak voltages using heavy filtration.

–**Soft beams** are produced at low peak voltages using less filtration.

D. X-ray beam quality

–The **quality** of an x-ray beam is specified as the **thickness of aluminum** (mm) that reduces the x-ray beam intensity by 50% (i.e., HVL).

–At 80 kVp, the legal minimum x-ray beam HVL in many states is 2.5 mm of aluminum.

–A lower HVL means that the beam has too many low-energy photons.

–Typical HVLs are 0.3 mm of aluminum in mammography (28 kVp), 1.5 mm of aluminum in xeroradiography (45 kVp), and 3 mm of aluminum in conventional radiography (80 kVp).

–Table 3-5 gives typical values of x-ray beam HVL for a three-phase generator as a function of peak voltage and beam filtration. These data show that HVL increases with increasing filtration.

V. Radiographic Contrast

A. Subject contrast

–**Subject contrast** is the difference in x-ray intensities **transmitted** through different parts of the patient.

–Subject contrast is affected by the incident photon energy, atomic number (Z), and density of the absorbers.

–The PE effect and Compton scatter are the primary factors contributing to the contrast seen in diagnostic x-ray images.

  –**PE effects** are generally important at low photon energies and produce high subject contrast. PE effects are also important when materials with high atomic numbers (e.g., calcium, iodine, barium) are present.

Table 3-5. Representative Half-Value Layers Showing the Effect of Filtration on Beam Quality

Peak Voltage (kVp)	Half-Value Layer (mm Al)	
	2.5 mm Al Filtration	3.5 mm Al Filtration
60	2.2	2.6
80	2.7	3.2
100	3.3	3.9
120	4.0	4.6

Note. Table shows values for a three-phase generator.

Compton scatter predominates at high photon energies where the PE effect is negligible.

B. Contrast agents

–Contrast agents including air, barium, and iodine are used to improve subject contrast.

–Barium is administered as a contrast agent for visualization on radiographic examinations for several reasons.

–The attenuation of barium is high because of its high atomic number (Z = 56) and physical density.

–The barium K-edge is 37 keV, which matches the photon energies used in fluoroscopy.

–Iodine (Z = 53, K-edge = 33 keV) is also an excellent contrast agent for similar reasons to those for barium.

–Iodinated contrast agents can be injected intravenously, but dilution in fluid and the osmolar limitations of intravascular fluids limit the achievable concentration.

–Air is a negative contrast agent and increases subject contrast because it is less attenuating than tissue.

C. Contrast and peak voltage

–Low photon energies result in high subject contrast because the PE effect is sensitive to the atomic number of the absorbing medium.

–High subject contrast, however, is difficult to record radiographically because of the limited dynamic range of film.

–Low kVp x-ray beams are rarely used in radiology because of limited penetration through patients.

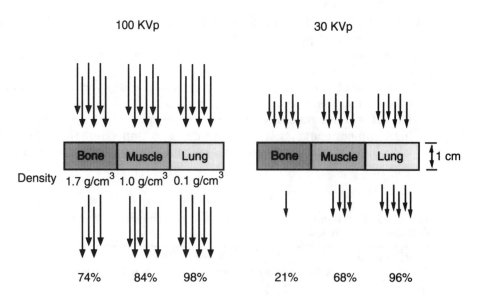

Figure 3-5. Subject contrast decreases with increasing photon energy. As energy increases, so does the ability of the x-ray to penetrate, resulting in less difference in x-ray attenuation between air and bone at high energies.

–High kVp x-ray beams have high mean x-ray energies and are more penetrating.

–Figure 3-5 shows how subject contrast depends on the kVp, showing that increasing kVp generally reduces subject contrast.

–Compton scatter becomes more important as the kVp is increased, and also reduces contrast.

 –At increased kVps, less x-ray tube output is needed to achieve a given level of patient penetration to result in a satisfactory radiographic image.

–Increasing kVp allows the x-ray output values (mAs) to be reduced and produce the same film density with reduced entrance skin exposures.

Review Test

1. Coherent scatter

(A) cannot occur at diagnostic x-ray energies
(B) is more important than Compton scatter
(C) produces scattered photons which degrade image quality
(D) increases patient dose
(E) none of the above

2. The threshold energy for pair production is

(A) there is no threshold
(B) 1.022 keV
(C) 5.11 keV
(D) 511 keV
(E) 1.022 MeV

3. Pair production interactions

(A) have a threshold energy of 511 keV
(B) are independent of atomic number (Z)
(C) are independent of photon energy
(D) generate electrons and positrons

4. Which of the following results in the total absorption of an x-ray photon?

(A) Coherent scatter
(B) Photoelectric effect
(C) Compton scatter
(D) Pair production
(E) All of the above

5. Photoelectric interactions cannot produce

(A) characteristic x-rays
(B) auger electrons
(C) photoelectrons
(D) positive ions
(E) scattered photons

6. The photoelectric effect will be a maximum for

(A) energies just above the atomic K-edge
(B) low Z materials
(C) high photon energies
(D) outer shell electrons
(E) atoms bound together in molecules

7. The energy (E) and atomic number (Z) dependence of the photoelectric effect varies approximately as

(A) Z^3/E^3
(B) E^3/Z^3
(C) Z/E
(D) E^2/Z
(E) $Z^3 \times E^3$

8. Compton interactions are most likely to result in

(A) 511 keV photons
(B) characteristic x-rays
(C) photoelectrons
(D) scattered photons with reduced energy
(E) internal conversion electrons

9. Which interaction dominates for 45 keV photons in water?

(A) Photoelectric effect
(B) Coherent scatter
(C) Compton scatter
(D) Photodisintegration
(E) Pair production

10. Pick the *most* appropriate interaction process—photoelectric effect (PE) or Compton scatter.

(A) Most important at low photon energies
(B) Dominant in tissue between 25 keV and 150 keV
(C) Scatter photons are produced
(D) Affected by absorption edges
(E) Occurs with inner shell (bound) electrons
(F) For visualization of barium and iodine contrast

11. True (T) or False (F). The linear attenuation coefficient (μ) for tissue in the diagnostic energy range

(A) decreases continuously with increasing energy
(B) may be used to estimate transmission of x-rays
(C) is expressed in units of g/cm^3
(D) gives mass attenuation coefficient when divided by the density (ρ)
(E) is proportional to the tissue thickness (±)

12. For an absorbing medium with thickness (t), the quantity $e^{-\mu t}$ is independent of

(A) incident photon intensity
(B) photon energy
(C) absorbing medium density
(D) absorbing medium atomic number

13. Match the following linear attenuation coefficients (μ cm^{-1}) at 50 keV with the material.

(A) Air
(B) Soft tissue
(C) Bone
(D) Lead

(i)   0.57 cm^{-1}
(ii) 88.6 cm^{-1}
(iii) 0.0002 cm^{-1}
(iv) 0.23 cm^{-1}

14. The mass attenuation coefficient is independent of

(A) photoelectric effect
(B) Compton scatter
(C) coherent scatter
(D) density of material (ρ)
(E) photon energy (E)

15. The half-value layer (HVL) for a material with a linear attenuation coefficient of 0.1 cm^{-1} is approximately

(A) 1 cm
(B) 1.4 cm
(C) 7 cm
(D) 10 cm

16. An x-ray beam is attenuated by three half-value layers. The x-ray beam intensity is reduced by a factor of

(A) 2
(B) 4
(C) 8
(D) 16
(E) 32

17. Filters remove the following radiation from an x-ray beam

(A) secondary
(B) low energy
(C) high energy
(D) leakage
(E) stray

18. The effective photon energy of an x-ray beam cannot be changed by

(A) tube current (mA)
(B) beam filtration
(C) tube voltage
(D) voltage waveform
(E) passage through a patient

19. Match the x-ray beam filter with the radiographic examination most closely associated with its usage.

(A) Routine radiography
(B) Film/screen mammography
(C) Chest radiography

(i)   Copper/aluminum
(ii) Molybdenum
(iii) Aluminum

20. The adequacy of the filtration of an x-ray tube may be determined by

(A) physical inspection
(B) x-ray tube documentation
(C) kVp measurement
(D) x-ray output measurement
(E) half-value layer measurement

21. Match the following beam quality and HVL.

(A) 0.3 mm Al
(B) 2.5 mm Al
(C) 3.5 mm Al
(D) 6 mm Al

(i)   Measured HVL on x-ray unit @ 80 kV
(ii) *Minimum* HVL @ 80 kV
(iii) Film/screen mammography unit HVL
(iv) HVL for chest x-ray unit @ 140 kV

22. The x-ray beam HVL does NOT depend on the

(A) radiation intensity
(B) peak kV
(C) voltage waveform
(D) filtration
(E) x-ray spectrum
(F) anode material

23. Increasing the x-ray tube voltage (kVp) will NOT increase

(A) x-ray beam intensity
(B) patient penetration
(C) beam half-value layer (HVL)
(D) beam filtration
(E) heat produced in the anode

24. The soft tissue contrast in chest radiographs performed at 140 kVp is primarily due to

(A) coherent scatter
(B) Compton scatter
(C) photoelectric effect
(D) pair production
(E) photodisintegration

25. The reason for high subject contrast on a barium enema examination is

(A) coherent scatter
(B) Compton scatter
(C) photoelectric effect
(D) pair production
(E) photodisintegration

Answers and Explanations

1–C. Coherent scatter results in scattered photons but *no transfer of energy,* and typically accounts for less than 10% of x-ray interactions in diagnostic radiology.

2–E. In pair production, a positron and electron are created where each has a rest mass energy of 511 keV.

3–D. In pair production, a photon is converted into an electron-positron pair. (The threshold is 1.022 MeV, above which the probability of an interaction increases with Z and with photon energy.)

4–B. Only the photoelectric effect results in the absorption of the incident x-ray photon.

5–E. Because the incident photon is absorbed, scattered photons are not produced. (Other products occur directly following PE interactions.)

6–A. The PE effect is always a maximum for photons with energies just above the K-shell binding energy. (The PE effect decreases with increasing photon energy and decreasing atomic number (Z) and does not depend on outer shell electrons or the molecular structure.)

7–A. The probability of the photoelectric effect increases rapidly as Z increases (Z^3) and decreases rapidly as E increases ($1/E^3$).

8–D. Lower-energy scattered photons (511 keV photons are annihilation radiation from positrons; characteristic x-rays are produced from inner-shell vacancies; photoelectrons are emitted following photoelectric absorption; internal conversion occurs with nuclear gamma ray emission).

9–C. Only the PE and Compton scatter are important in radiology. The PE and Compton effects are equal at 25 keV, with the PE more important at lower energies and vice versa.

10. A–PE; B–Compton scatter; C–Compton scatter; D–PE; E–PE; F–PE.

11. A–True; μ falls off very rapidly at low energies [E < 25 keV] and more slowly at higher photon energies; **B–True;** fractional transmission is $e^{-\mu t}$, where t is the thickness and μ is the attenuation coefficient at the effective [mean] photon energy; **C–False;** expressed in cm^{-1}; **D–True;** mass attenuation coefficient by definition is μ/ρ; **E–False;** μ is independent of tissue thickness (t) and is multiplied with t to compute the transmission $e^{-\mu t}$ factor.

12–A. The term measures the fractional transmission, which is independent of incident x-ray intensity (the attenuation coefficient [μ] is generally a function of photon energy [E], atomic number [Z], and density [ρ]).

13. A–iii; B–iv; C–i; D–ii (air is the least-attenuating material and lead the most attenuating).

14–D. By definition, μ/ρ, the mass attenuation coefficient, is independent of density (ρ).

15–C. The HVL is given by the expression $\ln_e 2/\mu$ (0.693/0.1 cm, or approximately 7 cm).

16–C. Each HVL reduces the intensity by 1/2, so the total intensity reduction is $(1/2)^n$ for n half-value layers and three half-value layers reduces intensity by a factor of 8.

17–B. Filters are used to remove the low-energy photons that increase the patient dose but do not contribute to the image.

18–A. Beam quality is independent of the tube current (mA), which primarily determines the x-ray beam output (intensity).

19. A–iii; B–ii; typically 30 μm molybdenum; **C–i;** chest x-rays performed at high kVps (120 to 140) are usually heavily filtered to reduce contrast and thereby permit visualization of lung/mediastinum.

20–E. Adequacy of x-ray tube filtration is determined by measuring the HVL, usually at 80 kVp, and ensuring it exceeds 2.5 mm Al.

21. A–iii; B–ii; C–i; D–iv. The higher the HVL, the higher the beam quality and mean energy.

22–A. The HVL expressed in mm Al only depends on the x-ray spectrum; it is thus independent of the intensity of the beam as measured by the exposure.

23–D. Beam filtration depends on the x-ray tube window and added filters, and is therefore independent of x-ray tube kV/mA.

24–B. Compton scatter is the primary interaction for soft tissues at high photon energy levels (> 25 keV or > 75 kVp).

25–C. The high atomic number of barium (Z = 56; K-edge 37 keV) results in strong absorption of the incident x-ray beam, and results in very high subject contrast.

4

Radiation Detection and Measurement

I. Radiation Units

A. Exposure

–**Exposure** is a source-related term used to express the intensity (i.e., amount) of radiation in an x-ray beam.

–Exposure measures the **ability of radiation to ionize air**.

–Exposure is the **total charge** liberated per unit mass of air when all the electrons liberated by the photon interactions are completely stopped in air.

–Exposure is measured in **coulombs per kilogram (C/kg)** in the SI system or in **roentgens (R)** in non-SI units: **1 R = 2.58 × 10^{-4} C/kg**.

–Exposure is only defined for photons with energies less than 3 MeV.

  –For monoenergetic 60-keV photons, an exposure of 1 R corresponds to a photon intensity of about 3×10^8 photons/mm^2.

–Exposure from an x-ray source obeys the **inverse square law** (see Chapter 2 V E) and decreases with the square of the distance from a source.

  –For example, increasing the distance between the source and measurement point by a factor of 2 reduces the exposure by a factor of 4.

B. Kerma

–**Kerma** stands for the *Kinetic Energy Released in the Medium*.

–Kerma is the **kinetic energy transferred** from uncharged particles (photons and neutrons) to charged particles (electrons and protons) when radiation interacts with matter.

–Kerma is specified in units of **joules per kilogram** (J/kg).

–Kerma in air or water may replace the roentgen as a measure of exposure in the SI system.

C. Absorbed dose

–**Absorbed dose** (*D*) measures the amount of radiation energy (*E*) absorbed per unit mass (*M*) of absorbing medium: ***D = E/M***.

–Absorbed dose is specified in **gray (Gy)** in the SI system and **rad** (radiation absorbed dose) in non-SI units.

–One gray is equal to 1 J of energy deposited per kilogram, and 1 rad is equal to 100 ergs of energy deposited per gram: **1 Gy = 100 rad; 1 rad = 10 mGy**.

–The absorbed dose in a radiation field depends on the absorbing medium that is placed into the radiation field.

–Therefore, the absorbing medium (e.g., air, soft tissue, bone) and its location (e.g., entrance skin, thyroid, spleen) should always be specified.

–Absorbed dose is not source-related as is exposure (R).

D. f-Factor

–The **f-factor** is the conversion factor between exposure and absorbed dose.

–The relation between absorbed dose (D) and exposure (X) is $D = f \times X$, where f is the roentgen-to-rad conversion factor, or **f-factor**.

–At diagnostic x-ray energies, the f-factor for air, muscle, and other soft tissue is close to 1. The f-factor for bone ranges from about 4 at low keV to almost 1 at high keV.

–Table 4-1 lists the f-factor for a range of photon energies and absorbing media.

E. Linear energy transfer

–**Linear energy transfer (LET)** represents the energy absorbed by the medium per unit length of travel (keV/μm).

–Uncharged radiation (photons and neutrons) **transfers energy** to the medium **via intermediate particles,** including photoelectrons (photons) and recoil protons (neutrons).

–For a given medium, LET is proportional to the square of the particle charge and is inversely related to particle kinetic energy. Thus, low-speed particles with multiple charges, such as slow-moving alpha particles, have the highest LET values.

–Neutrons, protons, alpha particles, and heavy ions are high LET radiations with values ranging from 3 to 200 keV/μm.

–Photons, gamma rays, electrons, and positrons are low LET radiations with values ranging from 0.2 to 3 keV/μm.

–High LET radiations are much more effective in producing biological damage than low LET radiation.

Table 4-1. f-Factor Values Used to Convert Exposure to Absorbed Dose

Photon Energy (keV)	Fat $\overline{Z} = 6.5$ $\rho = 0.92$	Muscle $\overline{Z} = 7.6$ $\rho = 1.04$	Bone $\overline{Z} = 12.3$ $\rho = 1.65$	Lithium Fluoride $\overline{Z} = 8.3$ $\rho = 2.7$
30	0.53	0.92	4.4	1.07
50	0.66	0.94	3.6	0.98
100	0.91	0.96	1.5	0.84
150	0.96	0.96	1.1	0.82

ρ = density (g/cm^3); $\overline{Z}$ = effective atomic number.

–Photoelectrons produced in tissue can produce hundreds of ion pairs.

–This deposited energy can break apart biologically important molecules such as DNA and cause cell function to be modified.

–When considering the biological effect of radiation, the total amount of energy absorbed (i.e., dose) and the effectiveness of this radiation at causing biological damage (i.e., LET) must be considered.

F. Dose equivalent

–**Dose equivalent** (H) attempts to quantify the biological damage arising from the deposition of ionizing radiation in tissues.

–Dose equivalent is primarily used in radiation protection.

–The dose equivalent is the absorbed dose (D) multiplied by the quality factor (QF) of the radiation, or $\boldsymbol{H = D \times QF}$.

–The **quality factor** depends on the radiation LET value.

–For low LET radiation sources (e.g., electrons, beta particles, x-rays, gamma rays), $QF = 1$; for high LET radiation sources (e.g., protons, neutrons, alpha particles), QF may be as high as 20.

–Dose equivalent is expressed in sievert (Sv) in the SI system and in rems (radiation equivalent man) in non-SI units: **1 Sv = 100 rem; 1 rem = 10 mSv**.

G. R's in radiology

–In diagnostic radiology and nuclear medicine, x-rays, gamma rays, and beta particles have low LET values and the quality factor (QF) equals 1.

–In this instance, exposure, absorbed dose, and dose equivalent are all approximately equal when using non-SI units (1 R ~ 1 rad ~ 1 rem).

–Although all three terms are often used interchangeably, they are conceptually different as shown in Figure 4-1.

–**Exposure (R)** refers to the ability of radiation to ionize air and is a source-related term.

–**Absorbed dose (rad)** refers to the energy absorbed and depends on the absorbing medium.

–**Dose equivalent (rem)** is a measure of the biological damage that is likely to result from the absorbed energy.

II. Film

A. Emulsions

–In diagnostic radiology, film is used for capturing, displaying, and storing radiographic images.

–Film consists of an approximately 10-µm thick **emulsion** supported by a mylar base, which is about 150 µm thick.

–Most films have an emulsion layer on both sides of the base.

–Additional layers can include a protective coating, antistatic, or anti-crossover layer.

–The emulsion contains **silver halide grains,** which can be sensitized by radiation or light to hold a latent image.

–Silver halide grains are typically 1 to 1.5 µm in diameter and contain 10^6 to 10^7 silver atoms. There are about 10^9 grains per cubic centimeter.

–Several light photons (approximately 4) must be absorbed to sensitize each grain.

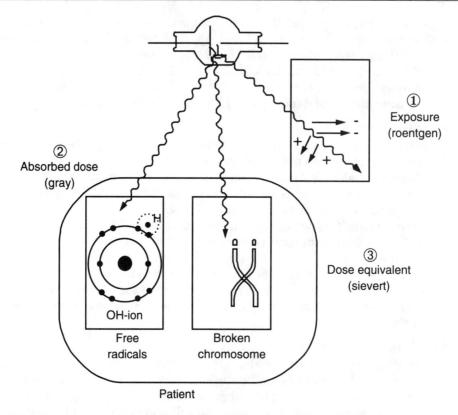

Figure 4-1. Exposure is a source-related term that refers to the ability to ionize air as shown in the ionization chamber (*1*). Absorbed dose refers to the radiation energy absorbed as shown in (*2*), where free radicals are being formed. Dose equivalent is used to quantify the biological damage resulting from ionizing radiation as shown in (*3*) where chromosome breaks have occurred.

–Absorbed light photons liberate electrons in the grain, which combine with positively charged silver ions (Ag^+). After exposure, grains have a few neutral silver atoms in the speck along with millions of Ag^+ ions.

B. Film development

–Sensitized grains are **reduced** in the developer by the addition of electrons.

–A **developed grain** results in a speck of silver that appears black on the film.

–Grains with no latent image are also developed but at a much slower rate.

–Film speed, contrast, and base and fog levels are all affected by developer chemistry and temperature.

–Increasing the developer temperature or development time increases the film contrast and density, but also increases fog.

–The development process is one of the most important aspects in producing good quality images.

C. Film processors

–Modern **film processors** automatically run film sequentially through the **developer, fixer,** and **washing solutions.**

–Developer temperatures typically range from 31°C to 35°C.

–Film is washed to remove all developer solution before proceeding to the fixing solution.

–The fixing solution contains acetic acid to inhibit further development and remove unexposed silver halide grains.

–After development and fixing, the film is washed to eliminate all chemicals and is dried by heaters or infrared lamps.

–The total **processing time** is typically **90 seconds** (25-second developer time, 21-second fixer time, 44-second washing and drying time).

–Dirty, uneven, or maladjusted rollers can leave lines or other artifacts (e.g., π lines) on the film. Static electricity can also cause severe film artifacts.

–Film processor quality control (QC) is essential in maintaining film image quality at a high level.

–Processor QC involves measuring developer temperature and monitoring the density and contrast of film exposed to a light source in a **sensitometer**.

D. Film density

–Film **blackening** is directly related to the number of photons that reach the film. Film blackening is normally measured using **optical density (OD)**.

–OD is defined by $\mathbf{OD = log_{10}(I_o/I_t)}$, where I_o is the light intensity incident on the film, and I_t is the light transmitted through the film.

–OD can be measured using a **densitometer**.

–**Transmittance** is the fraction of incident light passing through the film (transmittance = I_t/I_o).

–As OD increases, transmittance decreases.

–The useful range of film ODs is from about 0.3 (50% transmittance) to 2 (1% transmittance). Densities above about 2.2 require the use of a hot light.

–A logarithmic scale is used because a large density difference can be expressed on a small scale and because the physiologic response of the eye is logarithmic.

–The OD of superimposed films is additive, so two films with an OD of 1.0 (10% transmittance) superimposed would have an OD of 2.0 and transmit 1% of the incident light.

–Table 4-2 shows the relation between optical density and transmittance.

E. Characteristic curves

–The **characteristic curve** represents the relation between exposure and resultant film OD as shown in Figure 4-2.

–Characteristic curves are also known as **H and D curves**, named after Hurter and Driffield who first generated these curves in 1890.

–The **toe** is the low exposure region, and the **shoulder** is the high exposure region of the curve.

–**Base plus fog** level is the film blackening in the absence of any radiation exposure and typically ranges from 0.1 to 0.2 OD units.

–The maximum film density ranges from 2.5 to 3.0 OD units.

–Fast films require less radiation to achieve a given film density; slow films require more radiation.

Table 4-2. Percentage Transmittance and Resultant Value of Film Optical Density

Transmittance (T %)	Optical Density (OD)	Comments
100	0.0	
50	0.3	Base plus fog has a density of about 0.2
25	0.6	Lowest useful density in radiology
10	1.0	
5	1.3	Normally the region with highest film contrast
1	2.0	Higher densities require use of hot light
0.1	3.0	Typical maximum film density

$T = 100 \times (I_t/I_o)\%$; $OD = \log_{10}(I_o/I_t)$.

–The speed of a film is the inverse of the radiation exposure needed to produce a given net film density (e.g., 1.0). Thus, speed = 1/R, where R is the exposure required to produce the appropriate amount of film blackening.

F. Contrast and latitude

–Film contrast relates to the observed density difference for a given exposure difference incident on the film.

–Film contrast is **determined by** the **slope** of the characteristic curve.

–**Film gamma** is the **maximum slope** of the characteristic curve.

–**Gradient** is the **mean slope** between two specified film densities (normally 0.25 and 2.0 OD units). A high gradient (> 1.0) means that radiographic contrast is amplified.

–**Film latitude** is the **range of exposure levels** over which the film may be used.

–Film latitude and contrast are inversely related.

–A wide latitude film has a low gradient and low contrast.

–**Dynamic range** is the ratio of highest to lowest exposure that can be usefully detected and is approximately 40:1.

–Exposures outside this range are in the toe or shoulder region and, therefore, result in very low image contrast.

–Wide latitude films are used for chest radiographs.

–High-contrast single-emulsion films are used in mammography.

III. Solid-State Devices

A. Solid-state materials

–In solid crystals (e.g., NaCl), atoms are arranged in a regular three-dimensional structure.

–Whereas electrons in atoms are arranged in shells, electrons in crystals are arranged in **bands**.

–In solid-state devices such as diodes, only the two outer bands of electrons are important. These are called the (inner) **valence** and (outer) **conduction** band.

–The energy gap between the valence and conduction band is typically 1 to 3 eV and does not normally contain any electrons.

B. Solid-state dosimeters

–When x-ray energy is absorbed by the material, electrons are excited into

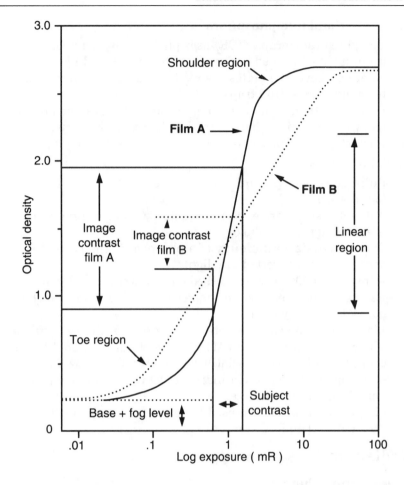

Figure 4-2. Characteristic curve showing relation between exposure and optical density for two different films. Film A has a higher contrast. Film B has a wider exposure latitude.

the conduction band and may be stored in **electron traps** for long periods. This property permits the amount of radiation incident on the solid-state device to be measured.

–Such solid-state materials may be used as **dosimeters** or **imaging devices**.

–To be useful, such solid-state material requires a mechanism for the electrons stored in the electron traps to be released.

–If the release mechanism is heat, the solid-state device is called **thermoluminescent**.

–If the release mechanism is light, then the solid-state device is called a **photostimulable phosphor**.

–Electrons released from these traps fall back to the valence band and emit their excess energy in the form of visible light photons with energies of 1 to 3 eV.

–These light photons can be detected and, thus, the amount of x-ray energy absorbed by the solid-state material can be measured.

C. Photostimulable phosphors

–Computed radiography (CR) uses photostimulable phosphor plates made of europium-activated barium fluorohalides ($BaF_2Fl:Eu$).

–After exposure, the plates are read out using low-energy laser light (red) to empty the electron traps.

–On stimulation, high-energy light (blue), which can be measured, is emitted, which is proportional to the incident x-ray exposure.

–Photostimulable phosphor plates can be erased using light and reused.

D. Scintillators

–**Scintillators** or **phosphors** are materials that emit light when exposed to radiation.

–Table 4-3 summarizes the characteristics of a number of scintillators used in diagnostic radiology.

–The **conversion efficiency** of a phosphor is the percentage of absorbed energy that is converted into light.

–Only 2% to 20% of the absorbed energy is converted to light.

–Radiographic screens are examples of scintillators in which the light output is detected by a film.

–Light output may also be detected by **photomultiplier tubes (PMTs)**.

–The output voltage from PMTs is directly proportional to the amount of energy absorbed by the scintillating material as shown in Figure 4-3.

–Sodium iodide (NaI) scintillation crystals are commonly used in nuclear medicine gamma cameras.

–Liquid scintillators are used to detect low-energy beta emitters such as ^3H (tritium) and ^{14}C (carbon).

IV. Radiation Measurements

A. Ionization chambers

–**Ionization chambers** detect ionizing radiation by measuring the (electron) charge liberated.

–The exposure (X) corresponds to a measurement of the total charge (Q) liberated ($X = Q/M$), where M is the mass of air in the chamber.

–Ionization chambers need a positive voltage at the collecting electrode (anode). This voltage attracts the liberated electrons.

–The applied voltage should be high enough to collect all the liberated electrons.

Table 4-3. Scintillators Used in Diagnostic Radiology

Material	Density (ρ) (g/cm^3)	Conversion Efficiency	Primary Light Emission	Application
ZnCdS:Ag	4.4	18%	Blue and green	Fluorescent screen*
NaI	3.7	12%	Blue	Nuclear medicine gamma camera
CsI	4.5	10%	Blue	Image intensifier
CaWO$_4$	6.1	3.5%	Blue	Old screen (pre-1970)
La$_2$O$_2$S:Tb	5.7	12%	Green	Rare earth screen
Y$_2$O$_2$S:Tb	4.9	18%	Blue	Rare earth screen

*Used in radiology for fluoroscopy before development of modern image intensifiers in the 1950s.

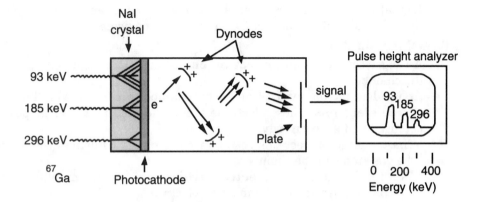

Figure 4-3. Incident photons are absorbed by the sodium iodide crystal, producing scintillations (light), which are converted to photoelectrons in the photocathode. These are accelerated and multiplied as they move between the charged dynodes toward the plate where they are detected. The pulse height analyzer determines signal strength as a function of energy.

–During radiography, a total charge of Q coulombs liberated in the chamber is collected and used to determine the radiographic exposure, which is expressed in roentgens (R) or coulombs per kilogram (C/kg).

–During fluoroscopy, there is a flow of charge liberated every second which corresponds to a current ($I = Q/t$) detected at the collecting electrode.

–A measurement of the rate of charge being liberated, which is equal to an electric current Q/t, corresponds to an exposure rate expressed in roentgens per second, minute, or hour.

–Figure 4-4 shows a typical ionization chamber used for measuring x-ray exposures.

–Ionization chambers are accurate dosimetry devices and are frequently

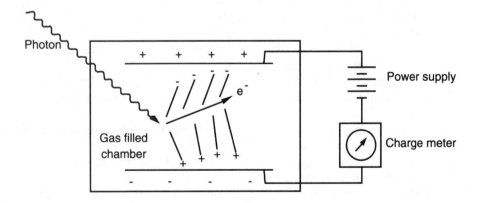

Figure 4-4. Exposure measured by an ionization chamber. The radiation ionizes air. The ions produced are attracted to the oppositely charged plates where they are detected and counted.

used to measure the output of x-ray tubes.

–Ionization chambers are used as **phototimers** in automatic exposure controls and in **dose calibrators** in nuclear medicine.

B. Geiger counters

–A Geiger counter is an **ionization chamber** with a high voltage across the chamber.

–An incident photon interacting in this chamber produces a small number of **free electrons**. These electrons are accelerated by the large positive potential and **gain energy**.

–These energetic electrons result in more electrons being ejected from the gas atoms in the chamber.

–As a result, there is an **electron avalanche,** or large amplification of the charge liberated by the incident electron.

–The large amplified output results in the "click" heard when using the Geiger counter.

–**Quenching gases** are added to Geiger counters to improve stability by minimizing the production of secondary discharges.

–Geiger counters are sensitive and are used to detect low levels of radioactive contamination.

–Geiger counters are too sensitive to measure diagnostic x-ray beams, which may have more than 10^7 photons/mm^2.

C. Film dosimetry

–Film may be used to measure the radiation exposure of radiation workers.

–The sensitivity of film to x-rays depends on photon energy.

–The response of film at 60 kVp is as much as 100 times higher than the response of film at 1 MeV (cobalt-60 energy levels) for the same radiation exposure.

–This enhanced sensitivity arises at the K-edge of the silver in film, which occurs at 25 keV.

–The mean photon energy of a 60-kVp x-ray beam is about 25 keV, and film response is a maximum at this peak voltage.

D. Thermoluminescent dosimetry

–Solid-state materials can store some of the absorbed x-ray beam energy in electron traps. In **thermoluminescent dosimeters (TLDs),** these electrons are released by the application of heat.

–The released electrons result in the emission of visible light.

–Heating TLDs after exposure results in a light output that is proportional to the radiation exposure.

–Lithium fluoride (LiF) is the TLD used in diagnostic radiology because its low atomic number ($Z = 8.3$) makes it reasonably tissue equivalent (see Table 4-1).

–The response of TLD as a function of photon energy is reasonably constant and much better than that of film.

–TLDs also have high dynamic ranges and can measure doses as low as 0.1 mGy (10 mrad) or as high as 10 Gy (1000 rad).

–TLDs are frequently used to measure patient exposures during radiographic examinations and may be used for **personnel dosimetry**.

Review Test

1. Exposure is the

(A) energy deposited from a photon beam to any material
(B) defined for charged particles below 3 MeV
(C) absorbed dose multiplied by the quality factor
(D) number of photons crossing unit area
(E) electrical charge liberated by photons in a mass of air

2. Measuring the total number of ions liberated in a specified mass of air by a beam of diagnostic x-rays would directly yield

(A) rad
(B) rem
(C) R
(D) ergs
(E) none of the above

3. The energy lost per unit length along the track of an alpha particle is a measure of

(A) ionization
(B) scintillation
(C) linear attenuation coefficient
(D) mass energy absorption
(E) linear energy transfer

4. The linear energy transfer (LET) of x-rays

(A) is greater than the LET for alpha particles
(B) is between 0.3 and 3 keV/mm
(C) is necessary for measuring exposure
(D) cannot be defined for energies > 2 MeV
(E) none of the above

5. To convert absorbed dose into dose equivalent, it is only necessary to know the value of the

(A) f-factor
(B) quality factor
(C) exposure level
(D) distance to the radiation source
(E) composition of absorbing material

6. The f-factor in diagnostic radiology

(A) is the roentgen-to-rad conversion factor
(B) is generally 1.0 for bone
(C) increases with photon energy
(D) is 20 for alpha particles and neutrons
(E) all of the above

7. Which of the following materials will receive the highest absorbed dose when exposed to 1 R of 80-kVp x-rays?

(A) Air
(B) Fat
(C) Muscle
(D) Bone
(E) Cannot be determined

8. Match the appropriate unit with the quantity it is used to measure.

(A) Dose equivalent
(B) Absorbed dose
(C) Activity
(D) Exposure

(i) C/kg
(ii) Gray
(iii) Becquerel
(iv) Sievert

9. The developer converts sensitized silver halide crystals to

(A) bromine
(B) acidic halide
(C) silver alkalide
(D) individual silver atoms
(E) metallic silver specks

10. In film processing, the fixer is used to

(A) modify the developer pH
(B) remove unexposed silver halide
(C) fix the silver to the emulsion
(D) remove the bromine
(E) reduce unexposed silver halide

11. Optical density is defined as

(A) ratio of transmitted to incident light
(B) ratio of incident to transmitted light
(C) logarithm of ratio of transmitted to incident light
(D) logarithm of ratio of incident to transmitted light

12. An area of a radiograph that only transmits 1% of the incident light intensity has an optical density of

(A) 0.3
(B) 1.0
(C) 2.0
(D) 3.0
(E) > 3.0

13. When a film with an optical density of 0.3 is placed on top of a film with an optical density of 0.5, the resultant optical density will be

(A) 0.2
(B) 0.8
(C) 1.0
(D) 1.5
(E) unable to be determined

14. Which of the following features may be determined from the characteristic film curve?

(A) Speed
(B) Gamma
(C) Base plus fog level
(D) Average gradient
(E) All of the above

15. A characteristic curve with a gradient of 3.0 would likely result in which of the following?

(A) Low radiation dose
(B) Low density
(C) Long processing time
(D) High contrast
(E) High base plus fog

16. Increasing which of the following temperatures is most likely to result in a high base plus fog level?

(A) Anode
(B) Developer
(C) Fixer
(D) Dryer
(E) Radiographic room

17. Increasing which film characteristic would most likely improve portable chest radiograph image quality?

(A) Speed
(B) Contrast
(C) Latitude
(D) Gradient
(E) None of the above

18. Which of the following CANNOT detect x-rays?

(A) Thermoluminescent dosimeter
(B) NaI crystal
(C) Charged couple device
(D) Photostimulable phosphor

19. True (T) or False (F). These detectors are used to determine the energy of incident gamma ray photons.

(A) Ionization chamber
(B) Geiger-Müller detector
(C) Scintillation crystal
(D) Thermoluminescent dosimeter

20. Match the following radiation detector with the most appropriate detector characteristics.

(A) Ionization chamber
(B) G-M detector
(C) Sodium iodide crystal
(D) Thermoluminescent detector

(i) Gives off light when heated
(ii) Used to measure x-ray tube output
(iii) Used to detect low-level ^{99m}Tc contamination
(iv) Used to identify radioisotopes

21. Which of the following does NOT emit light?

(A) Thermoluminescent dosimeters
(B) Photocathodes
(C) NaI scintillation crystals
(D) CR imaging plates

22. True (T) or False (F). The following radiation detectors normally make use of photomultiplier tubes.

(A) Sodium iodide crystal
(B) Thermoluminescent dosimeter
(C) X-ray system phototimer
(D) Ionization chamber
(E) Photostimulable phosphor

23. Quenching gases are used in

(A) ionization chambers
(B) proportional counters
(C) high pressure Xe detectors in CT
(D) ^{133}Xe ventilators
(E) Geiger-Müller counters

24. Gas-filled detectors are used to collect

(A) the total number of molecules in a given mass
(B) charged ions liberated by the radiation
(C) total light generated in a given mass
(D) heat released by absorbed radiation
(E) all of the above

25. Match the scintillator material with the conversion efficiency for converting absorbed x-ray energy into light.

(A) CsI
(B) CaWO$_4$
(C) Y$_2$O$_2$S:Tb

(i) 3.5%
(ii) 10%
(iii) 18%

Answers and Explanations

1–E. Exposure is given by the charge liberated in air by photons per unit mass and is expressed in C/kg (energy deposited per unit mass is absorbed dose; dose × QF is dose equivalent; and photons per unit area is fluence).

2–C. Exposure measured in roentgen (R) is the charge liberated per unit mass of air.

3–E. The linear energy transfer for alpha particles is high and equal to about 100 keV/μm.

4–B. The LET for x-rays is in the range of 0.3 to 3 keV/μm, is much lower than the LET for alpha particles, and has no direct relationship with measurement of x-ray exposure.

5–B. Dose equivalent (measured in sievert or rem) is the product of the absorbed dose (measured in gray or rad) and the quality factor. (Note that in radiology the quality factor is generally 1.0; thus the dose equivalent and absorbed dose are numerically equal.)

6–A. The f-factor converts exposure (roentgen) into absorbed dose (gray or rad). At diagnostic x-ray energies, f is approximately 1 for low Z materials like soft tissue and air, increases with atomic number Z, and is generally in the range of 3 to 4 for bone.

7–D. Bone will result in the highest dose since it has the highest f-factor (dose in bone will be about 4 rad since f for bone at 80 kVp will be about 4).

8. A–iv; B–ii; C–iii; D–i.

9–E. The sensitized grains, containing about 10^6 to 10^7 atoms, are reduced to specks of metallic silver which is black in appearance.

10–B. The fixer removes unexposed silver halide.

11–D. Film density, D, is given by $\log_{10}(I_o/I_t)$, where I_o is the incident light intensity, and I_t is the transmitted light intensity.

12–C. Logarithm$_{10}$(100) = 2.0.

13–B. 0.8. One advantage of the logarithmic scale is that film optical densities are additive.

14–E. All of the film characteristics listed may be obtained directly from the characteristic curve.

15–D. A gradient of 3 is a high contrast film and is likely to result in high image contrast (used in mammography).

16–B. Increasing the developer temperature will generally increase the observed film fog level.

17–C. Portable chest x-rays are done at low kVps, which increases contrast (high exposures in the lung region and low exposures in the mediastinum), and would most likely benefit from wide latitude films.

18–C. Charged couple devices (CCDs) are used to detect light (not x-rays), as in video camcorders. To use CCDs in radiology, a scintillator must be placed in front of the CCD to capture the x-rays and convert a fraction of the absorbed energy into light.

19. A–False; ionization chambers are used to measure the total output (mR) of an x-ray tube; **B–False;** G-M detectors give the same response irrespective of the energy of an absorbed photon; **C–True;** as used by gamma cameras in nuclear medicine; **D–False;** TLDs measure the total energy absorption, not the energy of single photons.

20. A–ii; physicists use ionization chambers to measure x-ray tube outputs in mR or mR/min; **B–iii;** G-M detectors are very sensitive and ideal for detecting low-level contamination in a nuclear medicine department; **C–iv;** NaI crystals coupled to a photomultiplier tube result in a signal that is proportional to the energy absorbed in the crystal, which is used for performing pulse height analysis to identify unknown radioisotopes; **D–i;** TLDs are read out by measuring the emitted light during heating.

21–B. Photocathodes absorb light photons and emit electrons.

22. A–True; B–True; photomultiplier tubes are used to detect the light emitted by thermoluminescent dosimeters as they are heated; **C–False;** ionization chambers or diodes are normally used; **D–False; E–True;** photomultiplier tubes are normally used to detect the light emitted by any x-ray detector.

23–E. Quenching gases are used in Geiger-Müller detectors to minimize the production of secondary discharges.

24–B. Charged ions liberated by the radiation.

25. A—ii; B—i; C—iii; (see Table 4-3).

5

Screen/Film Radiography

I. Intensifying Screens

A. Introduction

–**Intensifying screens** absorb x-ray photons and emit many more visible light photons, which then expose the film as shown in Figure 5-1.

–Intensifying screens improve the efficiency of radiographic imaging over use of film alone.

 –The use of intensifying screens decreases the mAs required for a given film density, resulting in a lower patient dose.

 –Shorter exposure times also decrease x-ray tube loading and image blur caused by patient motion.

–The **intensification factor** is the ratio of exposures, without and with intensifying screens, required to obtain a given film density and depends on the absorption and conversion efficiency of the screen.

 –The **absorption efficiency** refers to the percentage of x-ray photons absorbed in the screen.

 –The **conversion efficiency** refers to how many light photons are produced by each absorbed x-ray.

 –Typical intensification factors are 30 to 50.

B. Screens

–Phosphor layers in intensifying screens are typically 40 to 100 μm thick.

–The phosphor layer is supported by a thicker base.

–**Calcium tungstate ($CaWO_4$)** was used in intensifying screens until about 1970.

–Tungsten has a high K-shell binding energy (69.5 keV) compared to the mean photon energy levels normally used in diagnostic radiology; therefore, absorption is less than optimal.

 –For example, an examination performed at 100 kVp corresponds to a mean photon energy level of about 40 keV, which is well below the K-shell binding energy in the screen.

–**Rare earth screens** are "faster" than calcium tungstate because they have a higher absorption efficiency at the mean x-ray energies normally used in radiology.

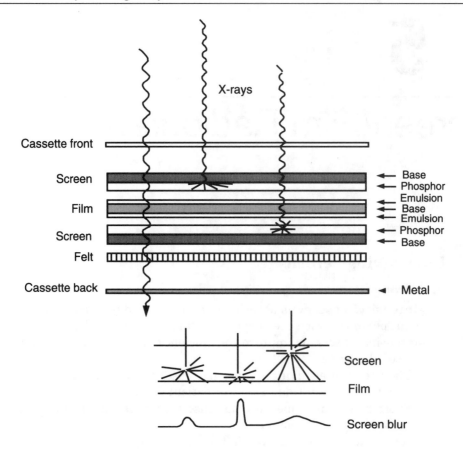

Figure 5-1. Cross section of a typical screen/film cassette containing double emulsion film and two screens.

–Rare earth screens also have a higher conversion efficiency.
–Table 5-1 summarizes the K-shell binding energy levels of the rare earth elements used in screens.

C. Screen/film speed

–The **speed of a screen/film combination** is inversely related to the exposure (1/R) required to produce a given density.

–As the speed increases, the exposure required decreases.

–The speed of a screen/film combination used in radiology ranges from approximately 50 to 800 and is normally expressed relative to a calcium tungstate standard assigned a speed of 100.

  –Screen speed increases with increasing screen thickness, absorption, and conversion efficiency.

  –Both screen and film must be specified when assigning speed to any screen/film combination.

–**High-speed screens** are generally thicker and have decreased spatial resolution.

  –Thick screens increase image blur as a result of increased diffusion of light in the screen before striking the film.

–**Detail screens** are thinner and, therefore, slower but have better spatial resolution.

Table 5-1. Elements Used in Screens

Element	Atomic Number (Z)	Density (ρ) (g/cm^3)	K-Shell Binding Energy (keV)
Yttrium (Y)	39	4.5	17
Barium (Ba)	56	3.5	37
Lanthanum (La)	57	6.1	39
Gadolinium (Gd)	64	7.9	50
Tungsten (W)	74	19.3	70

–Fast screen/film combinations are used for abdominal studies; slow films are used for extremity examinations.

D. Screen/film use

–Gadolinium oxysulfide (Gd_2O_2S) emits mainly green light, and lanthanum oxybromide (LaOBr) and calcium tungstate ($CaWO_4$) emit mainly blue light.

–The light output, that is, wavelength (λ) or color, of a screen and the sensitivity of the film must be matched (**spectral matching**).

–Table 5-2 lists a range of screen types used in radiology and their clinical applications.

–Intensifying screens can be significant sources of image artifact.

  –Scratches, stains, hair, dust, cigarette ash, and talcum powder are all potential sources of image artifacts.

  –As part of a quality control (QC) program, all screens should be regularly cleaned and evaluated for good screen/film contact.

E. Cassette

–The film and screens are held in a light-tight cassette.

–The screens are usually permanently mounted inside the cassette.

–A thin layer of foam backing holds the screen tightly against the film when the cassette is closed.

–The front of the cassette is made of a minimally attenuating material such as carbon fiber.

–The back of the cassette is made of lead to absorb x-rays and reduce backscatter, which degrades image quality.

–Dual-screen, dual-emulsion systems are used in most cases.

–The use of two screens improves x-ray absorption.

–Single-emulsion, single-screen systems are used for bone detail and mammography.

Table 5-2. Screen Characteristics and Common Clinical Applications

Screen Classification	Typical Composition	Limiting Resolution (lp/mm)	Clinical Uses
Film alone	. . .	>25	Extremity radiography
Mammography (Min-R)	Gd_2O_2S:Tb	~20	Mammography
Detail (100)	La_2O_2S:Tb	~12	Extremity radiography
Par (400)	La_2O_2S:Tb	~7	Chest imaging
Fast (600)	$BaPbSO_4$	~5	Abdominal imaging

F. Computed radiography

- –**Computed radiography (CR)** uses photostimulable phosphor (europium-activated barium fluorohalide) plates to capture x-ray exposure patterns.
- –The latent image on the phosphor plate is "read" using laser-stimulated light emission of electrons trapped in the phosphor during x-ray exposure.
  - –CR photostimulable phosphors are usually read out using approximately 2000 lines with 2000 data points on each line.
  - –The laser readout limits the achievable spatial resolution to approximately 2.5 line pairs per millimeter (lp/mm) for a 36 × 43 cm cassette.
- –Signals are digitized and stored in a computer.
- –Data can be processed in a variety of ways before being printed on film or displayed on a monitor.
- –With CR, the image capture, image storage, and image display functions are all separated, whereas they are all performed by the film in a screen/film combination.
- –CR is advantageous because it has a wide dynamic range of about four orders of magnitude of radiation exposure.
- –CR systems can produce diagnostic quality films with suboptimal x-ray techniques, which is ideal for performing portable x-ray examinations when phototiming cannot be used.

II. Scatter Removal

A. Scatter

- –**Scattered radiation** is undesirable in diagnostic radiology because it **reduces subject contrast**.
- –**Coherent scatter** is a **negligible** component of image degradation in diagnostic radiology.
- –Of paramount significance are the scattered photons resulting from **Compton scatter**.
- –The ratio of scatter to primary radiation exiting a patient can easily be 5:1 or greater.
  - –Scatter increases with increased field size (i.e., area of x-ray beam) and increased patient thickness.
  - –**Collimation** reduces the total patient mass irradiated and, therefore, reduces scatter.
- –At low peak voltage (kVp), there is more absorption due to the photoelectric effect and less Compton scatter.
  - –Lowering kilovoltage increases contrast but reduces penetration, increases patient dose, increases tube loading (mAs), and is generally not used to reduce scatter except in portable chest radiography when using a grid is difficult.

B. Air gaps

- –Air gaps between the patient and cassette reduce scatter, because the scattered photons are less likely to reach the screen/film receptor.
  - –However, by moving image receptors away from patients, magnification is introduced, a larger x-ray tube output is required, and focal spot blurring is increased.

–Air gaps are used for magnification radiography in **neuroradiology** and **mammography**.

–Air gaps are sometimes used in chest radiography. A long source-to-patient distance (3 m) compensates for loss of sharpness caused by focal spot size and minimizes magnification.

C. Grids

–**Antiscatter grids** are the most effective and practical method for **removing scatter** in diagnostic radiology.

–Grids are made up of many narrow parallel bars of lead or other highly attenuating material. X-rays pass between the strips, which are filled with low attenuation material.

–Grids are placed between the patient and the film.

–Figure 5-2 shows how grids reduce the amount of scatter radiation reaching the screen/film combination.

–The **grid ratio** is defined as the ratio of the strip thickness (h) along the x-ray beam direction to the gap (D) between the lead strips; that is, grid ratio is h/D.

–The **strip line density** is $1/(D + d)$ lines per unit length, where d is the strip thickness.

  –Grid ratios typically range from 4 to 16, and strip line densities from 25 to 60 lines per centimeter.

–**Focused grids** have diverging strips and must be used at specified focal distances.

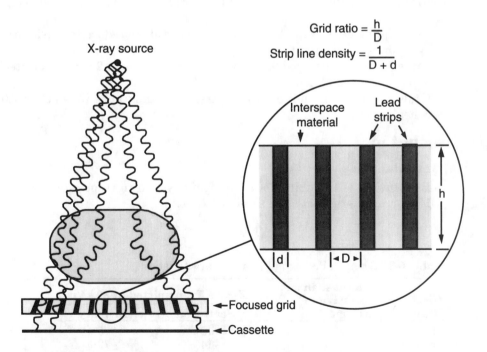

Figure 5-2. Grids reduce the amount of scattered radiation that reaches the film. The lead strips of a focused grid are designed to be parallel to the incoming beam.

–Most grids are placed in a Bucky and are called **reciprocating grids**.
–The grid moves during the exposure, spreading the image of the grid lines over the film and rendering them "invisible."

D. Grid characteristics

–**Primary transmission** is the percentage of incident primary radiation (not scattered) that passes through the grid.
–The **Bucky factor** is the ratio of radiation incident on the grid to the transmitted radiation and is a good indicator of the increase in patient dose due to the use of a grid.
–Typical values for the Bucky factor are 2 to 6.
–The **contrast improvement factor** is the ratio of contrast with a grid to contrast without a grid.
–A typical contrast improvement factor is approximately 2.
–Artifacts such as grid cutoff may be caused by improper alignment, the wrong focal spot to film distance for focused grids, and inverted grids.
–Increasing the grid ratio by either increasing the height of the lead strips or reducing the space between the lead strips increases image contrast.
  –Increasing the grid ratio also increases x-ray tube loading and patient exposure.
–Table 5-3 lists the principal radiographic characteristics of several common grids.

E. Clinical use of grids

–A **12:1** (30 lines/cm) ratio is common in a **reciprocating grid**.
–**Stationary grids** with low ratios of **6:1** and about 45 lines/cm are used with mobile x-ray units because a low grid ratio tolerates beam misalignments.
  –A high line density is used for stationary grids to reduce the visibility of grid lines on resultant radiographs.
–Grids are generally used for body parts greater than 12 cm thick or techniques above 70 kVp.
–Grids are generally not used for extremity radiographs in which scatter is negligible.

III. Resolution

A. Introduction

–**Resolution** is the ability of an imaging system to resolve two adjacent **high-contrast** objects as discrete entities.

Table 5-3. Common Radiography Grid Characteristics

Grid Ratio	Increase in mAs (relative to no grid)*	X-rays Transmitted at 80 kVp	
		Scattered	Primary
5:1	× 2	~18%	~75%
6:1	× 3	~14%	~72%
8:1	× 4	~10%	~70%
12:1	× 5	~5%	~68%

*Bucky factor.

–This may also be described by the terms **high-contrast resolution, blur, spatial resolution,** and **modulation transfer function**.

–**Focal spot size, screen thickness,** and **patient motion** are the most important factors that affect resolution. The relative importance of these factors is further influenced by image magnification.

B. Spatial frequency

–Resolution is often expressed in **line pairs per millimeter** (lp/mm), which is a measure of spatial frequency.

–A **line pair** includes an opaque space and radiolucent line.

–Large objects may be represented by low spatial frequencies and small structures by high spatial frequencies.

–**High-contrast resolution** is estimated using a parallel line bar phantom.

–One line pair per millimeter has 0.5 mm Pb bars separated by 0.5 mm of transparent material; 2 lp/mm has 0.25 mm Pb bars separated by 0.25 mm of transparent material, and so on.

–The **limiting resolution** is the maximum number of line pairs per millimeter that can be recorded by the imaging system.

–The human eye can resolve a maximum of 30 lp/mm and only about 5 lp/mm at a viewing distance of approximately 25 cm.

C. Screen blur

–**Screen blur** (unsharpness) is caused by light diffusion in the intensifying screen (see Figure 5-1).

–The image of a narrow line source is called a **line spread function (LSF)** and its width may be taken as a measure of resolution.

–Normally, width is measured at half the maximum value, termed **full width half maximum (FWHM)**.

–Thick screens have greater light diffusion in the screen and, therefore, wider LSFs.

–Thicker screens (fast screens) have improved x-ray absorption efficiencies and require decreased exposure times (lower patient doses), but have inferior resolution.

–Thin screens (slow screens) have poor x-ray absorption efficiencies, but excellent spatial resolution (detail screens).

–Resolution improves with increasing magnification, because the image is spread out over a large area and the impact of screen blur is reduced.

–Separation of the film from the screen increases blur.

–Parallax occurs with double emulsion film but is a minor contributor to image unsharpness.

D. Focal spot blur

–The blurred margin at the edge of objects is called the **penumbra**.

–The penumbra is the result of x-rays arriving from slightly different locations in the focal spot, because the focal spot is not a true point source but has a finite area.

–The resultant unsharpness is called **focal spot blur** or **geometric unsharpness**.

–Focal spot blur increases with magnification and focal spot size as shown in Figure 5-3.

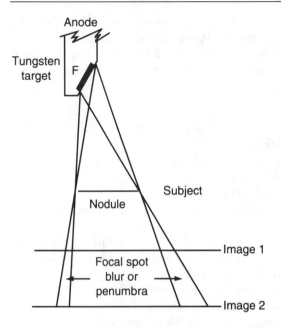

Figure 5-3. Focal spot blur increases as an object moves farther from the film and as focal spot size increases.

–Reducing the focal spot size increases the sharpness and definition of object edges by minimizing the penumbra.

–In magnification radiography, it is important to have very small focal spot sizes.

  –Magnification may be used in mammography to improve the visibility of microcalcification, but requires a 0.1-mm focal spot size to minimize geometric unsharpness.

  –Magnification is sometimes used in angiograms to improve the visibility of very small blood vessels (approximately 0.3-mm focal spot).

E. Motion blur

  –**Patient motion** introduces blur into a radiograph by smearing out the object in the exposed film.

  –Motion blur may be minimized by increasing the mA to reduce the exposure time.

  –Increasing mA may not be possible, however, because of limits on the focal spot loading of the x-ray tube.

  –Faster screens also decrease motion blur by allowing a shorter exposure.

F. Modulation transfer function

  –The **modulation transfer function (MTF)** is a curve that describes the resolution capability of an imaging system.

  –The **MTF** is the ratio of output contrast to input contrast in an imaging system. Each step in the imaging process can contribute to this loss of contrast.

  –The MTF of the imaging system is the product of the MTFs of the respective subcomponents.

  –If for a given spatial frequency, the MTF due to the focal spot is 0.9, due to motion is 0.8, and due to the screen is 0.7, then the **imaging system MTF** at this spatial frequency is the product of the individual components: $0.9 \times 0.8 \times 0.7 = 0.5$.

–Output contrast decreases as the spatial frequency (i.e., line pairs per millimeter) increases.

–At **low spatial frequencies,** the MTF is close to **1.0.**

–At **high spatial frequencies,** the MTF falls to **zero.**

G. Resolution in radiology

–The best spatial resolution is achieved when film is exposed directly without using a screen.

–Film resolutions up to 100 lp/mm are achievable, but only 1% of x-rays incident on the film are absorbed.

–In screen/film radiography, the screen MTF is normally the limiting factor in the imaging chain.

–In screen/film radiography, there is always a trade-off when magnification work is being performed.

–Focal spot MTF deteriorates with increasing magnification.

–Screen MTF, however, improves with increasing magnification.

–There is an optimum magnification value at which improvements in the focal spot MTF are offset by deterioration in the screen MTF.

–Table 5-4 summarizes representative values for limiting spatial resolution in diagnostic radiology.

IV. Noise

A. Introduction

–**Noise** is the random fluctuation of film density about some mean value following uniform exposure.

–Noise degrades image quality and limits the ability to visualize low-contrast objects.

–The major source of noise in radiography is the quantum nature of the x-ray photons used to generate the image.

B. Radiographic mottle

–**Radiographic mottle** describes the noise present in film images and has three distinct components: **screen mottle, film mottle,** and **quantum mottle**.

Table 5-4. Representative Values of Limiting Spatial Resolution

Imaging Technique	Resolution (lp/mm)
Film alone	25 to 100
Mammography	15 to 20
Screen/film (200 to 600 speed)	5 to 10
Photospot (100 or 105 mm)	~4
35-mm Cine	~3.5
Computed radiography (CR)	2.5 to 5.0
Digital subtraction angiography (DSA)	~2
Conventional fluoroscopy	~1
Computed tomography (CT)	~0.7
Magnetic resonance imaging (MRI)	~0.3
Ultrasound (axial resolution)	~0.2
Nuclear medicine (NM)	< 0.1

–**Screen mottle** is caused by nonuniformities in screen construction but is usually negligible in modern screens.

–**Film mottle** is caused by the grain structure of emulsions and is normally of little importance in screen/film radiography.

–**Quantum mottle** is caused by the discrete nature of x-ray photons and is the most important source of noise in radiography.

–In diagnostic radiology, the number of x-ray photons used to create a radiographic image is typically 10^5/mm^2.

–In conventional photography, the corresponding number of light photons required to expose a film is 10^9 to 10^{10}/mm^2.

–This difference in photon intensity explains why noise is generally negligible in conventional photography but is of paramount importance in radiology.

–The highest noise occurs in conventional fluoroscopy and the lowest noise occurs in detail radiography and mammography (Table 5-5).

C. **Quantum mottle**

–For a *uniform* x-ray exposure, adjacent areas of the film (measured in mm^2) have photon counts that randomly differ from the mean value N.

–The distribution of the number of photons in each square millimeter is described by **Poisson statistics**.

–In Poisson statistics, the **standard deviation (σ)** is given by the square root of the mean number of counts ($\sigma = \sqrt{N}$).

–Sixty-eight percent of the regions contain counts within one standard deviation of N ($N \pm \sqrt{N}$).

–Ninety-five percent have counts within two standard deviations of N ($N \pm 2\sqrt{N}$).

–Ninety-nine percent have counts within three standard deviations of N ($N \pm 3\sqrt{N}$).

–For example, for a uniform object imaged with an average of 100 photons per square millimeter [mean (N) = 100; $\sigma = \sqrt{N} = 10$], 68% of sampled areas are in the 90 to 110 range, 95% are in the 80 to 120 range, and 99% are in the 70 to 130 range.

–This random variation of photons incident on a radiation detector is known as **quantum mottle**.

–Quantum mottle is only dependent on the number of photons used to produce an image and decreases as the square root of radiation exposure increases.

Table 5-5. Representative Radiation Exposures Required at the Image Receptor to Produce One Image or Frame

Regular fluoroscopy	1 to 3 µR
Low noise fluoroscopy	5 to 10 µR
35-mm Cine	15 to 30 µR
Photospot film	100 to 200 µR
Fast screen/film radiography	100 to 500 µR
Detail film/screen radiography	500 to 1000 µR
Mammography	~5000 µR

D. Screen speed versus noise

–For screen/film combinations, there is normally a trade-off between speed and noise.

–In analyzing the relation between speed and noise, the key issue is to determine how many x-ray photons are required to produce the same optical density (OD).

–If screens are made thicker (faster), the resultant image noise remains the same because the same number of x-ray photons must be absorbed in the screen to produce the desired OD.

–If a more efficient phosphor, which emits more light per x-ray photon absorbed, is used, then fewer x-ray photons need to be absorbed in the screen to produce the desired OD and noise increases (i.e., fewer x-ray photons means more noise and vice versa).

–As conversion efficiency increases, so does quantum mottle.

–These two ways of increasing screen/film speed are shown in Figure 5-4.

–If speed is increased by the use of a faster film, fewer photons are required and noise increases.

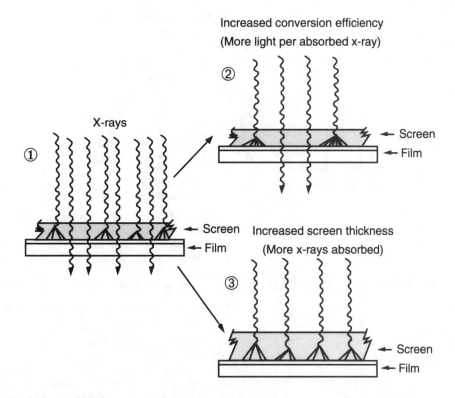

Figure 5-4. Relation between screen speed and noise. (*1*) A single emulsion film and screen with an absorption efficiency of 50%. (*2*) A screen with a higher conversion efficiency produces more light photons for each absorbed x-ray and dose is decreased. The resulting image is noisier because fewer x-rays are used to produce the same film blackening. (*3*) A thicker screen has a higher absorption efficiency, stops more of the incoming x-rays, and reduces dose. Noise is not increased because the same number of absorbed x-rays is used to produce the image.

Review Test

1. The primary reason that fast screen/film combinations reduce the patient dose is because they permit a reduction of the

(A) kVp
(B) mAs
(C) grid ratio
(D) focal spot size
(E) added filtration

2. When compared with calcium tungstate, rare earth screens generally result in a decrease of

(A) number of light photons per absorbed x-ray
(B) screen mottle
(C) speed
(D) patient dose
(E) all of the above

3. The number of scattered photons reaching a screen/film receptor decreases with increasing

(A) field size
(B) patient thickness
(C) kVp
(D) filtration
(E) grid ratio

4. The height of lead strips divided by the gap between these strips is called the grid

(A) focus
(B) range
(C) frequency
(D) ratio
(E) none of the above

5. High ratio grids generally result in an increase in the

(A) required mAs
(B) image contrast
(C) patient dose
(D) removal of scatter
(E) all of the above

6. Grids primarily attenuate which of the following types of photon arising from the patient?

(A) Compton scatter
(B) Coherent scatter
(C) Backscatter
(D) Characteristic x-rays
(E) All of the above

7. What effect will an air gap have on image contrast?

(A) Increase
(B) Reduce
(C) Eliminate
(D) None
(E) Unpredictable

8. Match the following grids with the application or characteristic.

(A) No grid
(B) 12:1, 30 lines/cm
(C) 6:1, 40 lines/cm
(D) 4:1, 60 lines/cm

(i) Portable examinations
(ii) Extremity radiography
(iii) Mammography grid
(iv) Common Bucky grid

9. The reason 12:1 grids are seldom used with portable radiography is because

(A) output of portable x-ray units is too low
(B) low kVp used is unable to penetrate grids
(C) accurate grid alignment is too difficult
(D) scatter is not important in portable x-rays
(E) air gaps are preferred to eliminate scatter

10. The modulation transfer function (MTF) does NOT generally

(A) describe the system resolution
(B) compare image to object contrast
(C) approach 1 at low spatial frequencies
(D) equal unity for perfect spatial resolution
(E) increase with increasing spatial frequency

11. Which of the following factors affect image sharpness?

(A) Focal spot size
(B) Motion
(C) Screen thickness
(D) Screen/film contact
(E) All of the above

12. True (T) or False (F). Geometric magnification

(A) requires more radiation at screen/film
(B) can improve system spatial resolution
(C) needs larger focal spot sizes
(D) increases the amount of scatter in the image

13. Increasing magnification WITHOUT changing focal spot size affects image detail (resolution) in a screen/film radiograph by

(A) reducing image blur
(B) not affecting image blur
(C) increasing image blur
(D) eliminating image blur
(E) not enough information provided

14. Poor screen/film contact will result in a significant loss of

(A) contrast
(B) magnification
(C) image detail
(D) x-ray absorption efficiency
(E) none of the above

15. Which of the following would most likely increase the spatial resolution of a screen/film combination?

(A) High grid ratio
(B) Slower film
(C) Thicker screen
(D) Thinner screen
(E) Faster film

16. Match the following radiographic imaging systems and limiting spatial resolution.

(A) General radiography screen/film
(B) No screen extremity radiography
(C) Photospot film
(D) Mammography

(i)   4 to 5 line pairs/mm
(ii)   5 to 10 line pairs/mm
(iii) 15 to 20 line pairs/mm
(iv) > 25 line pairs/mm

17. When a rare earth screen with three times the conversion efficiency and twice the absorption efficiency is substituted for a $CaWO_4$ screen, the patient dose would be expected to

(A) increase slightly
(B) stay the same
(C) be reduced by a factor of 2
(D) be reduced by a factor of 5
(E) be reduced by a factor of 6

18. A screen with a higher conversion efficiency, but the same x-ray absorption efficiency and screen thickness, will likely result in

(A) increased patient dose
(B) constant image noise
(C) reduced image noise
(D) loss of image detail
(E) none of the above

19. True (T) or False (F). The speed of an imaging system can be increased WITHOUT increasing the noise by using

(A) faster films
(B) phosphors with a higher conversion efficiency
(C) higher developer temperatures
(D) phosphor with higher absorption efficiency
(E) thicker phosphors

20. Quantum mottle is *primarily* determined by which one of the following factors?

(A) X-ray beam filtration
(B) Number of x-ray photons absorbed in screen
(C) X-ray photon energy
(D) Screen conversion efficiency
(E) Screen thickness

21. Reducing the temperature of a film processor from 95°F to 90°F, and keeping film density constant, will increase

(A) contrast
(B) fog
(C) quantum mottle
(D) screen blur
(E) patient dose

22. *Film* contrast, as opposed to *subject* contrast, is primarily affected by the

(A) kVp
(B) beam filtration
(C) presence of contrast agents (iodine, barium)
(D) tissue density differences
(E) film optical density level

23. Compared to a regular screen, a detail screen, of the same phosphor and same examination, will have a higher

(A) spatial resolution
(B) speed
(C) noise level
(D) grid ratio
(E) none of the above

24. The most likely reason a *phototimed* chest unit would produce dark PA radiographs is

(A) incorrect kVp selection
(B) incorrect mA selection
(C) automatic exposure control (AEC) is faulty
(D) grid has been left out
(E) reduced developer temperature

25. Raising kVp in screen/film radiography, while maintaining a constant film density, will generally increase the

(A) need for a high mA
(B) entrance skin dose
(C) scatter
(D) exposure time
(E) film processing time

26. Gastrointestinal (GI) tract contrast on film radiographs is NOT normally improved by

(A) infusion of barium
(B) reducing kV
(C) increasing mA
(D) tighter x-ray beam collimation
(E) increasing the grid ratio

27. Match the following problems and image quality defects.

(A) Poor screen/film contact
(B) Broken automatic exposure control (AEC)
(C) Bad rollers in processor
(D) High kVp

(i) Dark films
(ii) Reduced image contrast
(iii) Local area of decreased resolution
(iv) Line artifacts

28. Increasing x-ray beam filtration alone, while *keeping film density constant,* results in decreased

(A) subject contrast
(B) exposure times
(C) tube heat loading
(D) motion blur
(E) heel effect

29. Decreasing x-ray beam filtration alone, while *keeping film density constant,* results in increased

(A) maximum photon energy
(B) average photon energy
(C) entrance skin exposure
(D) importance of the Compton effect
(E) patient penetration

30. Match the "malfunction" with the *phototimed* x-ray result.

(A) Blown x-ray tube
(B) kVp set too low
(C) kVp set too high
(D) mA set too high
(E) Broken phototimer

(i) Film normal
(ii) Film too dark
(iii) Increased image contrast
(iv) Film uniformly clear
(v) Reduced image contrast

Answers and Explanations

1–B. The radiation exposure required to obtain the correct film density is significantly reduced with fast screen/film combinations permitting a large reduction in mAs.

2–D. Rare earth screens are faster because they absorb more x-rays and are more efficient at producing light, which allows the same film density to be obtained with less radiation; thus the patient dose decreases.

3–E. Higher grid ratios reduce the amount of scatter reaching the screen/film combination.

4–D. Grid ratio (h/D, where h is the height of the lead strip and D is the distance of the gap between these strips).

5–E. All the listed items are increased with higher ratio grids.

6–A. Grids attenuate both Compton and coherent scatter but most of the scatter reaching the screen/film receptor is Compton scatter.

7–A. Air gaps reduce scatter and thus will improve image contrast.

8. A–ii; minimum thickness and low kVp techniques reduce the effect of scatter; **B–iv; C–i; D–iii;** mammography is performed at low kVps and scatter is low, permitting the use of a 4:1 grid; a high strip line density minimizes their visibility on mammograms.

9–C. 12:1 grids are sensitive to misalignment problems; grids used for portable examinations are commonly about 6:1.

10–E. MTF generally *decreases* with increasing spatial frequency.

11–E. All of the listed items will affect image sharpness (resolution).

12. A–False; the radiation required to produce an optimal film density is solely determined by the screen and film, and is typically 0.5 mR, irrespective of magnification; **B–True;** magnification may reduce the relative importance of screen blur, as in magnification mammography; **C–False;** since magnification increases focal spot blur, it is essential that only small focal spot sizes are used if good resolution is to be achieved; **D–False;** magnification introduces an air gap which reduces the scatter.

13–E. Increasing the magnification will increase focal spot blur but improve screen resolution; additional information is required to evaluate which of these two opposite effects will be more important.

14–C. The gap between the screen and film will increase diffusion of light reaching the film and increase image blur.

15–D. Thin screens reduce the amount of screen unsharpness (blur).

16. A–ii; B–iv; direct film exposure normally introduces negligible blur; **C–i;** the image intensifier is the limiting factor and has a resolution of 4 to 5 line pairs/mm in an average magnification mode; **D–iii;** mammography screens are made very thin to minimize blur and permit visualization of microcalcifications.

17–E. There will be a sixfold reduction in patient dose since only 1/6 (i.e., $1/2 \times 1/3$) photons are required to generate the same amount of light in the rare-earth screen and produce the same film density as the $CaWO_4$ screen.

18–E. None of the above (patient dose is reduced; noise increases since less photons are required to produce the same amount of light; and image detail is the same since the screen thickness is not changed).

19. A–False; B–False; C–False; noise will increase because fewer photons are required to produce the same blackening; **D–True; E–True;** the number of light photons needed to blacken the film is the same, but the number incident on the screen is now fewer since the screen absorbs more of those incident on it; hence speed goes up but noise remains the same.

20–B. The primary factor is the number of x-ray photons used to create the image. (Note that although screen conversion efficiency and thickness affect the number of photons required to generate an image, these are secondary factors, not primary ones.)

21–E. Patient dose is increased because as the temperature is reduced, the film speed is reduced, requiring a greater exposure to produce the same amount of blackening.

22–E. Film contrast will be highest at density levels of about 1 and lowest in the over/underexposed regions (all other parameters affect subject contrast).

23–A. Spatial resolution will be increased because a thinner phosphor produces less screen blur.

24–C. The AEC would correct for faulty kVp/mAs settings and missing grids, whereas a low developer temperature produces light films.

25–C. Scatter generally increases with kVp (the importance of the photoelectric effect is reduced and Compton scatter increases).

26–C. mA normally will not increase image contrast, whereas all the other factors normally increase GI tract contrast.

27. A–iii; poor screen/film contact will increase blur in this region; **B–i;** a broken AEC will result in overexposures; **C–iv;** bad rollers will result in film artifacts; **D–ii;** high kVp reduces image contrast.

28–A. Subject contrast is always reduced as the average photon energy increases (exposure times, tube loading and motion blur increase, whereas the heel effect remains constant).

29–C. The entrance skin exposure is always increased as the kVp or filtration is reduced (the x-ray beam becomes less penetrating and more intensity is required to achieve the same exposure level at the screen/film).

30. A–iv; there will be no x-ray output, hence no film blackening; **B–iii;** reducing kV increases contrast; **C–v;** increasing kV always reduces contrast; **D–i;** with phototiming, the total exposure remains correct by reducing exposure time and therefore producing a normal film; **E–ii;** when the phototimer does not work, the x-ray exposure continues until the back-up timer switches the tube off, and thus the film will be overexposed.

6

Fluoroscopy

I. X-ray Image Intensifiers

A. Introduction

–An **image intensifier (II)** is used to convert incident radiation into a light image to be viewed, recorded, or photographed.

–An II consists of an evacuated glass, aluminum, or nonferromagnetic envelope that contains an **input phosphor, photocathode, electrostatic focusing lenses, accelerating anodes,** and **output phosphor** (Figure 6-1).

–IIs have diameters that range from 23 to 57 cm.

  –Large IIs (57 cm) cover large areas, such as the abdomen, and small IIs (23 cm) achieve high resolution in small regions, such as the heart.

  –In most modern IIs, field size can be reduced electronically using electrostatic focusing.

B. Image intensifier input phosphor

–The **input phosphor** absorbs x-ray photons and re-emits part of this absorbed energy as a large number of light photons.

–The input phosphor is typically a 200- to 400-µm thick **cesium iodide (CsI) screen**. Older fluorescent screens used copper-activated zinc cadmium sulfate (ZnCdS:Cu).

  –A CsI screen is better than a ZnCdS screen because it has vertically oriented crystals, which help channel the light, and a packing density that is three times that of ZnCdS.

  –CsI also has **twice the absorption** of incident x-rays as ZnCdS because the K-edges of the phosphor are closer to the incident x-ray energy [iodine, atomic number $(Z) = 53$, K-edge = 33 keV; cesium, $Z = 55$, K-edge = 36 keV].

–Like for intensifying screens, absorption is greater as the input phosphor thickness increases, but resolution is poorer because of light diffusion.

C. Image intensification

–Light photons emitted by the II input phosphor are absorbed by a **photocathode,** which emits photoelectrons.

–The photoelectrons are accelerated across the II tube by the anode (25- to

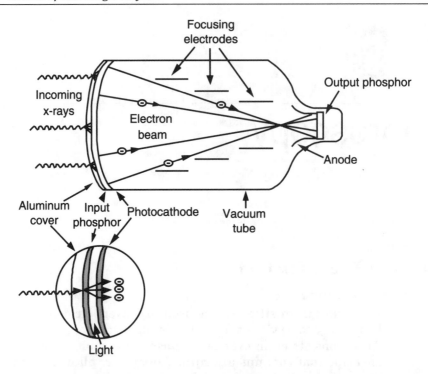

Figure 6-1. Incoming x-ray photons pass through the thin aluminum cover of the image intensifier and strike the input phosphor to produce light. The light strikes the photocathode, producing electrons, which are accelerated toward the anode by a 25-kV potential. Light is produced when the electrons strike the output phosphor.

35-kV potential) and focused onto the **output phosphor** by an electrostatic lens.

–These electrons, which now have energies of 25 to 35 keV, are absorbed by the output phosphor (ZnCdS:Ag) and emit a large number of light photons.

   –Thus, the pattern of incident x-ray intensities at the input phosphor is converted into an **intense pattern of light** at the output phosphor of the II.

–Table 6-1 lists the successive stages of interaction in an II and gives the corresponding efficiency for each stage.

D. Brightness gain

–The light image on the output of an II is brighter than that on the input phosphor; this increase is known as the **brightness gain (BG)**.

–The BG of an II equals the product of the **minification gain (MG)** and **flux gain (FG)**.

–**MG** is the increase in image brightness that results from reduction in image size from the input phosphor to the output phosphor: MG = $(d_i/d_o)^2$, where d_i is the input diameter and d_o is the output diameter.

   –The output phosphor is typically 2.5 cm in diameter; thus, for a 23-cm II, MG = $(23/2.5)^2$, or 85.

–**FG** is the increased number of light photons emitted from the output phosphor compared to the input phosphor.

–The FG is typically 50 to 100, so for each light photon emitted at the

Table 6-1. Efficiency for Each Stage of a Typical Image Intensifier Process

Image Intensifier Stage	Efficiency	Number per Incident 50-keV X-ray
Input phosphor (x-ray absorption)	50%	0.5 Photoelectrons
Input phosphor (light generation)	15%	1875 (2 eV) Light photons
Photocathode (electron emission)	10%	187 Photoelectrons
Output phosphor (electron absorption)	90%	170 Energetic electrons
Output phosphor (light generation)	10%	170,000 Light photons

input phosphor, there are 50 to 100 light photons emitted at the output phosphor.

E. Conversion factor

–The conversion factor is a modern method of measuring the gain or light output of the II.

–The **conversion factor** is the ratio of the **luminance** of the output phosphor measured in candelas per square meter (cd/m^2) to the input exposure rate measured in mR/s.

–A **candela** is a measure of luminance intensity or light brightness.

–The conversion factor of a modern 23-cm II is approximately 100 $cd/m^2/mR/s$.

–The exposure to the input phosphor must be increased when the field size is reduced to maintain a constant brightness level at the II output phosphor.

–The brightness of an II decreases with age.

F. Image intensifier image quality

–The central portion of an II image has a limiting **spatial resolution** of between 4 and 5 line pairs per millimeter (lp/mm).

–The resolution is reduced at the edges of the II.

–Table 6-2 gives typical values of resolution and light conversion factors for different-sized IIs.

–Fluoroscopy is performed at low doses, which means that relatively few x-rays are used to produce the image. This results in high **quantum mottle** (noise) levels.

–The **contrast ratio** of an II is defined as the ratio of periphery to central light intensities (output) when imaging a lead disc, which is one-tenth the diameter of the II input phosphor.

–A typical II contrast ratio is 20:1.

–Several factors contribute to the loss of contrast.

–Some x-ray photons pass through the input phosphor and photocathode and strike the output phosphor.

Table 6-2. Representative Values of Spatial Resolution and Conversion Gain for Cesium-based Image Intensifiers

Image Intensifier Diameter	Resolution (lp/mm)	Conversion Gain ($cd/m^2/mR/s$)
57 cm	3	600
33 cm	4	200
23 cm	5	100

–Some light produced at the output phosphor travels back to the photo-cathode and produces more electrons (**retrograde light flow**).

–Contrast is also reduced by **veiling glare,** which is the result of light scattered and reflected within the II and output window.

G. Image intensifier artifacts

–**Lag** is the continued luminescence after x-ray stimulation has stopped.

–Modern CsI tubes have a low lag time of about 1 ms, which is of little concern.

–**Pincushion distortion** (increased magnification at the periphery) is produced by all IIs as a result of inadequate electronic focusing.

   –Pincushion distortion is about 3% for 23-cm IIs and increases with II diameter.

–**Vignetting** is a fall-off in brightness at the periphery of the II field because the peripheral image is displayed over a larger area and has a lower BG from minification.

–Vignetting is typically less than 25%.

II. Television

A. Introduction

–Fluoroscopy systems use closed circuit television (TV) systems to view the image obtained on the II.

–A beam splitter allows two recording techniques, such as fluoroscopy and cine, to be used simultaneously.

–**TV cameras** convert light images into electric (video) signals that can be recorded or viewed on a monitor.

–Output images from IIs are focused onto a TV camera target using optical lenses.

–A diaphragm (aperture) is placed between the lenses to control the light intensity.

–The TV target is scanned with an electron beam in a series of horizontal lines to read the image light intensity.

–The display monitor converts video signals back into the "original" image for direct viewing.

B. TV scan modes

–In conventional TV systems, 262.5 odd lines (**1 field**) are first scanned, then 262.5 even lines (1 field) are **interlaced** to generate a full **frame** (sum of 2 fields) totaling 525 lines.

   –Interlacing prevents **flickering,** even though only 30 full frames are updated every second.

–In North America, conventional TV systems and display monitors read 30 frames per second, which corresponds to 60 fields per second.

–European TV systems generally use 625 lines and 25 frames per second (50 fields per second).

–European TV is not compatible with North American TV.

–Modern radiographic equipment generally uses 1000-line TV systems that may improve resolution by a factor of 2.

–If TV cameras are operated in a **progressive scan mode** rather than an interlaced mode, then each line is read sequentially.

–Progressive scan modes are used in digital systems and reduce motion artifacts.

C. Television camera types
–TV systems are classified as Vidicon or Plumbicon camera systems.
–**Vidicon TV cameras** reduce contrast by a factor of about 0.8, and TV monitors enhance the contrast by a factor of two.
–Vidicon systems improve the contrast of a fluoroscopy system compared with the contrast at the II output.
–Vidicon systems have high image lag, which improves the signal-to-noise ratio but results in some overlap of images.
–**Plumbicon TV cameras** have much less lag than Vidicon cameras.
–Low lag permits motion to be followed with minimal blur, but quantum noise is increased.

D. Television image quality
–The theoretical vertical resolution for a 525-line TV system and a 23-cm II is about 1 lp/mm.
–Only approximately 70% of this theoretical limit is achieved in practice.
–The ratio of measured to theoretical vertical resolution is called the **Kell factor,** which is normally 0.7.
–Horizontal resolution is determined by the **bandwidth** of the TV system and is normally equal to the vertical resolution.
–Fluoroscopy has a resolution of about 1 lp/mm, which is much poorer than screen/film, which has a resolution of better than 5 lp/mm.
–Resolution may be improved by using magnification modes, but the quality never achieves that of conventional radiography.

III. Fluoroscopic Imaging

A. Automatic brightness control
–Figure 6-2 is an overview of the complete fluoroscopic imaging system.
–The **automatic brightness control (ABC)** regulates the amount of

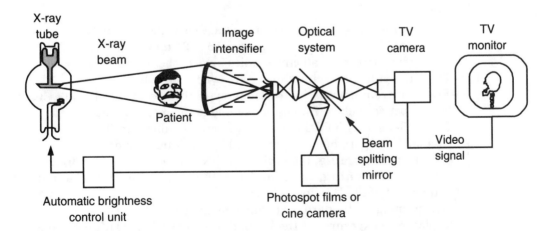

Figure 6-2. A typical fluoroscopy imaging system.

radiation incident on the II input phosphor (and the patient) to maintain a constant TV display.

–This is accomplished by changing the technique factors to maintain a constant light level at the II output phosphor.

–Fluoroscopy tube currents are low, between 1 and 5 milliamperes (mA), and x-ray tube voltages are normally between 70 and 90 kVp.

  –Peak voltage can be varied quickly, but tube current cannot because the current in the filament must be changed.

  –Changing the tube current permits the operator to select the peak voltage that gives the best image quality.

–The x-ray pulse width or duration can also be varied when pulsed exposures are used, such as in cardiac cine.

–Most modern systems use a combination of tube current and peak voltage variability to control image brightness.

B. Photospot films

–**Photospot films** record the image output of an II onto 70- and 105-mm roll film, or on 100-mm cut film.

–A series of mirrors and lenses focuses the image from the II output phosphor onto the film (see Figure 6-2).

–Photospot films have an exposure of about 100 µR per frame at the receptor, which is about three times lower than that required for conventional screen/film combinations.

–Other advantages of photospot film include the following:

  –There is no need to change the film as there would be to change a cassette.

  –The short exposure time (50 msec) reduces patient motion artifacts.

  –Rapid sequences up to 12 frames per second are possible.

  –Images can be recorded while viewing the II output (i.e., fluoroscopy images).

  –There is substantial film savings (80%).

  –Resolution of about 4 lp/mm can be achieved.

  –The disadvantage of photospot imaging is the small film size.

C. Cine

–A **cine film** is a series of photospot images obtained in rapid sequence.

–Cine uses 35-mm film and images are 18 × 24 mm.

–Ninety-five percent of all cine studies involve the heart.

–The x-ray pulses and cine shutter are synchronized.

–Framing frequency is in fractions or multiples of 30 (15, 30, 60, 90 frames per second; 30 frames per second is the most common).

–Figure 6-3 shows how the area of the rectangular film (35 mm) and the circular II output phosphors are used in two framing modes.

  –With **exact framing,** the II circle fits exactly within the film frame.

  –With **overframing,** the film frame fits within the II circle, and the outer part of the II image is "lost."

–Overframing is standard for cardiac imaging.

–Typical cine exposures at the II input are about 15 to 30 µR per frame.

–Ninety percent of the II output light goes to cine and 10% goes to the TV camera, which permits the operator to monitor the procedure.

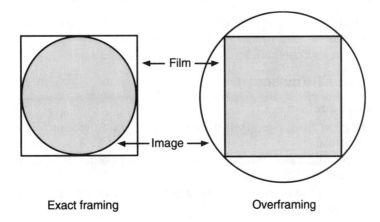

Exact framing   Overframing

Figure 6-3. With exact framing, the whole image is recorded, but only 79% of the film is used. With overframing, the entire film is used, but only 64% of the image is recorded.

    –Cine studies require the use of a grid-controlled x-ray tube, an optical distributor, and a synchronization circuit.

D. Radiation exposure

    –Entrance skin exposure rates in fluoroscopy typically range from 1 to 10 R/min.

    –The **maximum legal limit** for entrance skin exposure is generally **10 R/min**.

    –Fluoroscopy systems with a "high-dose" option normally have a 5 R/min dose limit in manual mode but no dose limit for high-dose options.

        –High-dose fluoroscopic options require special activation mechanisms as well as visible/audible indicators to show that the option is being used.

        –Indiscriminate use of high-dose fluoroscopy may result in very high doses and induce skin erythema or epilation.

    –Organ doses in fluoroscopy are considerably lower than skin doses because of the attenuation in soft tissue.

        –An AP entrance skin exposure of 1 R at the abdomen corresponds to an embryo/fetus absorbed dose of about 3 mGy (300 mrad).

    –Table 6-3 summarizes typical radiation doses for fluoroscopy, photospot filming, and cine modes of operation.

        –Patient exposures can be minimized by reducing fluoroscopy time and radiation field area.

Table 6-3. Representative Exposure Rates for a 23-cm Diameter Image Intensifier at the Phosphor Input and Patient Entrance

Fluoroscopy Operating Mode	Frame Rate (frames/sec)	Exposure Rate	
		Image Intensifier Input (μR/frame)	Patient Entrance (R/min)
Normal	30	3	4
High dose	30	9	12
Photospot	8	100	35
Cine	30	30	40

–Exposures may also be minimized by use of **last image hold,** which "freezes" the image on the monitor after the radiation exposure has been switched off.

IV. Digital Fluoroscopy

A. Introduction

–**Digital fluoroscopy** is a fluoroscopy system whose TV camera output is digitized.

–The digitized image can be enhanced before it is displayed on a TV monitor.

–Digital fluoroscopy images may be stored in a computer or printed using a laser camera.

–Digital fluoroscopy can replace conventional spot film imaging and photo-spot imaging.

–Digital fluoroscopy "spot" films are limited by their poor resolution, which is determined by the TV camera and is no better than about 2 lp/mm for a 1000-line TV system.

B. Digitized video images

–The TV output video signal of a fluoroscopy unit may be digitized and stored in a computer for further processing or subsequent display.

–Digitization is achieved using an **analog-to-digital convertor,** which samples the video signal from the camera and converts it to a discrete number that is stored in the computer.

–If the TV is a nominal 525-line system, one frame generally consists of 525^2 (250,000) **pixels** (picture elements).

–Each pixel needs either 1 byte (8 bits) or 2 bytes (16 bits) of space to record the signal level.

–Modern TV cameras may be operated in 1000-line mode, which results in a single frame having 1000^2 (1 million) pixels with an information content of either 1 or 2 Mbytes.

–Images may be acquired at up to 30 frames per second (525-line systems) or 7.5 frames per second (1000-line systems).

–TV cameras used in digital systems are selected to have low noise levels and high stability.

C. Digital subtraction angiography

–In **digital subtraction angiography (DSA)**, a fluoroscopically acquired digital **"mask" image** obtained without vascular contrast may be subtracted from subsequent frames obtained following contrast administration to generate a subtracted image showing only the contrast-filled vessels.

–Table 6-4 shows the typical exposure factors used in DSA imaging.

–DSA can detect low-contrast objects, so **less contrast agent** is needed.

–Although venous (rather than arterial) administration is possible, it is not used much because the reduced concentration of iodine contrast in the arteries produces images of poor quality.

D. DSA advantages

–Because DSA data are stored in a computer, the image appearance may be modified by changing displayed window/level settings.

Table 6-4. Typical Radiographic Techniques Used in a 23-cm Image Intensifier for Neuro-digital Subtraction Angiography

Parameter	Normal Range
Kilovolts	70 to 80 (kVp)
Milliamperes	100 to 250 (mA)
Pulse duration	30 to 100 (msec)
Acquisition rate	2 to 8 (frames/sec)
Image matrix size	512^2 or 1024^2
Entrance skin exposure	150 to 200 (mR/frame)
Input phosphor exposure	300 to 400 (µR/frame)

–Digital data also permit enhancement of images (e.g., unsharp masking enhances selected spatial frequencies).

–Digital data permit quantitative data to be obtained. For example, the mean rate of flow of iodine contrast through a vessel or the degree of vessel stenosis can be determined.

–DSA can be used to visualize contrast differences of less than 1% in x-ray transmission, whereas differences of 2% to 3% may often be missed with conventional screen/film combinations.

–DSA also allows less contrast to be used and allows images to be viewed immediately.

E. **Image quality in digital fluoroscopy**

–The resolution achieved is determined by the TV camera resolution and is typically no better than about 2 lp/mm for a 1000-line TV system.

–Image processing may offset the inferior spatial resolution performance of DSA.

–Because noise is randomly distributed in each image, the **noise level** in the final subtracted image **is higher** than in either individual image.

–**Frame integration** is the averaging or summing of several frames, which reduces the effect of random noise.

–DSA image quality may be degraded if the patient moves between acquisition of the mask frame and subsequent frames containing the contrast material.

–Corrections for patient motion may be made by computer manipulation of the digital images stored in memory.

–One method of **motion correction** is to incorporate spatial displacement of the mask frame.

–Another correction is to select a later frame for use as the mask (remasking).

Review Test

1. Match the following components of an image intensifier (II) system with their functions.

(A) Anode
(B) Input phosphor
(C) Photocathode
(D) Output screen

(i) Absorbs light and emits electrons
(ii) Absorbs x-rays and emits light
(iii) Absorbs electrons and emits light
(iv) Provides a positive voltage

2. The II input phosphor is made of

(A) NaI
(B) ZnCdS
(C) TLD
(D) CsI
(E) none of the above

3. The II output phosphor is made of

(A) NaI
(B) ZnCdS
(C) TLD
(D) CsI
(E) none of the above

4. The brightness gain of an II tube does NOT depend on the

(A) patient dose
(B) efficiency of the photocathode
(C) voltage across the II tube
(D) ratio of input to output screen sizes
(E) output phosphor conversion efficiency

5. Typical values for modern IIs do NOT include

(A) minification gains of 100
(B) flux gains of 50
(C) contrast ratios of 2:1
(D) brightness gains of 5000
(E) spatial resolutions of 5 line pairs per mm

6. Match the following operational parameters for II systems with the appropriate values.

(A) Accelerating voltage
(B) Entrance skin exposure rate
(C) Vignetting
(D) High contrast resolution

(i) 5 line pairs per mm
(ii) 20% loss of light intensity at field edges
(iii) 3 R/min
(iv) 25 kV

7. If the entrance skin exposure (ESE) rate of an II operated in the 30-cm mode is 1 R/min, the ESE rate in the 15-cm mode would be

(A) 1/4 R/min
(B) 1/2 R/min
(C) unchanged
(D) 2 R/min
(E) 4 R/min

8. If a 25-cm diameter II (2.5-cm output diameter) has a brightness gain of 5,000, then the flux gain is approximately

(A) 500
(B) 50
(C) 5
(D) unchanged
(E) cannot be determined

9. Changing the magnification mode of an image intensifier from 30 cm to 15 cm in fluoroscopy will normally increase

(A) entrance skin exposure rate
(B) distortion
(C) vignetting
(D) image brightness

10. The reason for interlacing two fields to form one frame in a conventional TV system is to reduce the

(A) patient dose
(B) motion artifacts
(C) input phosphor lag
(D) quantum mottle
(E) flicker

11. Vertical resolution of a standard North American TV is

(A) > horizontal resolution
(B) > European TV
(C) 0.7 × 30 frames per second
(D) 0.7 × 60 fields per second
(E) 0.7 × 262.5 line pairs

12. The *horizontal* resolution of a TV system is primarily determined by the

(A) image brightness
(B) bandwidth
(C) number of TV lines
(D) radiation exposure level
(E) focal spot size

13. The *vertical* resolution of a TV system is primarily determined by the

(A) image brightness
(B) bandwidth
(C) number of TV lines
(D) radiation exposure level
(E) focal spot size

14. In 35-mm cardiac cine, for a constant film density, patient entrance skin exposure is *reduced* by increasing the

(A) acquisition frame rate
(B) kV
(C) mA
(D) grid ratio
(E) focal spot size

15. Match the resolution with the viewing modes assuming the *same* image intensifier is used.

(A) 525-line TV
(B) Video cassette recorder
(C) 1025-line TV
(D) II output phosphor image

(i) 1.0 lp/mm
(ii) 1.2 lp/mm
(iii) 2.5 lp/mm
(iv) 5.0 lp/mm

16. The limiting spatial resolution in fluoroscopy can be improved by increasing the

(A) grid ratio
(B) II input size
(C) radiation dose level
(D) kV
(E) none of the above

17. Low contrast detectability in fluoroscopy images can be improved by increasing the

(A) focal spot size
(B) kVp
(C) x-ray beam filtration
(D) grid ratio
(E) fluoroscopy time

18. True (T) or False (F). Compared with radiographic film/screen exposures, fluoroscopy uses similar

(A) kVp
(B) mA
(C) exposure times
(D) added x-ray beam filtration
(E) grids

19. For *manual* technique fluoroscopy, image brightness at the output phosphor of an image intensifier is likely to be affected by all of the following parameters EXCEPT

(A) kVp
(B) mA
(C) patient thickness
(D) grid ratio
(E) exposure time

20. The major contributor to noise in a fluoroscopic image is variations in the

(A) input phosphor thickness
(B) accelerating tube voltage
(C) output phosphor thickness
(D) display screen brightness
(E) none of the above

21. Match the following fluoroscopy imaging procedures with the II input exposure per single "frame."

(A) Conventional fluoroscopy
(B) Screen/film imaging
(C) Photospot film imaging
(D) Last image hold viewing

(i) 0 μR
(ii) 2 μR
(iii) 100 μR
(iv) 300 μR

22. True (T) or False (F). In digital subtraction angiography (DSA)

(A) image intensifiers are used to create the images
(B) low noise TV cameras should be used
(C) a digital-to-analog converter samples the video signal
(D) spatial resolution is about 5 to 10 line pairs per mm
(E) image archival on optical disk is possible

23. The most important component affecting spatial resolution in DSA is the

(A) focal spot size
(B) II input phosphor thickness
(C) II output phosphor thickness
(D) digitization matrix
(E) computer CPU

24. True (T) or False (F). When compared with cine angiography, DSA

(A) uses a lower dose per frame
(B) has a lower spatial resolution
(C) uses lower frame rates
(D) has *inferior* detectability of contrast filled vessels

25. True (T) or False (F). Changing DSA matrix *alone* from 512 × 512 to 1024 × 1024 requires an increased

(A) acquisition frame rate
(B) analog-to-digital converter performance
(C) data storage requirement
(D) image processing time
(E) hard copy film processing time

Answers and Explanations

1. A–iv; anodes are positive and attract negatively charged electrons; **B–ii;** CsI input phosphors absorb x-rays and emit light; **C–i;** light from the input phosphor is absorbed (photoelectric effect) in the photocathode resulting in the emission of electrons; **D–iii;** electrons accelerated across the II strike the output phosphor and some of their energy is converted to light.

2–D. Virtually all IIs have input phosphors made from cesium iodide (CsI).

3–B. The output phosphor scintillator is made of zinc cadmium sulfide (ZnCdS).

4–A. The brightness gain is independent of exposure (i.e., patient dose). Brightness gain is a measure of how much light you get out of the II for a given light level at the input phosphor is the product of the minification gain and the flux gain.

5–C. Contrast ratios are typically 20:1; all the other values are representative of modern IIs.

6. A–iv; II accelerating voltages are in the range of 25 kV to 35 kV; **B–iii;** 3 R/min is a typical entrance skin exposure rate in fluoroscopy; **C–ii; D–i;** modern IIs have resolutions in the range of 4 to 5 line pairs/mm.

7–E. The irradiated input phosphor *area* is reduced by a factor of four, and the exposure level must be increased fourfold to maintain the same brightness level at the II output phosphor.

8–B. The brightness gain is the product of the flux gain and minification gain. Since the magnification gain is 100 ($25^2/2.5^2$), the flux gain must be 50.

9–A. Entrance skin exposure rate will increase by a factor of four since only 1/4 of the II is now absorbing x-rays, and the light level at the output phosphor has to remain constant.

10–E. When fields are displayed at a rate of 60/second (30 frames/second), there is no perception of flicker.

11–E. The 525 lines correspond to 262.5 line pairs but only 70% is achieved in practice (Kell factor of 0.7), resulting in a vertical resolution of 184 line pairs.

12–B. The bandwidth determines the horizontal TV resolution.

13–C. The number of TV lines is the primary determinant of the vertical TV resolution (525 lines in the United States; 625 lines in Europe).

14–B. Increasing the kV increases patient penetration and therefore reduces entrance skin dose for a constant II input dose level.

15. A–ii; typical resolution for a 23-cm II mode; **B–i;** the video system will introduce some degradation, thus the resolution is slightly less than normal fluoroscopy; **C–iii;** a 1,000-line TV will have a resolution twice that of a conventional 525-line fluoroscopy system; **D–iv;** the II output always has a better spatial resolution than the TV image.

16–E. By *reducing* the II size (field of view), the 525 lines are used to represent smaller distances and the number of line pairs "allocated" per mm increases.

17–D. Visibility of low contrast objects improves as scatter rejection improves, thereby increasing contrast.

18. A–True; patient penetration requirements are similar; **B–False;** fluoroscopy mA values are in the range 1 to 5 mA whereas in radiography, these are typically 100 mA; **C–False;** radiographic exposure times are typically tens or hundreds of milliseconds whereas fluoroscopy exposure times are seconds or minutes; **D–True; E–True;** grid ratios of about 10:1 are used for both fluoroscopy and radiography.

19–E. There is no "exposure time" in fluoroscopy since the x-ray beam is on all the time.

20–E. None of the above; variation in input x-ray photons (quantum mottle) is the dominant noise source in fluoroscopy.

21. A–ii; B–iv; screen/film exposure for a 400 speed system is about 0.3 mR; **C–iii;** photospot film needs about 1/3 dose of spot film exposures; **D–i;** there is no exposure during "last image hold."

22. A–True; B–True; C–False; analog-to-digital converters are used; **D–False;** limiting resolution is about 2 line pairs per mm for a 1000-line TV system; **E–True;** DSA systems require fast and high capacity disk drives up to about 50 MBytes.

23–D. The digitization matrix is the primary determinant of DSA spatial resolution performance (typical values are 512^2 or 1024^2).

24. A–False; DSA is about three times higher than cine (100 µR vs. 30 µR); **B–True;** 2.5 vs. 3.5 line pairs per mm; **C–True;** 7.5 vs. 30 frames per second; **D–False;** by subtracting frames with and without contrast, vessel visibility increases significantly.

25. A–False; acquisition frame rate is more likely to be reduced because the computer will be unable to cope with the extra data being acquired; **B–True;** there will be a fourfold increase in the digitization rate; **C–True;** a fourfold increase in data if the frame rate remains constant; **D–True;** there is more data to process; **E–False;** the hard copy filming time is not dependent on DSA matrix size.

7

Computers and Computed Tomography (CT)

I. Computers

A. Basics

–**Computers** use the **binary system**. A **bit** (binary digit) can be assigned one of two discrete values.

–One bit can code for 2 values, or 2 shades of gray, which correspond to white and black.

–n bits can code for 2^n values, or gray levels.

–**8 bits = 1 Byte; 2 Bytes = 1 word** (16 bits).

–A total of 256 shades of gray (2^8) can be coded for by 1 byte (8 bits).

–A total of 4096 shades of gray (2^{12}) can be coded for by 12 bits.

–Storage requirements for computers may be specified using kilobytes (kB) (10^3 Bytes), megabytes (MB) (10^6 Bytes), gigabytes (GB) (10^9 Bytes), or terabytes (TB) (10^{12} Bytes).

B. Image information

–**Pixels** are individual picture elements in a two-dimensional image.

–In digital images, each **pixel** is normally coded using either 1 or 2 Bytes.

–The total number of pixels in an image is the product of the number of pixels assigned to the horizontal and vertical dimensions.

–The number of pixels in each dimension is called **matrix size**.

–If there are 1024 (1 k) pixels in both the horizontal and vertical dimensions, then the image contains $1\ k \times 1\ k = 1\ M$, or 1024^2 pixels.

–Table 7-1 lists typical matrix sizes used in diagnostic radiology.

–The **information content** of images is the product of the number of pixels and the number of bytes per pixel.

–An image with a 512×512-pixel matrix and 1-Byte coding of each pixel requires 0.25 MB of memory ($512 \times 512 \times 1$).

–The same image obtained using 2-Byte coding of each pixel requires 0.5 MB of memory ($512 \times 512 \times 2$).

Table 7-1. Typical Matrix Sizes and Bytes per Pixel in Radiology

Modality	Matrix Size	Bytes per Pixel
Nuclear medicine	64^2 or 128^2	1 or 2
Magnetic resonance	128^2 to 256^2	2
Computed tomography	512^2	2
Ultrasound	512^2	1
Digital angiography	1024^2	2
Computed radiography	2048^2	2
Film digitizers	2048^2 or 4096^2	2
Mammography	4096^2 or 4096×6144	2

–A chest x-ray digitized to a 2 k × 2 k matrix using 2-Byte coding of each pixel ($2048 \times 2048 \times 2$) requires 8 MB of memory.

–Modern digital mammography systems are designed with matrix sizes between 4 × 4 k and 4 × 6 k pixels.

–With 2-Byte coding of each pixel, a single mammographic image would require 32 to 48 MB of memory.

C. **Computer hardware**

–Computer memories are **random access memory (RAM)** or **read only memory (ROM)**.

–**RAM** is temporary memory that stores information while the software is used.

–**ROM** is for storage only. Data in ROM cannot be overwritten.

–**Buffer memories** are normally considered a part of RAM and are used for video displays.

–A **central processing unit (CPU)** performs calculations and logic operations under the control of software instructions.

–**Parallel processing** occurs when several tasks are performed simultaneously.

–**Serial processing** refers to performing tasks sequentially.

–**Array processors** are hard-wired devices dedicated to performing one type of rapid calculation.

–Array processors are used in CT and magnetic resonance imaging where large numbers of calculations are needed to convert data into images.

D. **Computer software**

–Computers use **operating systems** to perform internal system bookkeeping activities such as storing files.

–A file is a collection of data treated as a unit.

–Examples of operating systems are DOS (for IBM personal computers), UNIX (for SUN computers), and VMS (for many mainframe computers). Macintosh computers use a proprietary operating system.

–**Computer software** provides instructions to the computer. Programs instruct the computer where input data are stored, how these data are to be manipulated, and where the results are to be placed.

–Most **computer programs** are written using high-level languages such as C, Pascal, COBOL, dBase, FORTRAN, or Basic.

–These high-level machine-independent languages are called **source code**.

–**Object code** or **machine language** is the machine-specific binary code instructions used by the CPU. It is difficult to write programs in object code.

–A **compiler** is a software program used to convert high-level language (source code) to machine language (object code).

E. Computer peripheral devices

–**Data storage devices** include hard disks, floppy disks, optical disks, optical jukeboxes, and magnetic tapes.

–Table 7-2 summarizes the data storage capabilities of various media.

–**Input devices** include keyboards, joysticks, light pens, trackballs, and touch screens.

–**Output devices** include cathode ray tube (CRT), monitors, laser film printers, and paper printers.

–Computers communicate via coaxial cables, telephone lines, magnetic tape transfers, microwaves, and fiber-optic links.

–A **modem** (modulator/demodulator) is used to transmit information over telephone lines.

–Figure 7-1 shows the peripheral devices associated with computers.

–Modern computers are linked using networks such as **Ethernet,** which may be used to transmit images to remote locations.

–**Baud rate** describes the rate of information transfer in bits per second.

–A baud rate of 9600 corresponds to 9600 bits/s or 1200 Bytes/s.

–Table 7-3 lists network options for transmitting images and the typical transmission times for a standard digitized chest x-ray (8 MB of information).

F. Picture archive and communications systems

–**Picture archive and communications systems (PACS)** are digital radiology systems that have the potential to eliminate the use of film.

–PACS are also called **image management and communications (IMAC)**.

–PACS require acquisition devices, computers, image archives, and image display stations.

–The components of a PACS must be connected by a digital communications network.

–Benefits of PACSs include the ability to manipulate data, compact storage, rapid image retrieval, and the ability to send images to remote locations.

Table 7-2. Typical Storage Capacities and Access Times for Computer Storage Media

Media	Storage Capacity	Access Time
Floppy disk	1 MB	~1 s
Hard disk	20 MB–2 GB	10 ms
Magnetic tape	600 MB–5 GB	10 s to a few minutes
Optical disk	600 MB–10 GB	16 ms
Optical jukebox	20 GB–3 TB	10–60+ s

$1 \text{ TB} = 10^3 \text{ GB} = 10^6 \text{ MB}$

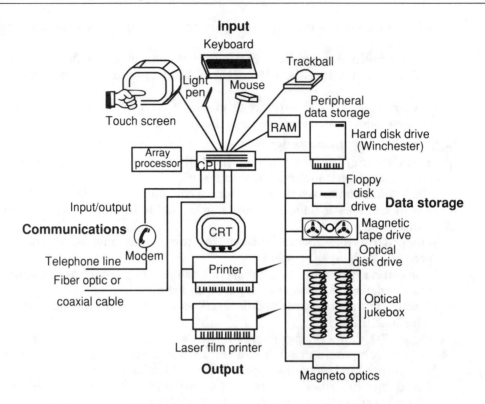

Figure 7-1. Input, output, memory, and communication devices used with computer systems.

–"Filmless" radiology departments include the OMSZ hospital in Vienna, the Hammersmith Hospital in London, the Veterans Administration Hospital in Baltimore, MD, and the United States Army Hospital in Madigan, WA.

II. Computed Tomography

A. Introduction

–**Computed tomography (CT)** is a **tomographic** imaging technique that generates cross-sectional images in the axial plane.
–**CT images** are maps of the relative linear attenuation values of tissues.
–CT x-ray techniques use a high kVp (120 to 140) with heavy filtration.
–For a fixed position of the x-ray tube, a **fan beam** is passed through the patient, and measurements of transmitted x-ray beam intensities are made by an **array** of detectors.
–Measured x-ray transmission values are called **projections**.
–CT images are derived by mathematical analysis of multiple projections.

B. Images

–**Field of view (FOV)** is the diameter of the area being imaged (e.g., 25 cm for a head).

Table 7-3. Types of Local Area Networks and Typical Time Required to Transfer a Digital Chest X-ray ($\equiv$ 8 MB Information)

Mode	Nominal Speed (Mb/s)	Chest X-ray Transfer Time
9600 Baud Modem (telephone)	0.01	~ 2 hours
Ethernet	10	~ 1 minute
Token ring	4–6	~ 1 minute
Fiber distributed data interface	125	< 10 seconds
Asynchronous transfer mode	600	< 1 second

–CT pixel size is determined by dividing the FOV by the matrix size. The matrix size used for CT is generally 512×512 (0.5 k).

–For example, pixel sizes are 0.5 mm for a 25-cm diameter FOV head scan (25 cm divided by 512) and 0.7 mm for a 35-cm FOV body scan (35 cm divided by 512).

–**Voxel** is a volume element in the patient. Voxel volume is the product of the pixel area and slice thickness.

–Figure 7-2 shows the relation among FOV, matrix size, voxel, and pixel.

–The **relative attenuation coefficient (μ)** is normally expressed in **Hounsfield units (HU),** which are also known as CT numbers.

$$HU_x = 1000 \times (\mu_x - \mu_{water})/\mu_{water}$$

–The 1000 in this equation determines the **contrast scale.**

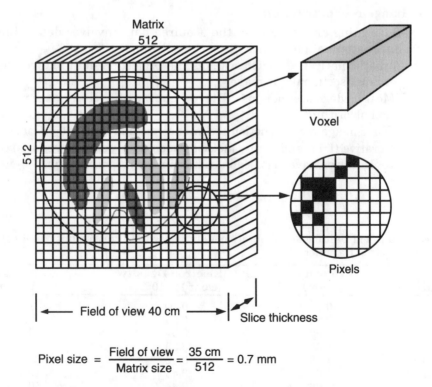

$$\text{Pixel size} = \frac{\text{Field of view}}{\text{Matrix size}} = \frac{35 \text{ cm}}{512} = 0.7 \text{ mm}$$

Figure 7-2. Relation among field of view, matrix size, voxel, and pixel in a computed tomography image.

–By definition, the HU value for water is 0, and the HU value for air is –1000.

–Table 7-4 lists typical HU values for a range of tissues.

–Because μ_x and μ_{water} are dependent on photon energy (keV), HU values depend on the kVp and filtration.

  –Therefore, HU values generated by a CT scanner are approximate and only valid for the effective kVp used to generate the image.

C. First- and second-generation scanners

–In 1972, the **EMI scanner** was the first CT scanner introduced into clinical practice.

–EMI scanners used a pencil beam and sodium iodide (NaI) detectors that moved across the patient (i.e., translated) and generated approximately 160 data points per projection on a point-by-point basis.

–The x-ray tube and detector were rotated 1 degree and another projection was obtained; 180 projections were obtained over a 180-degree rotation, taking approximately 5 minutes to generate a single image.

–This initial EMI design is called a **first-generation system**.

–**Second-generation scanners** also use translate–rotate technology but have multiple detectors and a fan-shaped beam.

–Second-generation scanners allowed larger rotational increments and faster scans, with a single section being generated in approximately 1 minute.

D. Image reconstruction

–Generating an image from the acquired data involves determining the linear attenuation coefficients of the individual pixels.

–A mathematical **algorithm** takes the projection data and reconstructs the cross-sectional CT image.

–Most modern scanners use **filtered back projection** image reconstruction algorithms.

–Older image reconstruction techniques include back projection.

–Iterative (trial and error) methods such as **algebraic reconstruction techniques** have also been used for image reconstruction.

Table 7-4. Hounsfield Unit for Representative Materials with Corresponding Values of Physical and Electron Densities

Material	Density (g/cm³)	Electron Density (e/cm³) × 10²³	Approximate HU Value
Air	< 0.01	< 0.01	–1000
Lung	0.25	0.83	–300
Fat	0.92	3.07	–90
Water	1.00	3.33	0
White matter	1.03	3.42	30
Gray matter	1.04	3.43	40
Muscle	1.06	3.44	50
Cortical bone	1.8	5.59	1000+

–Image reconstruction involving millions of data points may be performed in seconds using **array processors** (number crunchers).

–Different **filters** may be used in filtered back projection reconstruction, offering tradeoffs between spatial resolution and noise.

   –Some filters permit reconstruction of fine detail but with increased noise in the image such as in bone algorithms.

   –Algorithms such as those for soft tissue provide some smoothing, which decreases image noise but also decreases spatial resolution.

–The choice of the best filter to use with the reconstruction algorithm depends on the clinical task.

E. Image display

–Reconstructed images are viewed on CRT monitors or printed onto film using a laser printer.

–Each pixel is normally represented by 12 bits, or 4096 gray levels, which is larger than the display range of monitors or film.

–**Window width** and **level** are used to optimize the appearance of CT images by determining the contrast and brightness levels assigned to the CT image data (Figure 7-3).

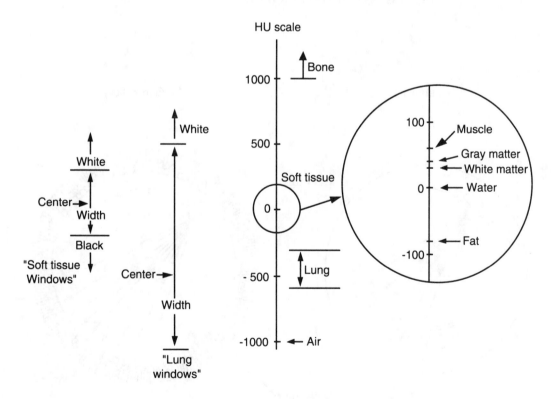

Figure 7-3. Window settings determine how the calculated tissue attenuation values are displayed. Window width determines the range from white to black. Window center defines the middle value.

–**Window level,** or center, is the CT number or HU value to be displayed as the medium intensity in the image.

–The window level is normally chosen close to the average HU value of the tissue of interest (e.g., 10 to 50 HU for soft tissue).

–**Window width** is the range of CT numbers displayed around the selected center and, therefore, determines the contrast.

–A narrow window width provides higher contrast than a wide window width.

–Window level and width settings allow the operator to emphasize the subtle density differences detected by CT and to record them on film.

–For example, selecting to view a CT image with a window width of 100 HU and a window level of 50 HU results in an image in which HU values of 0 or less appear black, HU values of 100 or more appear white, and HU values of 50 appear mid-gray.

–Window width and level settings only affect the displayed image, not the reconstructed image data stored in the computer.

III. Modern Computed Tomography Scanners

A. Third- and fourth-generation scanners

–**Third-generation scanners** use a rotating fan beam and detectors (rotate–rotate system) (Figure 7-4A).

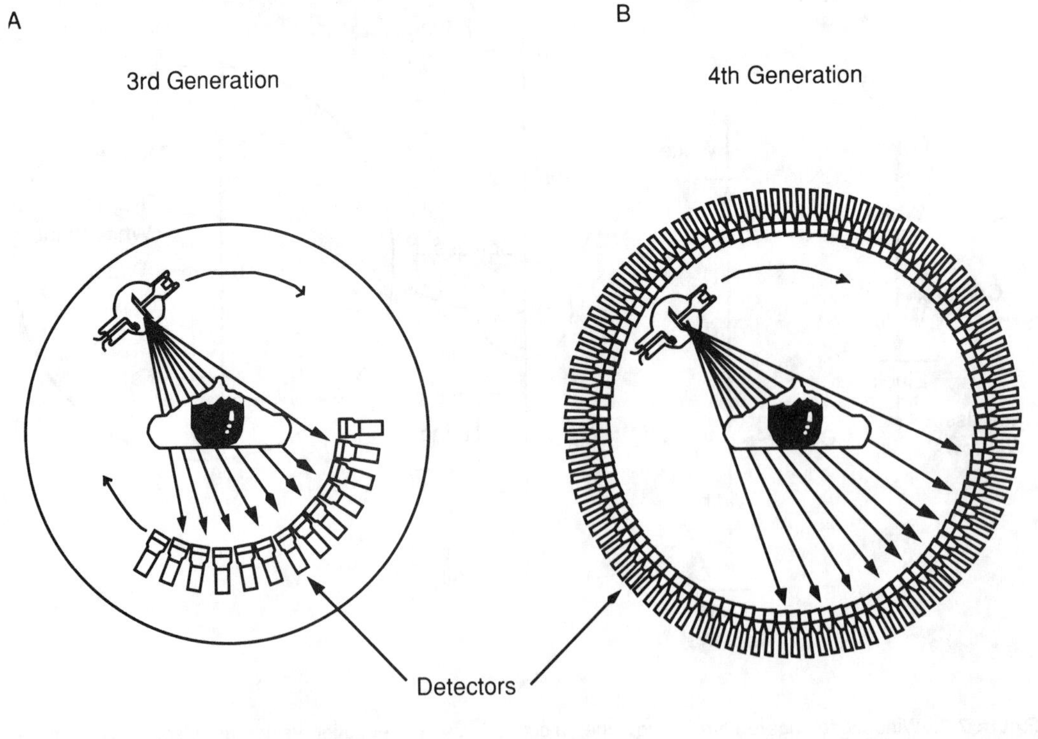

A

3rd Generation

B

4th Generation

Detectors

Figure 7-4. A, Third-generation CT scanners have a rotating tube and an array of detectors (rotate–rotate system). **B,** Fourth-generation CT scanners have a rotating tube and a fixed ring of detectors (rotate–fixed system).

–**Fourth-generation scanners** have a rotating tube and fixed ring of detectors (up to 4800) in the gantry (rotate–fixed system) (see Figure 7-4*B*).

–Third- and fourth-generation scanners can typically acquire a single section in 1 or 2 seconds.

–The imaging performance of third- and fourth-generation CT scanners is approximately equal.

–The cables that supply high voltage to the CT x-ray tube limit rotation to one revolution.

–Most modern CT scanners make use of **slip ring** technology in which high voltage is supplied to the tube through contact rings in the gantry. With slip ring scanners, the x-ray tube can rotate in one direction indefinitely.

–Slip ring scanners are fast and can scan several sections in a single breath hold.

B. X-ray tubes and collimators

–Heat loading on CT x-ray tubes is generally high, requiring high anode heat capacities.

–Modern systems have x-ray tube capacities of more than 2 megajoules.

–CT tubes have focal spots of approximately 1 mm.

–High performance CT x-ray tubes may cost $50,000 or more.

–The beam is collimated as it exits the tube and again before it strikes the detectors.

–**Collimation** defines the section thickness and reduces scatter.

–Adjustable collimators allow section thickness to range between 1 and 10 mm.

–The heavy filtration used with CT scanners typically produces a beam with an aluminum half-value layer (HVL) of approximately 10 mm.

C. Solid-state detectors

–Scintillation crystals produce light when x-ray photons are absorbed.

–When coupled to a light detector (photomultiplier tube or photodiode), an electric signal proportional to the incident radiation intensity is produced.

–The most common material used in solid-state detectors is **cadmium tungstenate** ($CdWO_4$), which is an efficient x-ray detector.

–Only solid-state detectors are used for fourth-generation scanners, which require thin detectors because of the detection geometry.

D. Gas detectors

–**Xenon gas** ionization detectors consist of a gas-filled chamber with anodes and cathodes maintained at a potential difference.

–Incident x-ray photons ionize the gas, producing electron–ion pairs.

–The current produced is proportional to the intensity of incident radiation.

–Gas detectors can only be used in third-generation scanners.

–Gas detectors are usually maintained at a high pressure (25 atm) to increase x-ray detection efficiency.

–Gas detectors are more stable than solid-state detectors.

E. Fifth-generation scanners

–**Fifth-generation scanners** use an electron gun that deflects and focuses a fast-moving electron beam along a 210-degree arc of a large diameter tungsten target ring in the gantry.

–The x-ray beam produced is collimated to traverse the patient and strike a detector ring.

–Multiple detector rings permit the simultaneous acquisition of multiple image sections.

–There are no moving parts, which allows images to be obtained in as little as 50 to 100 ms, thereby decreasing motion artifacts.

–Fifth-generation scanners are useful in cardiac imaging and in patients unable to cooperate for routine studies that require breath holding (e.g., pediatric and trauma patients).

F. Helical computed tomography

–Slip ring CT scanners may be used in a **helical (spiral) mode**.

–Unlike conventional CT scanners in which the x-ray tube rotates around a stationary patient one section at a time, in helical CT the patient is moved along the horizontal axis as the x-ray tube rotates around the patient.

–The x-ray beam central ray entering the patient follows a helical path during the CT scan.

–The relation between patient and tube motion is called **pitch,** which is defined as the table movement during each revolution of the x-ray tube (measured in millimeters) divided by the collimation width (measured in millimeters).

–For example, for a 5-mm section thickness, the patient may move 10 mm during the 1 second it takes for the x-ray tube to rotate through 360 degrees, and the pitch would thus be equal to 2.

–Image reconstruction is obtained by interpolating projection data obtained at selected locations along the patient axis.

–Images can be reconstructed at any level and in any increment but always have a thickness equal to the collimation used.

–The ability to rapidly cover a large volume in a single breath hold eliminates respiratory misregistration and reduces the volume of contrast agent required.

IV. Image Quality and Radiation Dose

A. Introduction

–Image quality may be characterized in terms of **contrast, noise,** and **spatial resolution**.

–In general, image quality involves tradeoffs between these three factors and patient radiation dose.

–Artifacts encountered during CT scanning can degrade image quality.

B. Contrast

–**CT contrast** is the difference in the HU values between tissues. This contrast generally increases as kVp decreases but is not affected by mA or scan times.

–CT contrast may be artificially increased by adding a contrast medium such as iodine.

–Image noise may prevent detection of low-contrast objects such as tumors with a density close to the adjacent tissue.

–The **displayed image contrast** is primarily determined by the CT window width and window level settings.

C. Noise

–CT noise is determined primarily by the number of photons used to make an image (**quantum mottle**).

  –When a detector receives a total count of 100 photons, the standard deviation is $\sqrt{100}$, or 10 (i.e., 10% of the mean).

  –A total of 68% of repeat measurements are within 1 standard deviation of the mean (i.e., between 90 and 110 counts).

  –If the count is increased to 1000, the standard deviation is 32 ($\sqrt{1000}$), or 3.2% of the mean; if the count is 10,000, the standard deviation is 100 ($\sqrt{10,000}$), or 1% of the mean.

–Quantum mottle decreases as the number of photons increases.

–CT noise is generally reduced by increasing the kVp, mA, or scan time, if all other parameters are constant.

–CT noise is also reduced by increasing voxel size (i.e., by decreasing matrix size, increasing FOV, or increasing section thickness).

–The typical noise with a modern CT system is approximately 5 HU (i.e., 0.5% difference in attenuation coefficient).

D. Resolution

–**Spatial resolution** is the ability to discriminate between adjacent objects and is a function of pixel size.

–If the CT FOV is d and the matrix size is M, then the pixel size is d/M.

  –For a typical head scan with an FOV of 25 cm and a matrix of 512 pixels, the pixel size is 0.5 mm.

  –Because two pixels are required to define a line pair (lp), the best achievable spatial resolution is 1 lp/mm.

–Typical resolution in CT scanning ranges from 0.7 to 1.5 lp/mm.

–In plane (axial) resolution may be improved by operating in a **high resolution mode** using a smaller FOV or a larger matrix size.

–Factors that may also improve CT spatial resolution by reducing image blur include smaller focal spots, smaller detectors, and more projections.

–Resolution perpendicular to the section is dependent on slice thickness and is important in sagittal and coronal reconstructions.

E. Radiation dose

–The dose profile in a CT scanner is not uniform along the patient axis and may vary within any irradiated section.

–Typical maximum doses for a single section are 40 mGy (4 rads) for a head scan or 20 mGy (2 rads) for a body scan.

–Doses at the patient surface may be higher than the dose at the center of the patient.

  –In head scans, the surface to center ratio is approximately 1:1.

  –In body scans, the surface to center ratio is approximately 2:1.

–Because of scattered x-rays, the CT section dose profile is not perfectly square but has tails that extend beyond the section edges.

–Tissues beyond the section are thus exposed to radiation.

–When contiguous sections are scanned, the cumulative radiation dose in a section may be as high as twice the radiation dose associated with a single section.

–Manufacturers specify doses using the **computed tomography dose index (CTDI),** which is the integral of the axial dose profile for a single CT slice divided by the nominal slice thickness.

–Although the CTDI can be readily measured, it is not directly related to patient risk.

F. Radiation risks

–Patient risk is related to the total energy imparted (deposited) in the patient.

–Patient risk is calculated by summing doses to all irradiated organs weighted by their relative radiosensitivities.

–Such a weighted patient dose is the **effective dose equivalent (H_E).**

–H_E for head scans is approximately 2 mSv (200 mrem).

–H_E for body scans is approximately 5 to 15 mSv (500 to 1500 mrem).

–If all other factors are constant, patient risks generally increase with increases in the number of slices, slice thickness, scan time, kVp, and mA values, because more energy is imparted into the patient.

–The **effective dose (E)** is conceptually similar to H_E, but makes use of more recent values of organ radiosensitivity weighting factors.

–Quantitative values of H_E and E are similar for most CT examinations.

G. Artifacts

–CT scanners may have **artifacts** in the reconstructed images.

–**Partial volume artifact** is the result of averaging the linear attenuation coefficient in a voxel that is heterogenous in composition.

–Partial volume artifact increases with pixel size and section thickness.

–Random or unpredictable motion (e.g., if the patient sneezes) produces **streak artifacts** in the direction of motion.

–In high-density structures, such as metal implants, the detector may record no transmission.

–In these cases, the reconstruction algorithm generates streaks adjacent to the high-density structures.

–**Beam hardening artifacts** or "cup" artifacts are caused by the polychromatic nature of the x-ray beam (beam hardening).

–As the lower energy photons are preferentially absorbed, the beam becomes more penetrating and results in lower computed values of the attenuation coefficient (HU).

–Beam hardening artifacts are most marked at high-contrast interfaces such as between dense bone in the skull and the brain where dark streaks (lower HU values) occur.

–**Ring artifacts** may arise in third-generation systems if a single detector is faulty or miscalibrated.

–Artifacts caused by equipment defects are rare on modern CT systems.

Review Test

1. Match the following number of bits with the information below.

(A) 1
(B) 8
(C) 10
(D) 12
(E) 16

(i) 2 bytes
(ii) 1 byte
(iii) 1024 gray scale levels
(iv) 2 gray scale levels
(v) 4096 gray scale levels

2. If all 8 bits in a byte are set to 1, then the decimal number is

(A) 8
(B) 255
(C) 1023
(D) too big to store in a word
(E) none of the above

3. Match each of the following computer hardware items with the corresponding performance characteristics.

(A) RAM
(B) Floppy disk
(C) CPU
(D) Optical disk jukebox
(E) ROM

(i) Performs logical and arithmetic operations
(ii) Storage device *loses* information when power goes out
(iii) Storage that *cannot* be overwritten
(iv) Can have online storage capacity of 1 TeraByte
(v) Can be erased if brought close to an MR scanner

4. True (T) or False (F) to the following definitions regarding digital computers.

(A) *Byte* always consists of 8 bits
(B) *File* is a collection of data treated as a unit
(C) *Microprocessor* is a single integrated circuit
(D) *Modem* maintains the power supply to computers
(E) *PACS* stands for picture archival and communications system

5. True (T) or False (F). Input devices for a computer include

(A) keyboard
(B) trackball
(C) laser printer
(D) light pen
(E) array processor
(F) touch screen

6. Parallel processing

(A) involves running several tasks simultaneously
(B) requires an array processing
(C) cannot be performed in machine code
(D) requires the sharing of peripheral devices
(E) all of the above

7. Computers can communicate with each other using all the following communication channels EXCEPT

(A) coaxial cables
(B) telephone lines
(C) fiber optic cables
(D) microwave links
(E) high-frequency generators

8. Components found in a PACS are likely to include

(A) digital acquisition devices
(B) digital archives
(C) diagnostic display stations
(D) patient data base
(E) all of the above

9. How many megabytes (MB) are required to store each of the following images?

(A) NM – $128 \times 128 \times 1$ byte
(B) MR – $256 \times 256 \times 2$ byte
(C) US – $512 \times 512 \times 1$ byte
(D) CT – $512 \times 512 \times 2$ byte
(E) DSA – $1,024 \times 1,024 \times 2$ byte
(F) CR – $2,048 \times 2,048 \times 2$ byte

10. The measured x-ray transmissions from a single CT fan beam through a patient is called a

(A) filter
(B) back-projection algorithm
(C) tomographic slice
(D) primary beam
(E) projection

11. Which image reconstruction algorithm is used most often in current commercial CT scanners?

(A) 2-Dimensional Fourier transform
(B) 3-Dimensional Fourier transform
(C) Back projection
(D) Filtered back projection
(E) Algebraic reconstruction algorithm

12. CT collimators are

(A) variable for different section thicknesses
(B) not necessary for helical scans
(C) usually made out of plexiglass
(D) bow-tie shaped
(E) cooled using fans

13. Which of the following detectors could NOT be used in CT scanners?

(A) Silver bromide grains
(B) $CdWO_4$
(C) Xenon gas
(D) NaI crystals

14. Match the following matter with the corresponding CT numbers (Hounsfield units).

(A) Fat
(B) Gray matter
(C) Water
(D) Bone
(E) Lung

(i) −400
(ii) −90
(iii) 0
(iv) 40
(v) 1000

15. Anode heat loading on a CT x-ray tube increases with all of the following EXCEPT

(A) kV
(B) mA
(C) scan time
(D) section thickness
(E) number of sections

16. Match the following generation CT scanners with the correct detector.

(A) First-generation scanner
(B) Third-generation scanner
(C) Fourth-generation scanner

(i) Pencil beam
(ii) Stationary detector array
(iii) Rotating detector array

17. Fourth-generation CT detectors are frequently made of

(A) low-pressure air ionization chambers
(B) Geiger tubes
(C) $CdWO_4$
(D) high-pressure Xenon
(E) all of the above

18. Use of intravascular contrast when performing a single CT section will significantly increase the

(A) HU of blood vessels
(B) required kVp
(C) required mA
(D) patient dose
(E) image noise

19. The CT image display contrast

(A) must be selected prior to the x-ray exposures
(B) may be altered after the CT scan
(C) does not modify the appearance of the CT image
(D) can be used to change the HU values of image data
(E) none of the above

20. True (T) or False (F). If a CT display is set at a window width of 100 and a window center of 50, the

(A) HU value of water changes to 50
(B) white matter will look gray
(C) fat will look black
(D) water will look black
(E) bone will look white
(F) lung will look white

21. CT laser film printers

(A) significantly improve spatial resolution
(B) modify the CT numbers
(C) record < 1 kB of image data
(D) require double-sided emulsion film
(E) none of the above

22. In helical CT scanning all of the following apply EXCEPT

(A) continuous slip ring is required for the x-ray tube
(B) cannot be performed with bow-tie filters
(C) higher x-ray tube heat capacity is needed
(D) partial volume effects will increase

23. CT scanner spatial resolution improves with an increase of

(A) focal spot size
(B) detector elements size
(C) kV and mA
(D) scan time
(E) reconstruction matrix size

24. Tissue characterization by CT number is difficult because of the dependence of CT number on all the following EXCEPT

(A) beam hardening
(B) tissue heterogeneity
(C) mAs
(D) partial volume effects
(E) kVp

25. The visibility of small high-contrast structures in CT images will most likely improve with increase of

(A) patient dose
(B) scan time
(C) image matrix size
(D) slice thickness
(E) kV

26. The visibility of large low-contrast structures in CT images may improve with an increase in

(A) filtration
(B) mAs
(C) matrix size
(D) display window width
(E) size of film image

27. Image noise is affected by the following

(A) section thickness
(B) reconstruction algorithm
(C) patient thickness
(D) mAs
(E) all of the above

28. Partial volume artifacts in CT are generally reduced when

(A) section thickness increases
(B) scanning time is increased
(C) image matrix size increases
(D) fifth-generation scanners are used
(E) small focal spot sizes are used

29. Which of the following is LEAST likely to be a source of CT image artifacts?

(A) Anode wobble
(B) Faulty detectors
(C) Metallic implants in patient
(D) Limited sampling of projection data
(E) Radiofrequency source close to the CT scanner

30. Ring artifacts in a third-generation CT scanner are caused by

(A) kVp drift
(B) tube arcing
(C) faulty detector element
(D) patient motion
(E) all of the above

Answers and Explanations

1. A–iv; 1 bit can be either on (black) or off (white) and thus 2 gray scale levels; **B–ii;** 1 byte is 8 bits; **C–iii;** gray levels is given by 2^n where n is the number of bits (for $n = 10$, 2^{10} is 1024); **D–v;** $2^{12} = 4096$; **E–i;** 2 bytes (1 word) = 16 bits.

2–B. When all bits are set to 0, the number is 0. Since there are 2^8 or 256 levels, the maximum level is 255.

3. A–ii; RAM (random access memory) requires a power supply to maintain stored data; **B–v;** floppy disks use magnetic media to store information which is lost whenever a large magnetic field is applied; **C–i;** CPU = central processing unit; **D–iv;** the amount of image information generated by a radiology department in a year is about 1 terabyte and could be stored in an optical jukebox; **E–iii;** ROM = read only memory.

4. A–True; B–True; C–True; they are commonly known as "chips"; **D–False;** Modulator/demodulator (modem) is used to transmit information on telephone lines; **E–True;** with a PACS, hospitals could be totally "filmless" and thereby be more efficient in storing and transmitting radiologic images.

5. A–True; B–True; C–False; it is an output device; **D–True; E–False;** it is a hardware component used by the CPU to perform specific calculations as in CT image reconstruction; **F–True**.

6–A. Serial processing performs tasks sequentially, whereas parallel processing has tasks running at the same time.

7–E. High-frequency generators are used to produce high voltages across x-ray tubes.

8–E. All the listed items are key components of any picture archive and communications system (PACS).

9. A–1/64 MB (1/8 k × 1/8 k × 1 B); **B–1/8 MB** (1/4 k × 1/4 k × 2 B; **C–1/4 MB** (1/2 k × 1/2 k × 1 B); **D–1/2 MB** (1/2 k × 1/2 k × 2 B); **E–2 MB** (1 k × 1 k × 2 B); **F–8 MB** (2 k × 2 k × 2 B).

10–E. A projection is a profile of transmitted x-ray intensities through the patient at any given location of the x-ray tube, with up to 1000 projections acquired and used to reconstruct the CT image.

11–D. Filtered back projection is currently used on virtually all commercial CT scanners to reconstruct images from projection data.

12–A. The collimators are located at the x-ray tube and detectors and have a variable width (1 to 10 mm), which defines the CT section thickness.

13–A. Silver bromide grains are used in film emulsion and cannot be used in CT.

14. A–ii; fat is –90 HU; **B–iv;** gray matter is 40 HU; **C–iii;** water is 0 HU by definition; **D–v;** bone is 1000 to 4000 HU; **E–i;** lung is mostly air and measures –300 to –600 HU.

15–D. Section thickness selection does not directly affect x-ray heat loading.

16. A–i; first-generation CT scanners used a pencil x-ray beam that moved along a line to obtain a projection before being rotated to obtain the next projection; **B–iii;** in third-generation CT scanners, the detector array and x-ray tube both rotate; **C–ii;** in fourth-generation CT scanners, the detector array is stationary.

17–C. Most fourth-generation CTs use solid state detectors such as $CdWO_4$. Gas detectors are *only* used in third-generation scanners.

18–A. Intravenous contrast increases the density and atomic number of blood and tissues. This increases x-ray attenuation and thereby the resultant HU value.

19–B. Changing the display contrast (window center and width) alters the *appearance* of the CT image, but not the reconstructed image data (HU).

20. A–False; window/level changes cannot change HU values, only their appearance on a screen or film; **B–True;** white matter will be in the middle of the display range; **C–True;** all HU values < 0 will look black and fat has a value of about –90; **D–True; E–True;** all HU values >100 will look white; **F–False;** lung will look black.

21–E. None of these statements is true.

22–B. Most modern CT scanners use bow-tie filters to equalize the radiation level incident on the x-ray detectors, including helical scanners.

23–E. Spatial resolution improves with an increase in reconstruction matrix size, assuming that there are enough detectors along the projection and an adequate number of projections are obtained.

24–C. mAs will have no effect on CT numbers, but will affect the precision with which they are measured (noise).

25–C. Increasing image matrix size improves spatial resolution and is most likely to improve the detectability of small high-contrast objects.

26–B. Low-contrast objects are difficult to see because of noise, and increasing the mAs increases the number of photons used and hence reduces CT image noise.

27–E. All of the listed factors generally affect the image noise.

28–C. A larger image matrix size improves spatial resolution and hence is likely to reduce "volume averaging" known as the partial volume effect.

29–E. Radiofrequency sources are unlikely to have any effect on the x-ray detection and therefore should produce no artifacts.

30–C. A faulty detector reading on third-generation scanners gives rise to ring artifacts. The closer the artifact to the image center, the more central the detector element that is faulty in the linear detector array.

8

Nuclear Medicine

I. Radiopharmaceuticals

A. Production of radioactivity

–**Radionuclides** may be produced in a nuclear reactor by adding neutrons to nuclides (e.g., ^{59}Co + neutron $\rightarrow$ ^{60}Co).

–Radionuclides produced in a generator generally decay by a beta minus process.

–Radionuclides may be produced in **cyclotrons** where protons or deuterons are added to stable nuclides (e.g., ^{201}Hg + deuteron $\rightarrow$ ^{201}Tl + 2 neutrons).

–Cyclotron-produced radionuclides generally decay by either a beta plus process (^{15}O) or electron capture (^{123}I).

–Radionuclides may also be produced as **fission products** of heavy nuclides.

–In nuclear medicine, **generators** are often used to produce radionuclides for clinical use.

–^{99m}Tc is obtained from the parent ^{99}Mo in a generator, and ^{113m}In is obtained from a ^{113}Sn generator.

–Both ^{99m}Tc and ^{113m}In decay by isomeric transition.

–Table 8-1 lists the key characteristics of common radionuclides used in nuclear medicine.

B. Radiopharmaceutical characteristics

–**Radiopharmaceuticals** are designed to mimic a natural physiologic process.

–The evaluation of function rather than anatomy sets nuclear medicine studies apart from other imaging studies.

–Nuclear medicine diagnostic studies use **gamma rays** (produced in the nucleus of an atom) rather than x-rays.

–To minimize the patient radiation dose, radiopharmaceuticals should do the following:

–Have a short half-life that is compatible with the duration and objectives of the nuclear medicine study.

Table 8-1. Characteristics of Common Radionuclides

Nuclide	Photons (keV)	Production Mode	Decay Mode	Half-life $(T_{1/2})$
^{67}Ga	93, 185, 296, 388	Cyclotron	EC	78 hours
^{99m}Tc	140	Generator	IT	6 hours
^{111}In	173, 247	Cyclotron	EC	68 hours
^{123}I	159	Cyclotron	EC	13 hours
^{125}I	27, 36	Reactor	EC	60 days
^{131}I	364	Fission product	β	8 days
^{133}Xe	80	Fission product	β	5.3 days
^{201}Tl	70, 167	Cyclotron	EC	73 hours

β = beta decay; EC = electron capture; IT = isomeric transition.

–Produce monochromatic gamma rays with energies between 100 and 300 keV.

–Minimize production of particulate radiation such as beta particles, internal conversion electrons, and Auger electrons.

–Be nontoxic and contain no chemical or radionuclide contaminants.

–Localize in the organ or tissue of interest.

–Ideally, radionuclides should be readily and economically available.

C. Radiopharmaceutical localization

–Radiopharmaceutical **localization mechanisms** include the following:

  –**Active transport** such as thyroid uptake scanning with iodine.

  –**Compartmental** localization such as blood pool scanning with human serum albumin, plasma, or red blood cells.

  –**Simple exchange** or **diffusion** such as bone scanning with pyrophosphates.

  –**Phagocytosis** such as liver, spleen, and bone-marrow scanning with radiocolloids.

  –**Capillary blockade** such as lung scanning with macroaggregate (8 to 75 μm) or organ perfusion studies with intra-arterial injection of macroaggregates.

  –**Cell sequestration** such as spleen scanning with damaged red blood cells.

D. Technetium (^{99m}Tc) generator

–The technetium generator consists of an alumina column loaded with ^{99}Mo. ^{99}Mo decays to ^{99m}Tc.

–Saline is passed through the column to elute the ^{99m}Tc. The ^{99}Mo is not soluble in saline and, therefore, remains in the column.

–A wet generator contains saline at all times.

–Saline must be added to a dry generator when ^{99m}Tc is needed.

–^{99m}Tc decays by isomeric transition with 88% emitted as 140-keV gamma rays. The remainder of energy is emitted as internal conversion electrons, characteristic x-rays, and Auger electrons.

–The ideal gamma energy of 140 keV, convenient half-life of 6 hours, and ready availability from a generator make ^{99m}Tc the most popular radionuclide in nuclear medicine.

–^{99m}Tc is used in approximately 80% of all nuclear medicine examinations.

–Pertechnetate ($^{99m}TcO_4$) is produced directly from ^{99}Mo using a saline eluant.

–The half-life of ^{99}Mo is 67 hours, which allows the generator to remain useful for approximately 1 week (~2.5 half-lives).

–**Transient equilibrium** between the parent (^{99}Mo) and daughter (^{99m}Tc) is reached in approximately 4 half-lives (24 hours).

–**Secular equilibrium** occurs after approximately 6 half-lives in generator systems in which the half-life of the parent is much greater (100 times) than that of the daughter.

E. Imaging radiopharmaceuticals

–Oral or intravenous administration of pertechnetate results in uptake in the thyroid, salivary glands, and stomach.

–^{99m}Tc may be used to label a wide range of biological entities including diethylenetriaminepentaacetic acid (DTPA), iron complexes, macroaggregated albumin (MAA), polyphosphate, red blood cells, and sulfur colloid (SC).

–As an example, SC is available as a commercial kit containing 0.3-mm particles.

–After SC is injected, approximately 70% localizes in the liver within 10 to 20 minutes; the remainder is distributed in the spleen and bone marrow.

–Radioiodine is used for thyroid imaging and to evaluate thyroid function (uptake), and labeled Hippuran is used to evaluate kidney function.

–Radioactive gases (e.g., ^{133}Xe) may be used in lung perfusion imaging.

–Other radiopharmaceuticals used in nuclear medicine include ^{51}Cr-labeled red blood cells, ^{67}Ga-labeled citrate to detect tumor and infection, and ^{111}In-labeled leukocytes to detect acute infections.

II. Nuclear Medicine Instrumentation

A. Gamma cameras

–**Gamma cameras (Anger cameras)** are the most common imaging devices used in nuclear medicine (Figure 8-1).

–**Scintillation crystals** absorb incident photons and produce light.

–Most crystals are made of sodium iodide (NaI) and are 10 mm thick.

–The **intrinsic sensitivity** or **efficiency** of a crystal is the percentage of incident gamma rays detected.

–Table 8-2 summarizes how photopeak detection efficiency increases with increasing detector thickness and decreases with increasing photon energy.

–As crystal thickness increases, sensitivity generally increases, but resolution decreases.

–Light output from the NaI crystal is detected by an array of **photomultiplier tubes (PMTs)**.

–Gamma cameras typically use 37, 61, or 91 PMTs.

–A special coupling epoxy resin is used to improve contact between the NaI crystal and photomultiplier tubes and, therefore, improve light transmittance.

–Signals from PMTs generate information about where each photon interacted (**spatial data**).

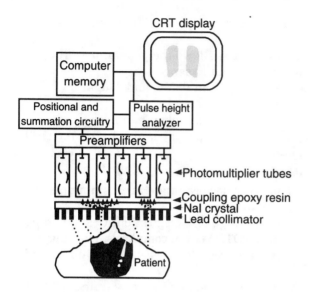

Figure 8-1. Components of a gamma camera.

–The position of the gamma ray is determined by the relative strength of the signal received by several PMTs.

–Gamma camera resolution increases as the size of the PMTs decreases and as the number of PMTs increases.

–Images are built up count-by-count with between 500,000 and 1 million data points per image.

–Occasionally, images are not required and an uptake probe is used which only counts activity.

B. Detected energy spectrum

–The energy spectrum detected by the scintillation crystal (NaI) includes several important features as shown in Figure 8-2.

–The **main photopeak** is produced when an incident gamma ray is completely absorbed in the crystal (photoelectric effect).

–An **iodine escape peak** occurs at approximately 30 keV below the photopeak and is the result of iodine characteristic K-shell x-rays that escape the crystal.

Table 8-2 Sodium Iodide (NaI) Crystal Photopeak Detection Efficiency

Photon Energy (keV)	Photons Detected (%) by NaI Crystal with Detector Thickness of:		
	5 mm	10 mm	25 mm
100	94	100	100
140*	72	92	100
200	32	54	85
300	12	22	46
500	3	6	15

*99mTc

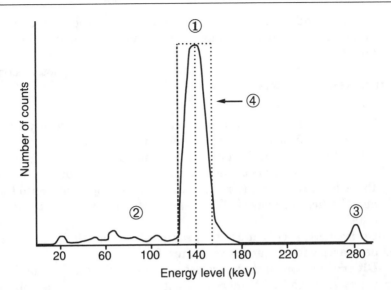

Figure 8-2. Technetium spectrum and photopeak window settings. The photopeak (*1*) is the result of complete absorption of ^{99m}Tc gamma rays in the crystal. The iodine escape peak, Compton scatter events, and secondary x-rays from lead occur below this (*2*). The sum peak (*3*) is the result of two photons being simultaneously absorbed in the crystal and counted as one. The area within the dashed line (*4*) shows the acceptance range of a pulse height analyzer (PHA) set at 140 keV with a 20% window.

–**Scatter events** in the NaI crystals occur where the energy of the scattered electron is absorbed in the crystal but the scattered photon escapes.

–The **Compton edge** represents the maximum energy transferred to a scattered electron in the Compton process.

–Lower energy photons absorbed by the NaI crystal are generated by Compton scattering of gamma rays in tissue.

–**Pulse pile-up** events occur when the energy of two photons is registered simultaneously.

C. Pulse height analysis

–A **pulse height analyzer (PHA)** is an electronic device used to determine which portion of the detected spectrum is to be used for creating the nuclear medicine image (see Figure 8-2).

–The PHA is placed between the detector and counting portion of the camera system (see Figure 8-1).

–The PHA can be set to allow only certain photon energy levels to be counted, thus decreasing the contribution of Compton scatter and pulse pile-up to the resultant image.

–The PHA allows the operator either to set the upper and lower energy limits or to set a peak energy level and associated window.

–The window, measured by percent, determines the acceptable range of energy levels around the peak for subsequent counting.

–For example, a peak of 140 keV with a 20% window accepts photon energy levels ranging from 126 to 154 keV (see Figure 8-2).

—A wide window accepts more photons and produces an image more quickly, but it includes more scatter photons, which degrade image quality.

—Ideally, only photopeak events that correspond to a photoelectric absorption event in the crystal are accepted.

D. Collimators

—Collimators are used to provide spatial information by only allowing photons arriving from certain directions to reach the crystal.

—Collimators are typically made of lead and contain multiple holes (Figure 8-3). The lead strips between the holes are called **septa**.

—**Parallel hole** collimators project the same object size onto the camera, and the field of view (FOV) does not change with distance (see Figure 8-3A).

—**Converging collimators** produce a magnified image, and FOV decreases with distance (see Figure 8-3B).

—**Diverging collimators** project an image size that is smaller than the object size, and FOV increases with distance from the collimator (see Figure 8-3C).

—**Pinhole collimators** generate a minified or magnified image depending on the distance of the object from the collimators. The image is inverted and the FOV increases rapidly as the observer moves away from the pinhole (see Figure 8-3D).

E. Collimator performance

—The resolution of a collimator is expressed as the **full width half maximum (FWHM)** of a line source.

—Collimator sensitivity is low with approximately 10^{-4}, or only 0.01%, of the emitted photons being detected.

—Most collimators involve a trade-off between spatial resolution performance and sensitivity.

—Resolution is increased if the size of the holes is reduced (thicker septa) or the collimator is made thicker.

—These same changes decrease the number of photons reaching the crystal, thus reducing system sensitivity.

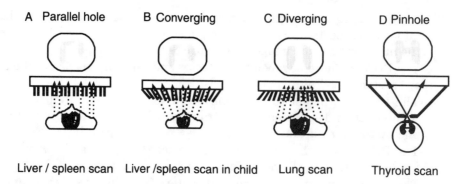

| A Parallel hole | B Converging | C Diverging | D Pinhole |

| Liver / spleen scan | Liver /spleen scan in child | Lung scan | Thyroid scan |

Figure 8-3. Collimators used in nuclear medicine. **A,** Parallel hole collimator used for routine imaging. **B,** Converging hole collimator magnifies the image. **C,** Diverging hole collimator reduces image size. **D,** Pinhole collimator.

–The thinner the septa, the more scatter penetrates and reduces the resultant image contrast.

–Parallel hole collimators are classified for high-sensitivity (i.e., low resolution), general purpose, and high-resolution (i.e., low sensitivity) uses.

–**High-sensitivity** collimators are thinner and transmit approximately twice as many 140-keV photons as the all-purpose collimator.

–**High-resolution** collimators transmit approximately half as many photons as the all-purpose collimator.

–Table 8-3 summarizes the variation of resolution as a function of distance from the source to the collimator.

III. Image Quality

A. System resolution

–An image of a line source of activity is known as the **line spread function**.

–Measurement of the FWHM of the line spread function is a common measure of resolution in nuclear medicine.

–**System resolution (R)** depends on the intrinsic resolution of the gamma camera (R_i) and resolution of the collimator (R_c).

–System resolution is $R = \sqrt{R_i^2 + R_c^2}$.

–**Intrinsic gamma camera resolution** is degraded with increased detector thickness because of increased light diffusion in the NaI crystal.

–Intrinsic resolution is typically between 3 and 5 mm.

–FWHM values in nuclear medicine are approximately 10 mm with an all-purpose collimator and 7.5 mm with a high-resolution collimator in a typical patient examination.

–Resolution is degraded if the PMTs separate from the crystal.

–Resolution may also be measured using a bar phantom pattern.

B. Image contrast

–Contrast in nuclear medicine images is generally high because the radiopharmaceuticals localize well in the organ of interest.

–Some radioactivity is always found in other tissues, and photons from this activity generate undesirable **background counts,** which degrades image contrast.

–The ratio of organ-specific uptake to unwanted uptake in other tissues is called the **target to background ratio**.

–Contrast is also affected by **septal penetration** and **scatter.**

–When images are printed on film or displayed on a monitor, image contrast is also affected by the characteristic curve of the film or monitor.

Table 8-3. Typical Full Width Half Maximum Resolution Values for Different Types of Clinical Collimators

Distance from Collimator (cm)	Spatial Resolution (mm) as FWHM		
	High Resolution	All-Purpose Collimator	High Sensitivity
0	2	3	5
5	5	7	10
10	8	10	15
15	12	14	20

C. Image noise

–Random noise degrades image quality and may be classified as **random** or **structured**.

–Random noise or **quantum mottle** is a result of the low number of photons used to create a typical nuclear medicine image and is a major factor in image quality.

  –Noise is the primary reason why nuclear medicine images are generally of low quality.

  –If too few counts are recorded, the high quantum mottle can reduce lesion detectability.

–**Structured noise** includes nonuniformities in the gamma camera and is a minor contributor to overall noise.

  –Most modern gamma cameras use computers to perform corrections for nonuniformities, thereby reducing the significance of structured noise.

  –Overlying objects in the patient (e.g., uptake in the gastrointestinal tract when imaging the kidneys) can also result in structured noise.

D. Artifacts

–Gamma camera artifacts are caused by many different sources.

–Damaged collimators can cause significant uniformity problems.

–Patient motion is a common source of artifacts.

–Metal objects worn by the patient produce photopenic areas that may mimic pathologic cold lesions.

–**PMT failure** may also produce a cold defect.

–**Off-peak images** contain excessive Compton scatter and occur when the PHA window is outside the main photopeak.

–**Edge packing**, or increased brightness at the edge of the crystal, is due to internal reflection of light at the edge of the crystal and absence of PMTs beyond the crystal edge.

–**Cracked crystals** produce linear defects in the image.

IV. Dosimetry

A. Half-lives

–**Physical half-life ($T_{1/2}$)** is the time required for a radionuclide to decay to half its original activity.

–The **decay rate**, or activity, of a source is the number of disintegrations occurring each second.

–Lambda (λ) is the **decay constant,** and activity equals $N \times \lambda$, where N is the number of atoms in the sample.

–The activity of a source decays exponentially as $e^{-\lambda \times t}$, where t is time expressed in the same units as λ: $T_{1/2} = 0.693/\lambda$.

–The **biological half-life (T_b)** is determined by the clearance of the radionuclide from the organ, tissue, or body.

–The **effective half-life (T_e)** of a radionuclide in any organ encompasses both radioactive decay and biological clearance.

–The relation between $T_{1/2}$, T_b, and T_e is as follows:

$$1/T_e = 1/T_b + 1/T_{1/2}$$

–If a radionuclide has a physical half-life of 6 hours and a biological half-life of 3 hours, then $1/T_e = 1/6 + 1/3$, and $T_e = 2$ hours.

–Figure 8-4 illustrates the exponential decay of a radionuclide.

–The effective half-life is always less than either the physical or biological half-life as shown in Figure 8-5.

–If either the biological or physical half-life is much longer than the other, the effective half-life approximates to the shorter of the two.

B. Cumulative activity

–The total number of nuclear transformations in an organ or tissue is called **cumulative activity**.

–Cumulative activity is the area under a curve of activity in an organ or tissue plotted as a function of time.

–The **average life** of a radioactive nucleus is **1.44 × $T_{1/2}$** or $1/\lambda$.

–The cumulative activity of a radionuclide source also equals the product of the average life and the initial radioactivity (see Figure 8-4).

–In the SI system, the number of transformations is expressed in becquerel-seconds (Bq-s) as 1.44 × initial activity in organ (Bq) × $T_{1/2}$ (s).

–In non-SI units, the number of transformations is expressed in microcurie-hours (μCi-hours) and is calculated as 1.44 × initial activity (μCi) in organ × $T_{1/2}$ (hours).

–Values of cumulative activity in organs and tissues of interest in nuclear medicine dosimetry are obtained empirically for each radiopharmaceutical by monitoring the time course of activity.

–Cumulative activity values are often different for normal patients and patients with certain diseases.

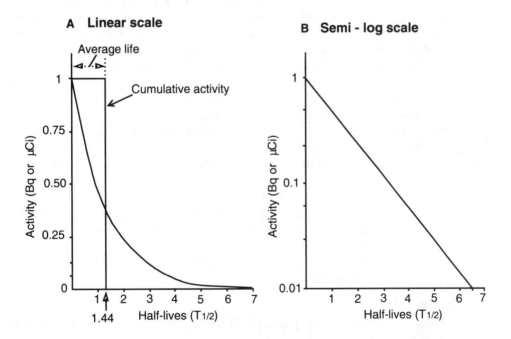

Figure 8-4. A, Physical half-life ($T_{1/2}$) is the decay of radioactive substances. The cumulative activity of a radiopharmaceutical is equal to the area under the curve, which is also the product of the average life (1.44 times the half-life) and the initial activity, as shown by the shaded box. **B,** Radioactive decay is exponential and can be plotted as a straight line on a semi-log scale.

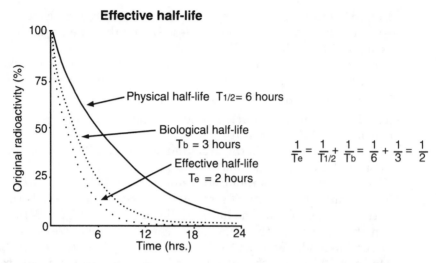

Figure 8-5. The effective half-life (T_e) of a radiopharmaceutical is a function of the biological elimination (T_b) and the physical half-life ($T_{1/2}$).

C. Dosimetry method

–The radiation dose (D) to any organ or tissue is obtained by dividing the total energy absorbed (E) in the organ by the organ mass (M).

–Absorbed dose $D = E/M$ gray (Gy).

–A source organ has an uptake of a radionuclide, which results in a total of A nuclear transformations (cumulative activity).

–The energy absorbed in Ã target organ for each type of radiation per single nuclear transformation in the source organ is obtained from the product of three terms: 1) the average number of radiation emissions per transformation, 2) the average energy associated with each emission, and 3) the fraction of this energy deposited in the organ of interest.

–The total energy deposited in the target organ is then obtained by summing over all the radiations emitted by the nuclide.

–Dividing the absorbed energy by the target organ mass gives the **"S" factor**, which is the absorbed dose in a target organ per unit of cumulative activity in a source organ.

–The S factor is dependent on organ shape, size, and the location of the radioactivity.

–S factor units are rad 1 µCi-hr (Gy 1 Bq-s).

–Calculated S factors for radionuclides used in nuclear medicine for numerous source or target organs and tissues are available in the scientific literature.

–Table 8-4 summarizes the method used to determine organ and tissue doses in nuclear medicine.

D. Patient doses

–For ^{131}I located in the thyroid, the S factor giving the dose to the thyroid is 22 mrad/µCi-hr.

–If 1 µCi remains in the thyroid for 1 hour (i.e., 1 µCi-hr is the number of transformations or cumulative activity), then the resultant thyroid dose is 22 mrad (0.22 mGy).

Table 8-4. Factors Used to Compute Organ Dose*

Term	Equation	Units SI	Non SI	Comments
Absorbed dose	$D = E/M$	Gy	rad	Target organ of mass (M) absorbs energy (E)
Absorbed energy	$E = \tilde{A} \times \Sigma_i\,(n_i \times E_i \times \phi_i)$	J	erg	n_i radiations of energy (E_i) per nuclear transformation of nuclide; ϕ_i is fraction of energy absorbed in target organ; summation (Σ) is over all radiations
Cumulative activity	$\tilde{A} = A_o \times 1.44 \times T_e$	Bq-s	μCi-hour	A_o is the initial activity in source organ with effective half-life of T_e
S factor	$S = \Sigma_i\,(n_i \times E_i \times \phi_i)/M$	Gy/Bq-s	rad/μCi-hour	Obtained from standard tables for each nuclide and selected source and target organs
Absorbed dose	$D = S \times \tilde{A}$	Gy	rad	S factor is dose in target organ per unit cumulative activity (A) in source organ

*Administered radionuclide has an initial activity (A_o) in a source organ and irradiates a selected target organ.

-If 20 mCi of ^{99m}Tc is administered to a patient and uniformly distributed in the body with no biological clearance, the value of cumulated activity is $1.44 \times 20{,}000 \times 6$ μCi-hr.

-The ^{99m}Tc S factor is 2×10^{-3} mGy per μCi-hr, where both the source and target organs are the whole body.

-The patient's whole body dose is thus $1.44 \times 20{,}000$ μCi $\times$ 6 hours $(T_{1/2}) \times (2 \times 10^{-3})$ mrad $\times$ (S factor), which equals 350 mrad (3.5 mGy).

-The maximum organ doses from nuclear medicine procedures are approximately 50 mGy (5 rad).

-Normally, more than one organ or tissue receives a significant radiation dose in nuclear medicine studies.

-The **effective dose equivalent (H_E),** combines all the organ doses with their relative radiosensitivities:

-$H_E = \Sigma_i\, w_i \times H_i$, where H_i is the dose equivalent to organ i, which has a relative radiosensitivity of w_i.

-H_E is the best indicator of patient risk in nuclear medicine.

-The mean H_E value for most examinations is approximately 5 mSv (500 mrem) [Table 8-5].

V. Quality Control

A. Generator quality control

-If the Tc generator is damaged, ^{99}Mo or alumina can break into the saline elute.

-Alumina interferes with the proper formation of ^{99m}Tc radiopharmaceutical kits.

-Color indicator paper is used to test for alumina breakthrough.

Table 8-5. Effective Dose Equivalent (H_E) from Radiopharmaceuticals Used in Nuclear Medicine

Procedure	Radiopharmaceutical	Administered Activity MBq (mCi)	H_E per Procedure mSv (mrem)
Brain	^{99m}Tc Gluconate	750 (20)	7.5 (750)
Bone	^{99m}Tc Pyrophosphate	750 (20)	6 (600)
Liver/spleen	^{99m}Tc Sulphur colloid	200 (5)	2 (200)
Biliary	^{99m}Tc HIDA	200 (5)	4.5 (450)
Cardiac (MUGA)	^{99m}Tc Red blood cells	750 (20)	5.5 (550)
Cardiac	^{99m}Tc Pyrophosphate	600 (15)	3.5 (350)
Cardiac	^{201}Tl Thallus chloride	75 (2)	7 (700)
Lung	^{99m}Tc MAA	150 (4)	2.5 (250)
Renal	^{99m}Tc DTPA	600 (15)	6 (600)
Inflammation	^{67}Ga Gallium citrate	200 (5)	20 (2000)
Thyroid uptake	^{131}I Sodium iodide	0.2 (0.05)	1.2 (120)
Thyroid scan	^{99m}Tc Pertechnetate	200 (5)	2.5 (250)
Thyroid uptake	^{123}I Sodium iodide	7.5 (0.2)	0.55 (55)
Infection	^{111}In leukocytes	2 (0.05)	1.2 (120)

DTPA = diethylenetriaminepentaacetic acid; HIDA = hepato-iminodiacetic acid; MAA = macroaggregated albumin; MUGA = multiple gated acquisition.

- —Molybdenum has a half-life of 67 hours and gamma ray energy levels of 740 and 780 keV.
- —Molybdenum breakthrough results in an unnecessary and high radiation dose to the patient.
  - —A **dose calibrator** is used to determine the content of ^{99}Mo each time the generator is eluted.
- —A lead shield blocks the ^{99m}Tc gamma rays, allowing ^{99}Mo gamma rays to be counted.
- —The legal limit for molybdenum breakthrough is 5.5 kBq (0.15 µCi) of ^{99}Mo per 37 MBq (1.0 mCi) of ^{99m}Tc.

B. Radiopharmaceutical quality control

- —**Radionuclide purity** is the presence of unwanted radionuclides in the sample and is checked using a well counter to search for unwanted energy levels. For example, ^{123}I may contain ^{124}I, and ^{201}Tl may contain ^{202}Tl.
- —**Radiochemical purity** is the chemical purity of the isotope and is checked by thin-layer chromatography. For example, there may be free pertechnetate in ^{99m}Tc labeled DTPA.
  - —**Chromatography** separates compounds that are soluble in saline.
- —For example, free pertechnetate is soluble in saline, but sulfur colloid is not.
- —**Chemical purity** refers to the amount of unwanted chemical contaminants in the agent.
- —**Sterility** means that the radiopharmaceutical is free of any microbial contamination.
- —Even if a preparation is sterile, it may still contain **pyrogens**, which may cause a reaction if administered to a patient.
  - —All sterility and pyrogenicity tests should be performed before the agent is administered to patients.
  - —Although such tests are not feasible with each dose for short-lived radionuclides (e.g., ^{99m}Tc), they should be performed periodically to ensure satisfactory sterility and apyrogenicity.

C. Gamma camera quality control

–The photopeak window of the PHA is checked daily by placing a small amount of a known radioisotope in front of the camera.

–**Field uniformity** is the ability of the gamma camera to reproduce a uniform distribution of activity.

–Differences in the PMT response and transmission of light in the crystal contribute to nonuniformity.

  –Nonuniformities of greater than 10% are unacceptable for clinical imaging.

  –Modern cameras have a uniformity of better than 2% between adjacent areas.

–Field uniformity is checked daily by placing a uniform flood source in front of the camera.

  –**Extrinsic floods** are obtained with the collimator in place.

  –**Intrinsic floods** are performed without the collimator.

  –An **uncorrected flood** is obtained with the computer correction circuitry turned off.

–**Resolution** (i.e., the ability to separate two points) and **linearity** (i.e., the ability to accurately image a straight line) are checked weekly using a bar phantom without a collimator.

D. Dose calibrator quality control

–A **dose calibrator** is an ionization chamber used to measure the activity of a radioisotope dose in MBq (mCi).

–Each dose is measured in a dose calibrator before injection into the patient.

–**Constancy** (i.e., precision) is checked daily by measuring two standardized long half-life sources (e.g., ^{57}Co, ^{137}Cs).

–Day to day measurements should vary by less than 5%.

–**Accuracy** is checked at installation and annually using calibrated sources.

–**Linearity** is checked quarterly by measuring the decay of ^{99m}Tc over 72 hours or more, or by using calibrated shields.

VI. Nuclear Medicine Tomography

A. Single photon emission computed tomography

–Single photon emission computed tomography (SPECT) provides computed tomographic views of the three-dimensional distribution of radioisotopes in the body.

–Parallel hole collimators are commonly used for SPECT imaging.

  –Hybrid converging and parallel hole collimators offer superior resolution and sensitivity performance and are sometimes used for brain SPECT.

–In SPECT, the gamma camera rotates 180 degrees or 360 degrees around the patient, acquiring data that allow tomographic images to be generated. Typically, 64 or 128 projections are taken.

  –Scan profiles from these projections are used as inputs for filtered-back projection reconstruction algorithms to compute tomographic images.

  –Transverse, sagittal, and coronal views can be generated.

—Problems in SPECT relate to obtaining quantitative information and long acquisition times.

—To obtain quantitative information, corrections need to be made for scatter and attenuation.

B. SPECT performance

—**Multiheaded cameras** are used to increase system sensitivity and reduce scan times.

—The use of **elliptical orbits** (i.e., body contouring) for gamma camera travel around the patient allows the distance to the patient to be minimized, thus improving sensitivity and resolution.

—The resolution associated with SPECT is generally poorer than for planar imaging because of the need to use high-sensitivity collimators to obtain an adequate number of counts in each projection image.

—The major benefit of SPECT is the improved contrast that results from the elimination of overlapping structures.

—SPECT studies are susceptible to image artifacts caused by nonuniformities and by axis of rotation misalignment.

—Common clinical applications of SPECT include thallium studies for myocardial ischemia or infarctions and cerebral blood flow.

C. Positron emission tomography physics

—**Positron emission tomography (PET)** makes use of short-lived positron emitters such as ^{11}C ($T_{1/2}$ = 20 minutes), ^{13}N ($T_{1/2}$ = 10 minutes), ^{15}O ($T_{1/2}$ = 2 minutes), ^{18}F ($T_{1/2}$ = 110 minutes).

—Most short-lived radioisotopes require a cyclotron for production, although rubidium (^{82}Rb, $T_{1/2}$ = 75 s) can be obtained from a generator.

—^{18}F in the form of fluorodeoxyglucose is the most commonly used agent.

—PET is based on the simultaneous detection of the two 511-keV annihilation photons produced when a positron loses its kinetic energy and combines with an electron (Figure 8-6).

—**Annihilation coincident detection** or simultaneous detection using coincident circuitry allows extrapolation to locate the emission site.

—Collimators are used to define planes and limit the number of coincidence counts, but are not needed for localization of photons.

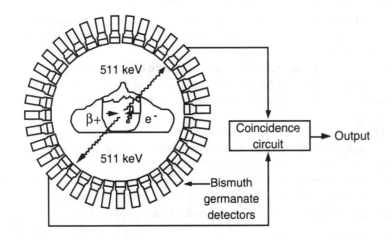

Figure 8-6. Positron emission tomography.

–**Bismuth germanate** detectors are usually used.

–The spatial resolution of commercial PET systems (FWHM) can approach 5 mm.

–Images are generated using filtered-back projection algorithms.

D. PET imaging

–A wide range of radiopharmaceuticals may be used for PET imaging, including fluorodeoxyglucose (^{18}F), used to study metabolism, and ammonia (^{13}N), used to study perfusion.

–PET studies may produce absolute quantitative information on processes such as perfusion and metabolism.

–Because a collimator is not required, PET images normally have a large number of counts (and low noise).

–Serial studies may be performed because of the short half-life of PET radionuclides.

–The major limitation of PET is the large cost of building a PET imaging center with an on-site cyclotron and radiopharmaceutical production facilities.

–Most facilities use PET as a research tool, and the clinical role of PET imaging remains uncertain.

Review Test

1. Match the origination of the radionuclide with the most appropriate decay mode.

(A) Bombarding with neutrons in a reactor
(B) Bombarding with protons in a cyclotron
(C) Mining pitchblende

(i) Alpha emission
(ii) Beta minus emission
(iii) Beta plus emission

2. True (T) or False (F). Radioactive equilibrium

(A) is secular when the half-life of the parent >> half-life of the daughter
(B) requires about 6 half-lives for secular equilibrium to be established
(C) is transient if the half-life of the parent is > half-life of the daughter
(D) for a ^{99}Mo/^{99m}Tc generator may be termed transient
(E) is established in 24 hours for a ^{99}Mo/^{99m}Tc generator

3. For ^{99m}Tc decaying to ^{99}Tc, all of the following are true EXCEPT

(A) the half-life of ^{99m}Tc is 67 hours
(B) the half-life of ^{99}Tc is 2.1×10^5 years
(C) activity is $N \times \lambda$ (N = number of atoms; λ is decay constant)
(D) $\lambda = 0.693/T_{1/2}$ where $T_{1/2}$ is the half-life

4. If 100 mCi ^{99m}Tc is "milked" from a ^{99}Mo generator (at equilibrium) at 9 A.M. on Monday, then

(A) the activity of ^{99}Mo is 50 mCi at 3 P.M. on Monday
(B) 80 mCi ^{99m}Tc can be "milked" at 9 A.M. on Tuesday
(C) 50 mCi ^{99m}Tc can be "milked" at 9 A.M. on Sunday
(D) the generator can no longer be used for ^{99m}Tc production

5. The "ideal" radiopharmaceutical for imaging an organ in nuclear medicine studies would have

(A) a short half-life
(B) no particulate emissions
(C) rapid clearance from the blood stream
(D) photons with an energy of about 150 keV
(E) all of the above

6. The radiation level adjacent to the one-week-old ^{99}Mo/^{99m}Tc generator depends on all of the following EXCEPT the

(A) initial activity of ^{99}Mo
(B) number of times the generator was milked
(C) amount of Pb shielding around the generator
(D) amount of ^{99}Mo remaining
(E) distance from the generator

7. Technetium-99m generators CANNOT be

(A) produced in a cyclotron
(B) used to dispense more than 1 Ci
(C) shipped by air
(D) purchased by licensed users
(E) used for more than 67 hours

8. Match the following half-lives with the appropriate radionuclide.

(A) 2 minutes
(B) 110 minutes
(C) 13 hours
(D) 67 hours
(E) 8 days

(i) Fluorine-18
(ii) Molybdenum-99
(iii) Iodine-123
(iv) Iodine-131
(v) Oxygen-15

9. Gamma camera crystals

(A) are made of cesium iodide
(B) convert ~95% of gamma ray energy to light photons
(C) are generally 100 μm thick for good resolution
(D) have lead backing to minimize backscatter
(E) have a high probability of absorbing 140 keV photons

10. The pulse height analyzer in a gamma camera system

(A) increases the detector efficiency
(B) analyzes the total energy deposited in crystal
(C) corrects the count rate losses due to "dead time"
(D) performs a coincidence detection analysis
(E) increases the count rate

11. Match the typical resolution at full width half maximum (FWHM) with the detection system.

(A) Gamma camera (intrinsic)
(B) Gamma camera (low-energy all-purpose collimator)
(C) Gamma camera (high-resolution collimator)
(D) PET

(i)   3 mm
(ii)   5 mm
(iii) 7.5 mm
(iv)   10 mm

12. For each clinical application, match the best collimator.

(A) Thyroid imaging
(B) Pediatric study
(C) Lung scan
(D) Liver scan

(i)   Diverging
(ii)   Parallel hole
(iii) Converging
(iv)   Pinhole

13. For parallel hole collimators, which of the following improves as the distance from the face of the collimator is increased?

(A) Resolution
(B) Sensitivity
(C) Energy resolution
(D) Imaging time
(E) None of the above

14. Nuclear medicine images acquired using a computer typically have

(A) 500,000 to 1,000,000 counts
(B) matrix sizes of 64×64 or 128×128
(C) 256 gray scale levels
(D) 4 to 16 kBytes of image data
(E) all of the above

15. In general, gamma camera system resolution with a parallel-hole collimator

(A) is determined at full width half maximum (FWHM)
(B) includes an intrinsic resolution of about 3 mm
(C) depends on collimator sensitivity
(D) deteriorates with distance from the collimator
(E) all of the above

16. The system resolution of a gamma camera with a parallel hole collimator improves with increased collimator

(A) hole size
(B) thickness
(C) diameter
(D) distance to patient
(E) sensitivity

17. Thyroid imaging studies can be performed with all of the following EXCEPT

(A) ^{99m}Tc pertechnetate
(B) NaI uptake probe
(C) ^{123}I
(D) parallel hole collimator
(E) pinhole collimator

18. A circular cold spot artifact in a gamma camera image could NOT be the result of

(A) a cracked NaI crystal
(B) a metallic object on the patient
(C) a defective photomultiplier tube
(D) an incorrect photopeak energy setting of the PHA

19. Match the following half-life relationships.

(A) T_b is very long
(B) T_b is very short
(C) T_b and $T_{1/2}$ are equal
(D) T_b and $T_{1/2}$ are both very long

(i)   Negligible loss of activity
(ii) $T_e = T_b$
(iii) $T_e = T_b/2$
(iv) $T_e = T_{1/2}$

20. When ^{99m}Tc is administered to a patient, which of the following CANNOT contribute to the patient dose?

(A) Auger electrons
(B) Beta particles
(C) Internal conversion electrons
(D) Gamma rays
(E) Characteristic x-rays

21. Which of the following statements regarding radioiodine and the fetal thyroid are true?

(A) Inorganic iodine crosses the placenta
(B) Iodine can concentrate in fetal thyroids
(C) The highest risk is in the second and third trimesters
(D) Fetal thyroid is not present before week 10 of pregnancy
(E) All of the above

22. True (T) or False (F). For patients undergoing typical nuclear medicine procedures

(A) effective dose equivalents are about 5 mSv (500 mrem)
(B) the dose is lower than a chest x-ray examination
(C) maximum organ doses are about 50 mGy (5 rad)
(D) the effective dose equivalents are similar to PET studies
(E) increasing the NM imaging time increases the dose

23. An ideal therapeutic radionuclide (e.g., ^{32}P) would have

(A) high uptake in the organ of interest
(B) high-energy beta decay
(C) no high-energy gamma rays
(D) a long biologic half-life in the organ of interest
(E) all of the above

24. Match the following image characteristics with the appropriate equipment.

(A) Edge packing
(B) Linearity
(C) Uniformity
(D) Distortion

(i) Damaged collimator
(ii) Flood source
(iii) Line bar phantom
(iv) Periphery of gamma camera

25. Low-level radioactive wastes, such as tubing and swabs contaminated with ^{99m}Tc, may be monitored with

(A) Geiger-Müller counters
(B) film badge dosimeters
(C) thermoluminescent dosimeters
(D) ionization chambers
(E) do *not* need to be monitored

26. Match the radionuclide impurity with the corresponding radioactive material.

(A) ^{123}I capsules
(B) ^{99m}Tc pertechnetate
(C) ^{67}Ga
(D) ^{201}Tl

(i) ^{99}Mo
(ii) ^{124}I
(iii) ^{202}Tl
(iv) None

27. True (T) or False (F). Single photon emission computed tomography (SPECT) normally requires

(A) positron emitting radioisotopes
(B) gamma camera rotation
(C) coincidence detection
(D) pulse height analysis
(E) filtered back projection reconstruction algorithms
(F) sampling of activity in patient's blood

28. For SPECT, all the following are true EXCEPT

(A) 64 or 128 projections are obtained
(B) it takes about 20 minutes to perform
(C) corrections are usually made for patient motion
(D) images show relative radioisotope concentrations
(E) image quality is affected by scatter

29. Advantages of PET over conventional gamma camera imaging include

(A) a wider choice of molecules that may be labeled with positron emitters
(B) better resolution
(C) lower image noise
(D) rapid decay of radiopharmaceutical
(E) all of the above

30. PET imaging systems

(A) need high-energy parallel hole collimators
(B) cannot handle very high count rates
(C) suffer from significant attenuation losses
(D) detect annihilation photons in coincidence

Answers and Explanations

1. A–ii; adding neutrons to nuclei results in excess neutrons which leads to beta minus decay; **B–iii;** adding protons to nuclei requires them to lose their excess positive charge by positron emission or electron capture; **C–i;** ^{226}Ra is an alpha emitter which decays to form radon (^{222}Rn).

2. A–True; B–True; C–True; D–True; E–True.

3–A. The half-life of ^{99m}Tc is 6 hours. The parent of ^{99m}Tc, ^{99}Mo has a half-life of 67 hours.

4–B. It takes about 24 hours for transient equilibrium to be established between the ^{99}Mo/^{99m}Tc. The activity of ^{99}Mo will be 80 mCi since it decays with a half-life of 67 hours.

5–E. An ideal radiopharmaceutical would have all of these properties.

6–B. Elutions only affect the amount of ^{99m}Tc in the generator and since the ^{99m}Tc photon energy (140 keV) is very low, this will not contribute significantly to the measured radiation level *outside* the shielded generator.

7–A. ^{99}Mo may be produced in a reactor or from fission products, but cannot be produced in a cyclotron since ^{99}Mo is a beta emitter, requiring the addition of neutrons, not protons.

8. A–v; B–i; C–iii; D–ii; E–iv.

9–E. A typical NaI crystal thickness of 10 mm absorbs over 90% of the 140 keV photons via the photoelectric effect.

10–B. The pulse height analyzer measures the total energy deposited in the photon interaction and "accepts" only photopeak interactions that correspond to a photoelectric interaction with the full photon energy.

11. A–i; B–iv; C–iii; D–ii.

12. A–iv; thyroid studies are normally performed using pinhole collimators to improve resolution; **B–iii;** converging collimator is used in pediatric studies to magnify the image; **C–i;** diverging collimators minify the image and permit both lungs to be visualized in a single image; **D–ii;** liver scans are normally performed with an all-purpose or high-resolution parallel hole collimator.

13–E. None of these factors improve. In clinical practice, it is important to minimize the patient–collimator distance.

14–E. All of the statements are true.

15–E. All of the statements are true.

16–B. Increasing collimator thickness improves resolution but reduces sensitivity.

17–B. An uptake probe measures the total amount of activity in the thyroid but does not generate any kind of image.

18–A. A cracked NaI crystal would give rise to a linear artifact, not a circular one.

19. A–iv; B–ii; C–iii; D–i. All of these follow from the definition of effective half-life $1/T_e = 1/T_{1/2} + 1/T_b$.

20–B. There are no beta particles associated with ^{99m}Tc.

21–E. All of the statements are true.

22. A–True; B–False; typical H_E for a PA chest x-ray is 20 µSv (2 mrem); **C–True; D–True;** although positron emitters are much shorter lived, they deposit much more energy per decay, and these two factors cancel each other out; **E–False;** patient dose is determined by the amount of activity administered, and "imaging" time is irrelevant to patient dose.

23–E. All these characteristics are desirable in a *therapeutic* radionuclide because they maximize the organ dose and minimize external radiation hazards from gamma rays.

24. A–iv; edge packing is observed at the edge of nuclear medicine images; **B–iii;** line bar phantoms are used to ensure that the image is as straight as the object; **C–ii;** gamma camera uniformity is assessed using flood sources; **D–i;** distortion may result from a damaged collimator.

25–A. Geiger-Müller counters are generally used to monitor low-level waste because of their high sensitivity, portability, and immediate responses.

26. A–ii; B–i; ^{99}Mo may be eluted from the column; **C–iv;** ^{67}Ga is produced in a cyclotron from ^{67}Zn and has no radiochemical impurities; **D–iii.**

27. A–False; positron emitters are required for PET imaging; **B–True;** projections are normally obtained through 360 degrees around the patient; **C–False;** annihilation radiation in *PET* is obtained using coincidence detection; **D–True;** this is required to minimize the amount of scatter accepted; **E–True;** filtered back projection algorithms are used in SPECT; **F–False;** this is occasionally done in PET to obtain absolute quantitative physiological data.

28–C. Patient motion correction is not normally performed for SPECT imaging. Digital subtraction angiography imaging software sometime permits corrections to be made for patient motion.

29–E. All of the statements are generally true in PET imaging.

30–D. Two 511 keV photons are emitted 180 degrees apart, which are detected by a coincidence circuit.

9

Radiation Protection

I. Biological Basis

A. Introduction

- –Ionizing radiation can induce detrimental biological effects in organs and tissues by producing ions and depositing energy that may damage important molecules such as **DNA**.
  - –**Free radicals** are chemically reactive molecules with unpaired electrons that are produced by ionizing radiation and can damage tissue.
  - –Chromosome breaks and aberrations are examples of biological damage caused by radiation.
- –The amount of biological damage produced depends on the total energy deposited (dose) and on the type of radiation.
  - –Alpha particles are generally more effective at producing biological damage than beta particles, x-rays, or gamma rays for the *same* amount of energy (dose) deposited in the tissue.
- –The radiobiological **LD$_{50/60}$** is the lethal dose that will kill 50% of the population in 60 days.
  - –The estimated LD$_{50/60}$ from a single dose ranges from 3 to 5 Gy (300 to 500 rad).
- –Data on the detrimental effects of radiation come from studies on atomic bomb survivors, radiation workers, and radiation therapy patients.

B. Cells and radiation effects

- –Metabolic functions of cells occur in the cytoplasm.
- –Genetic information is found in the cell nucleus.
- –Human cells are either **germ cells,** which are involved in reproduction, or **somatic cells**.
- –Cell division of reproductive cells is called **meiosis**.
- –**Mitosis** is the process of cell division in somatic cells.
  - –The stages of somatic cell division include **prophase, metaphase,** which is the most radiosensitive phase, **anaphase, telophase,** and **interphase,** which is the resting stage.
- –The **DNA** molecule carries the code needed for cell metabolism and is exactly duplicated when the cell divides.

–**Genes,** which are the units of heredity, are small segments of the DNA molecule that determine cell characteristics.

–Radiation may induce a break in the DNA molecule, or it may damage a section of the DNA molecule, which could result in genetic or somatic damage.

–A change in the genetic code (mutation) of a germ cell can affect future generations.

–At high doses, radiation can cause **cell death,** defined as the loss of reproductive capacity.

–Lymphoid tissue and rapidly proliferating tissues, such as spermatids and bone marrow stem cells, are relatively radiosensitive.

–Cells with higher oxygen content are generally more sensitive to radiation.

–Nerve cells are the least radiosensitive cells.

–Radiation can cause damage to cells directly or, more commonly, indirectly by producing ions.

C. Deterministic effects

–At high doses [i.e., doses > 0.5 Gy (50 rad)], radiation effects are called **deterministic** (or nonstochastic) and generally result from cell death.

–Deterministic effects are characterized by a **threshold dose,** below which the effect does not occur (Figure 9-1).

–Deterministic effects include skin erythema (reddening), cataract induction, epilation (hair loss), and induction of sterility.

–The prodromal symptoms of acute radiation syndrome (anorexia, nausea, vomiting, and diarrhea) begin at 1 to 2 Gy (100 to 200 rad).

–Table 9-1 lists approximate threshold doses for deterministic effects in man.

–Cataract formation is dependent on the total dose and on the time over which this dose is delivered.

–Cataracts may be induced at acute doses as low as 2 Gy (200 rad) and as soon as 6 months after exposure.

–Radiation-induced cataracts occur in the posterior part of the lens.

–Sperm count can be decreased with 0.15 to 0.3 Gy (15 to 30 rad), but sterility requires 3 to 4 Gy (300 to 400 rad) in women and 5 to 6 Gy (500 to 600 rad) in men.

–Lymphocytes are the most radiosensitive cells in the blood and decreased cell counts have been observed after doses of less than 1 Gy (100 rad).

–One important goal of radiation protection is to *prevent* the occurrence of deterministic effects.

D. Stochastic effects

–At low doses [i.e., doses < 0.5 Gy (50 rad)], the **stochastic effects** of **carcinogenesis** and **genetic damage** are of primary importance.

–**Stochastic** means random or probabilistic.

–The severity of radiation-induced stochastic effects is *independent* of the radiation dose.

–The radiation dose only affects the *probability* of the stochastic effect occurring (as dose increases, the chance of the effect occurring increases).

–The existence of any threshold doses for stochastic effects is unknown and controversial.

A

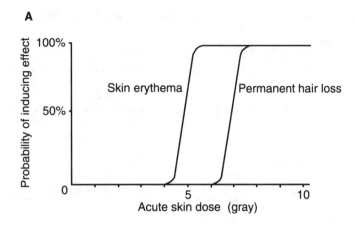

B

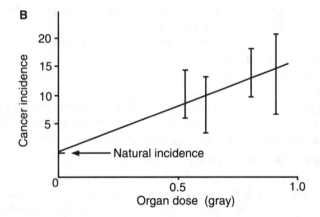

Figure 9-1. Representative dose response curves for stochastic and deterministic effects.

–For radiation protection purposes, stochastic effects are assumed to have **no threshold** (see Figure 9-1).

–Stochastic risks are dependent on sex and age at exposure.

–Radiation protection is designed to *minimize* the radiation dose and, therefore, the corresponding stochastic radiation risk.

II. Radiation Risks

A. Radiation-induced cancers

–Effects on the exposed individual, such as cancer induction, are called **somatic effects**.

–**Cancer induction** is the largest risk of radiation exposure at doses normally encountered in radiology.

–Bone marrow, gastrointestinal tract mucosa, breast tissue, gonads, and lymphatic tissue are the most susceptible to radiation-induced malignancy.

–Cancer risks from radiation exposure are generally higher for children than for adults.

–Radiation may induce both benign and malignant tumors.

Table 9-1. Approximate Threshold Doses for Deterministic Radiation Effects in Man (Acute Exposure)

Target organ	Dose Gy (rad)	Results
Whole body	50 to 100 (5000 to 10,000)	Death from cerebral edema (1 to 2 days)
Whole body	7 to 50 (700 to 5000)	Death from gastrointestinal failure (3 to 4 days)
Whole body	2 to 7 (200 to 700)	Death from infection due to hematopoietic failure (4 to 6 weeks)
Skin	7 (700)	Permanent alopecia (temporary alopecia at doses in excess of about 3 Gy, or 300 rad)
Skin	5 (500)	Erythema
Sperm cells	5 to 6 (500 to 600)	Permanent azospermia
Eye lens	2 (200)	Cataract induction

–Cancer induction has a latency of only a few years for leukemia, but is considerably longer for solid tumors.

–Radiation therapy once used to treat acne and tonsilitis has been linked to brain tumors and thyroid cancer.

–Radiation-induced thyroid cancer is more likely in children and women than in men.

–Evidence of the carcinogenic effects of radiation exposure has been observed in follow-up studies of ankylosing spondylitis patients, radium dial painters, uranium miners, and atomic bomb survivors.

B. **Cancer risk estimates**

–In *International Commission on Radiological Protection (ICRP) Publication 26 (1977)*, the fatal cancer radiation risk was estimated to be 1.25% per sievert (Sv) [125 per 10^6 per rem] for whole-body exposure.

–Recent revisions of radiation risk by the United States National Academy of Sciences Committee on the Biological Effects of Ionizing Radiation (BEIR), United Nations Scientific Committee on the Effects of Atomic Radiation (UNSCEAR), and ICRP increase the radiation-induced fatal cancer risk by a factor of between 2 and 3 [**4% per sievert** (100 rem) depending on the exposed population].

–This increase is primarily because of the adoption of a **relative risk model** for cancer induction in which radiation increases the natural incidence of cancer by a constant fraction.

–Previously, an **absolute risk model** was used in which radiation induced a given (absolute) number of cancers in the exposed population.

–The *BEIR V* report published in 1990 introduced a **linear response** paradigm, application of a **relative risk model**, and **new estimates of radiation doses** received by atomic bomb survivors.

C. **Genetic risks**

–Before 1950, **genetic effects** were considered the most important risk of radiation exposure.

–Genetic effects (i.e., effects on future generations because of chromosome mutations) are the result of radiation exposure to the gonads.

–There is virtually no epidemiological evidence of the genetic effects of radiation in humans, and current risk estimates are based on animal experiments.

–Genetic effects depend on the demographics of the exposed populations, with older populations having lower risks than younger populations for the same exposure.

–For a working population, the genetic risk (i.e., serious genetic effects in the next two generations) was estimated to be 0.4% per sievert (i.e., 40 per 10^6 per rem) gonadal radiation according to *ICRP Publication 26*.

–The **genetically significant dose (GSD)** from diagnostic x-rays is an index of potential genetic damage to a population based on gonadal exposure and chances of reproduction.

  –The GSD is the dose that, if delivered to an entire population, would produce the same effect as that produced by gonadal doses to individuals.

D. Fetal risks

–The **fetal risk** when exposing pregnant women depends on the gestation period.

–The most likely result of a major radiation exposure during the first 10 days postconception is early intrauterine death.

–The fetus is most vulnerable to radiation-induced congenital abnormalities during the first trimester, specifically, 20 to 40 days after conception.

  –Radiation-induced microcephaly is the most likely abnormality, occurring at 50 to 70 days postconception and growth and mental retardation occurring at 70 to 150 days postconception.

  –The greatest effect after 150 days postconception is an increased risk of childhood malignancies.

–The risk of congenital abnormalities is negligible when exposure is below approximately 10 mGy (1 rad) and is considered small when exposure is up to 0.1 Gy (10 rad) when compared with the normal risks of pregnancy.

  –In the United States, a congenital abnormality occurs in approximately 5% of live births, which makes the impact of medical x-rays difficult to evaluate.

–At doses greater than 0.1 Gy (10 rad), the risk of congenital malformation increases.

  –An abortion to avoid the possibility of radiation-induced congenital anomalies is considered only when doses exceed 0.1 Gy (10 rad).

–For a dose of 10 mGy (1 rad) in the second or third trimester of gestation, the risk of childhood leukemia may be increased by as much as 40%.

III. Radiation Protection

A. Organizations

–The **ICRP** was founded in 1928 and issues periodic recommendations on radiation protection.

  –*ICRP Publication 26 (1977)* is the basis of most current regulations in the United States and other countries.

  –*ICRP Publication 60 (1990)* defines updated recommendations, but is not expected to become law for more than a decade.

–The **UNSCEAR** also issues reports on radiation risks.

–The **International Commission on Radiological Units and Measurements (ICRU)** advises on issues such as measurement units in radiology.

–The **BEIR committee** periodically reviews the risks from radiation.

–In 1990, the BEIR committee issued *BEIR V* report, which contains updated radiation risk estimates.

–In the United States, the foremost radiation protection body is the **National Committee on Radiological Protection and Measurements (NCRP),** which advises federal and state regulators on radiation protection.

–The **Nuclear Regulatory Commission (NRC)** is responsible for the rules and regulations regarding nuclear materials.

–Specific rules and regulations are compiled in Parts 19 and 20 in Chapter 10 of the *Code of Federal Regulation (CFR)*.

–Approximately 30 states are known as **agreement states** and arrange with the NRC to self-regulate medically related licensing and inspection requirements for nuclear materials. The remaining 20 states are regulated directly by the NRC.

–Each state is responsible for regulations pertaining to x-ray imaging equipment.

B. Occupational exposure

–Dose limits can refer to individual organs or to uniform whole-body irradiation.

–Individual organ dose limits include doses to the eye lens, extremities, and other tissues.

–**Controlled areas** have significant dose equivalent exposure rates [up to 1 mSv (100 mrem) per week] and must be supervised by a **radiation safety officer**.

–Table 9-2 summarizes recommended dose limits for occupational exposure as outlined in *NCRP Publication 91 (1987)* and *ICRP Publication 60 (1990)*.

–**Occupational dose limits** exclude exposures from medical procedures and natural background.

–People who may receive more than 25% of the expected dose limits of a radiation worker should be monitored.

–The actual exposures to radiology department staff is relatively low.

–The typical annual effective dose equivalent exposures are approximately 0.2 mSv (20 mrem) for x-ray technologists, 1.5 mSv (150 mrem) for radiation therapy technologists, and 2 mSv (200 mrem) for nuclear medicine technologists.

C. Pregnant workers

–For radiation protection purposes, the fetus is normally considered to be a member of the public.

–Pregnant radiation workers are monitored by a dosimeter worn on the abdomen under the lead apron to ensure fetal dose limits are not exceeded.

–A measured dose of 2 mSv to the surface of the abdomen is normally considered equivalent to 1 mSv to the fetus.

Table 9-2. Recommended Occupational Dose Limits

Dose Limit	NCRP 91 (1987)	ICRP 60 (1990)
Whole body	50 mSv/y (5 rem/y)	20 mSv/y (2 rem/y)
Lens of the eye	150 mSv/y (15 rem/y)	150 mSv/y (15 rem/y)
Other organs (e.g., hands, skin)	500 mSv/y (50 rem/y)	500 mSv/y (50 rem/y)
Lifetime whole body	$10 \times (N–18)$ mSv (N–18 rem)	< 0.8 Sv (40 years) [< 80 rem]
Fetus (monthly)	0.5 mSv (50 mrem)	N/A
Fetus (9 months)	5 mSv (500 mrem)	1 mSv (100 mrem)

N = age in years of exposed radiation worker.

–Table 9-2 lists recommended dose limits to the fetus for pregnant radiation workers.

D. Nonoccupational exposure

–Dose limits for members of the **public** are generally a factor of 10 lower than those for occupational exposure.

–*NCRP Publication 91* (1987) recommends a dose limit for whole-body exposure of 5 mSv/year (500 mrem/year) and for individual organs, 50 mSv/year (5 rem/year).

–*ICRP Publication 60* (1990) recommends reducing the whole-body dose limit for members of the public from 5 mSv/year (500 mrem/year) to 1 mSv/year (100 mrem/year).

–Radiation facilities should be designed so no one receives a radiation exposure in excess of these annual dose limits.

–In practice, the conservative nature of most shielding calculations ensures that actual doses to members of the public from medical x-ray facilities are low.

IV. Patient Doses

A. Patient skin doses

–The radiation dose received by a patient is frequently specified in terms of the **entrance skin exposure** or **entrance skin dose**.

–The entrance skin dose for a typical chest radiograph is 0.1 to 0.2 mGy (10 to 20 mrad); for an anteroposterior (AP) skull radiograph, 1.5 mGy (150 mrad); for an abdominal radiograph, 3 Gy (300 mrad); and for a lateral lumbar spine radiograph, 10 mGy (1 rad) with a 400-speed system.

–A useful rule of thumb is that a technique of 100 kVp and 100 mAs produces an exposure of approximately 1 R at a distance of 1 m.

–Skin doses are generally easy to measure or calculate, but they are poor indicators of patient risk.

–For a given entrance skin dose, it is possible to estimate individual organ doses for many common radiologic examinations from published data of the ratios of skin to organ doses.

–Entrance skin doses are generally lower than the deterministic threshold doses for epilation (approximately 3 Gy, or 300 rad) and skin erythema (approximately 5 Gy, or 500 rad).

–Interventional neurological and cardiac procedures requiring long fluoroscopy times (hours) and large numbers of film may induce deterministic effects such as epilation.

B. Integral dose and dose-area product parameters

–The **integral dose** measures the total amount of energy in millijoules (mJ) imparted to a patient and may be considered a crude estimate of patient risk.

    –Approximately 1 mJ of energy is imparted for a chest x-ray, and approximately 100 mJ of energy is imparted for a head CT examination.

–Another measure of patient exposure is the **dose-area product (DAP),** which is the product of the entrance skin dose and cross-sectional area of the x-ray beam (exposed area).

    –For example, the entrance skin dose for chest x-rays is approximately 0.1 mGy (10 mrad) and the x-ray beam area is approximately 1000 cm^2, resulting in a dose-area product of approximately 100 mGy-cm^2 (10,000 mrad-cm^2).

–Integral dose and DAP are a useful means of providing relative risks to patients undergoing *similar* types of radiographic examination.

C. Effective dose and effective dose equivalent parameters

–Most medical radiologic exposures result in a nonuniform dose distribution within the patient.

    –For example, the entrance skin dose for an AP abdominal radiograph may be approximately 3 mGy (300 mrad), the exit skin dose approximately 0.03 mGy (3 mrad), and the scattered dose at the thyroid less than 0.003 mGy (0.3 mrad).

–The **effective dose equivalent (H_E)** and **effective dose (E)** add the doses of *all* exposed organs to give an estimate of the total risk to a patient exposed during a radiographic procedure.

–H_E is a weighted sum of the doses to all the exposed organs and tissues in the body: $H_E = \Sigma_i\, w_i \times H_i$, where H_i is the dose equivalent to organ i that has a weighting factor of w_i.

–H_E is the uniform whole-body dose, resulting in the same risk as the nonuniform dose.

–E is conceptually similar to H_E but uses improved organ-weighting factors.

–Figure 9-2 shows the range of dose parameters that may be used to specify the radiation received by the patient.

D. Patient doses

–H_E is probably the best indicator of the radiation risk to a patient from a diagnostic radiologic procedure.

–Table 9-3 summarizes representative H_E values in radiology.

–There are likely to be large variations for any individual depending on the technique, factors used, total number of films taken, fluoroscopy time, and so on.

–H_E may be compared directly with regulatory dose limits and natural background levels, which are normally given in terms of H_E.

–E values are similar to H_E values for most diagnostic procedures.

E. Patient protection

–Patient doses should be minimized whenever possible and the **ALARA** (as low as reasonably achievable) principle should always be followed.

Chest radiograph

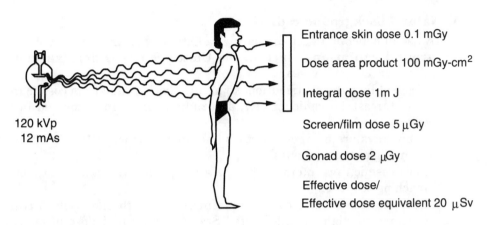

Entrance skin dose 0.1 mGy

Dose area product 100 mGy-cm^2

Integral dose 1m J

Screen/film dose 5 μGy

Gonad dose 2 μGy

Effective dose/
Effective dose equivalent 20 μSv

120 kVp
12 mAs

Figure 9-2. Measures of radiation received by a patient undergoing a PA chest examination.

—Careful attention to close collimation reduces the exposed area, thus minimizing patient risk.
—Gonadal shielding should be used if the patient is of reproductive age, if the gonads lie in or near the primary beam, and if the shield does not interfere with the examination.
  —For example, a gonadal shield can usually be used for a unilateral hip examination.
—**Patient exposure** is proportional to mAs and kVp squared, and is inversely related to the square of the distance from the focal spot.
—A short focus-to-skin distance increases the patient entrance skin dose.
  —This distance should always be greater than 38 cm in fluoroscopy.
—Correct phototiming of exposures prevents overexposure of films and eliminates the need to perform repeated films.
—Rare earth intensifying screens reduce the required exposures significantly and should always be used.

Table 9-3. Typical Effective Dose Equivalent (H_E) Values in Radiology

Procedure	H_E mSv (mrem)
PA chest x-ray	0.01–0.05 (1–5)
Skull x-ray	0.1–0.2 (10–20)
Abdominal x-ray	0.6–1.7 (60–170)
Barium exam	3–8 (300–800)
Head CT	2–4 (200–400)
Body CT	5–15 (500–1500)
Nuclear medicine	2–10 (200–1000)

V. Population Doses

A. Natural background radiation

–A useful benchmark for comparing radiation exposure is **natural background radiation,** which in the United States is approximately 3 mSv/year (300 mrem/year).

–Table 9-4 lists the contributions to natural background from cosmic radiation, terrestrial radioactivity, and radionuclides incorporated in the body.

–Cosmic rays are energetic protons and alpha particles (10^{10} to 10^{19} eV), which originate in galaxies.

 –Most cosmic rays interact with the atmosphere, with fewer than 0.05% reaching sea level.

 –Because exposure to cosmic rays increases with elevation, a transcontinental flight in the United States results in a dose of approximately 20 µSv (2 mrem), a transatlantic flight results in 30 to 50 µSv (3 to 5 mrem), and space travel results in approximately 10 µSv/hour (1 mrem/hour).

–Natural background radiation varies with location, and values greater than the average listed in Table 9-4 are possible.

 –In Leadville, Colorado, for example, an additional 0.9 mSv (90 mrem) per year of radiation are attributed to the higher cosmic background at an elevation of 3000 m.

 –Leadville also has elevated levels of terrestrial radioactivity on the Colorado plateau, which results in an additional dose of approximately 0.7 mSv (70 mrem) per year.

B. Radon

–The biggest contribution to natural background is from domestic **radon.**

–Radon (^{222}Rn) is a radioactive gas formed during the decay of radium.

–Radium (^{226}Ra) is a decay product of uranium found in the soil and has a half-life of 1620 years.

–Radon is an alpha emitter, which has a half-life of approximately 4 days.

–The progeny of radon are also radioactive and include two short-lived beta emitters and two short-lived alpha emitters.

–Radon daughters attach to aerosols and are deposited in the lungs, thereby permitting the bronchial mucosa to be irradiated and inducing **bronchogenic cancer.**

Table 9-4. Typical Annual Radiation Exposure in the United States

Source	mSv/y (mrem/y)
Radon	2 (200)
Cosmic rays	0.3 (30)
External (gamma rays)	0.3 (30)
Internal (e.g., ^{40}K, ^{14}C)	0.4 (40)
Man-made products	0.1 (10)
X-ray and nuclear medicine studies	0.5 (50)
Total	3.6 (360)

—The average concentration of radon outdoors is 4 to 8 Bq/m^3 (0.1 to 0.2 pCi/L); indoors, the average is 40 Bq/m^3 (1 pCi/L).

—Remedial action is recommended at levels in excess of 160 Bq/m^3 (4 pCi/L).

C. Population medical doses

—Approximately 300 million diagnostic medical procedures (x-ray, nuclear medicine, and dental) are performed in the United States each year.

—The effective dose equivalent (H_E) from the x-ray and nuclear medicine studies averaged over the population (*per caput* dose) are approximately 0.4 mSv (40 mrem) and 0.14 mSv (14 mrem) per year, respectively.

—Countries such as Japan and Russia have higher *per caput* doses from medical exposure, approximately 1.5 mSv (150 mrem) per year.

—In the United States, the **GSD** from diagnostic x-rays and nuclear medicine studies is approximately 0.25 mSv (25 mrem) and 0.02 mSv (2 mrem) per year, respectively.

—Diagnostic procedures using ionizing radiation are the highest source of man-made radiation exposure (see Table 9-4).

—The highest contributor to medical exposure is CT, which is a relatively high-dose procedure (see Table 9-3) whose use has grown substantially over the last two decades.

VI. Dose Limitation Methods

A. Protection in radiography

—The principle methods of controlling radiation exposure are decreasing exposure time, increasing distance from the radiation source, and using appropriate collimation and shielding (Figure 9-3).

—Because both primary and scattered radiation fall off as the inverse square of the distance, doubling the distance reduces the exposure level by a factor of 4.

—As a general rule, the scatter dose level from patients at 1 meter is approximately 0.1% of the entrance skin dose.

—For example, during fluoroscopy, the patient entrance skin exposure rate is approximately 3 roentgens per minute (R/min), and the operator exposure at 1 m is approximately 3 mR/min.

—Leakage radiation from the tube housing should be less than 0.1 R/h at a distance of 1 m.

—During fluoroscopy, workers should not be in the room if not necessary.

—Radiation workers should never hold a patient for a study.

—A parent or relative should be instructed to position the patient and should be given a lead apron to wear.

—When performing portable examinations, the operator should stand at least 2 m away from the patient.

B. Operator shielding

—Lead is an effective protective barrier (i.e., it has a high attenuation coefficient) because of its high density and high atomic number.

—Lead aprons used in diagnostic radiology should have 0.25 mm or 0.5 mm equivalents of lead.

—A 0.5-mm lead apron reduces radiation exposure by at least a factor of 10.

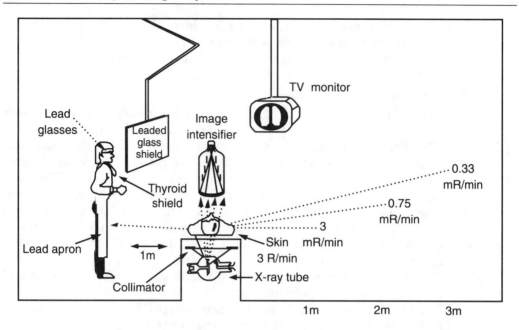

Figure 9-3. Radiation protection aspects of fluoroscopy.

–Individual organs not protected by lead aprons, such as the eye lens or thyroid, may receive much higher doses during fluoroscopy.

–Leaded glass can significantly reduce the dose to the eye.

–A thyroid shield can significantly reduce the dose to the neck.

–Protective gloves should have a lead equivalence of 0.25 mm.

C. Room shielding design

–The design of radiation facilities should always incorporate the **ALARA** principle.

–Design of barriers in radiology departments depends on factors such as **workload** (W), which is how often the machine is in operation (mA min/week), **use factor** (U) (fraction of time that radiation points in a specified direction), **occupancy factor** (T) (fraction of time people work on the other side of the barrier), and **distance** (D) from the source to the barrier.

–The design of shielding must also take into account the **exposure output** in mR/mAs for primary, scattered, and leakage radiation (Figure 9-4).

–A primary protective barrier absorbs primary radiation.

–A secondary barrier protects workers from scattered radiation.

–For primary barriers, the use factor is 1 for the floor, 1/16 for the walls, and 0 for the ceiling.

–The use factor for stray radiation is 1 and for scattered radiation is 0.1.

–Occupancy factors are generally 1 for offices and laboratories, 1/4 for corridors and restrooms, and 1/16 for waiting rooms and outside areas used by pedestrians.

–In practice, the shielding used for most x-ray installations is 1.6 mm (1/16 inch) of lead in the walls.

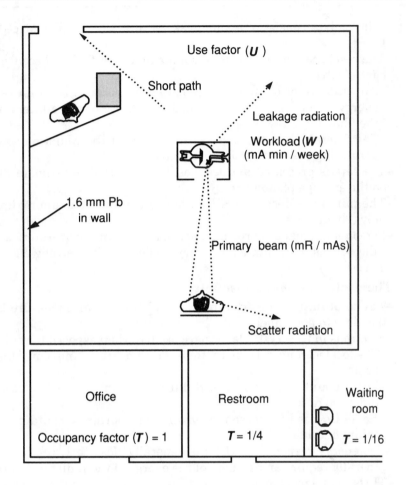

Figure 9-4. Room shielding needs are calculated based on the intensity of primary, scatter, and leakage radiation.

—In designing x-ray facilities, there should be no **short paths** such as gaps between doors.

—Shielding is normally required to extend at least 2 m from the floor.

VII. Personnel Dosimetry

A. Film dosimetry

—Personnel monitoring devices are worn to ensure that workers receive doses below the appropriate dose limit and to monitor radiation safety practices.

—Monitoring devices are normally worn for a month.

—Film badges are the most common and least expensive monitoring device.

–Film badges consist of a small case with a piece of film placed between filters.

–The response of film to x-rays is a maximum at 25 keV because of the K-edge of silver.

  –An estimate of photon energy is needed because the film response is energy-dependent and is obtained by the use of three filters in front of the film.

  –The filters assess the penetrating power of the radiation source, thus permitting the energy to be estimated.

–The film is processed and the density measured to estimate dose based on the average photon energy.

–The minimum dose that a film badge can detect is approximately 0.2 mSv (20 mrem).

–Personal film badges provide a permanent record of operator exposure.

–Film badges have limited accuracy because of their strong energy dependence.

B. Thermoluminescent dosimetry

–**Thermoluminescent dosimeters (TLDs)** can also measure the radiation dose to personnel.

–Electrons in the crystal lattice are excited when exposed to radiation.

  –These electrons return to their ground state and emit light when heated.

  –The amount of light released during heating is used to estimate the radiation dose.

–The TLDs used in personnel monitoring normally contain crystalline lithium fluoride (LiF).

–The energy response of TLDs is generally close to 1, thus TLDs do not generally require an estimate of the energy of the radiation source.

–TLDs can be used to detect a wide range of radiation dose levels.

–The detection limit for a TLD is approximately 0.2 mSv (20 mrem).

C. Pocket ionization chamber

–Pocket ionization chambers are shaped like large pens.

–As a result of the ionization produced in the chamber, a charged capacitor is discharged when exposed to radiation.

–Pocket ionization chambers can provide immediate readings.

–The typical sensitivity range of a pocket ionization chamber is 0 to 200 mR.

–Pocket ionization chambers are easily recharged and reused.

–Pocket ionization chambers, however, are not very accurate because of their mechanical frailty (e.g., may be dropped on the floor).

Review Test

1. Radiation doses in diagnostic radiology are likely to result in a significant

(A) increase of temperature
(B) number of chromosome breaks
(C) production of ionization
(D) number of cell membranes broken
(E) number of cells killed

2. The most radiosensitive cells are the

(A) bone marrow cells
(B) neuronal cells
(C) keratinized skin cells
(D) kidney parenchymal cells

3. Radiobiological $LD_{50/60}$ is the dose that

(A) kills 50% of the population
(B) kills 50 members of the population
(C) kills 60% within 50 hours
(D) kills 50% within 60 days
(E) kills e^{-1} of the population within 60 days

4. Match the radiation dose with the appropriate effect for an acute whole-body exposure.

(A) 1 Gy (100 rad)
(B) 5 Gy (500 rad)
(C) 10 Gy (1000 rad)
(D) 100 Gy (10,000 rad)

(i)   Gastrointestinal tract
(ii) Central nervous system
(iii) Depressed lymphocyte count
(iv) Hematopoietic system

5. What is the threshold *acute* radiation x-ray dose for the following deterministic effects?

(A) Cataract induction
(B) Low lymphocyte count
(C) Permanent azoospermia
(D) Skin erythema

6. Stochastic effects of radiation

(A) include carcinogenesis
(B) have a threshold of 50 mSv/year
(C) have a dose dependent severity
(D) involve cell killing
(E) can be recognized as caused by radiation

7. Match the following studies of radiation-induced cancers with their associated cancers.

(A) Radiation therapy for ankylosing spondylitis
(B) Chest fluoroscopy for tuberculosis
(C) Radium dial painters

(i)   Osteosarcoma
(ii) Leukemia
(iii) Breast cancer

8. Radiation-induced thyroid neoplasms

(A) are more common in women
(B) may be malignant or benign
(C) are more common in children per unit dose
(D) have a long latent period
(E) all of the above are true

9. True (T) or False (F). The 1990 report of the National Research Council on the health effects of low-level radiation (*BEIR V*) used

(A) linear dose–response models
(B) new doses for the A-bomb survivors
(C) a relative risk model
(D) data on lung cancers caused by domestic radon
(E) a threshold dose for carcinogenesis

10. Match the stage of gestation in humans with the effect most likely produced by a 50 rad (0.5 Gy) dose (based on animal studies).

(A) Preimplantation (0 to 10 days postconception)
(B) Early organogenesis (20 to 40 days postconception)
(C) Late organogenesis (50 to 70 days postconception)
(D) Early fetal period (70 to 150 days postconception)
(E) Late fetal period (150 days postconception to term)

(i)   Small head size (microcephaly)
(ii) Gross malformation
(iii) Early intrauterine death
(iv) Growth and mental retardation
(v)   Increased risk of childhood malignancy

11. A fetal radiation dose of 10 mGy (1 rad)

(A) is very unlikely during any diagnostic exam
(B) is less than annual natural background
(C) could occur during 1 minute of fluoroscopy
(D) would suggest the need for a therapeutic abortion
(E) would kill the fetus

12. Match the following *whole body* doses with the corresponding regulatory limits.

(A) 1 mSv/yr (100 mrem/yr)
(B) 5 mSv/yr (500 mrem/yr)
(C) 20 mSv/yr (2 rem/yr)
(D) 50 mSv/yr (5 rem/yr)
(E) No limit

(i) Patients undergoing diagnostic x-ray examinations
(ii) Regulatory limit for the public
(iii) Regulatory limit for radiation workers
(iv) ICRP 60 proposed limit for the public
(v) ICRP 60 proposed limit for radiation workers

13. Radiation protection standards recommended by the National Council on Radiation Protection and Measurements (NCRP) are based on all the following EXCEPT

(A) the ALARA principle should be used
(B) there are no risks below certain radiation levels
(C) unnecessary exposures are not permitted
(D) the major health risk is carcinogenesis
(E) the fetus is treated as a "member of the public"

14. Regulatory dose limits for a diagnostic radiology technologist include the following doses

(A) Chernobyl disaster
(B) high altitude airplane flight
(C) domestic radon
(D) screening mammograms
(E) none of the above

15. During the entire gestation period, the fetus of an occupationally exposed technologist, by law, should receive

(A) no occupational radiation exposure
(B) less than 50 mSv (5 rem)
(C) only low LET radiation exposure
(D) no exposure during weeks 7–15
(E) none of the above

16. A "non-agreement" state

(A) has no nuclear power generating facilities
(B) can abolish dose limits for occupational exposure
(C) has responsibility for regulating radioactive materials
(D) is regulated by the Nuclear Regulatory Commission
(E) has not agreed to nuclear waste disposal sites

17. Match the following radiation quantities with the appropriate units.

(A) Exposure
(B) Dose–area product
(C) Absorbed dose
(D) Integral dose
(E) Effective dose equivalent

(i) mSv
(ii) mJ
(iii) mR
(iv) mGy
(v) mGy-cm^2

18. Match each of the following entrance skin doses with the relevant x-ray examination.

(A) 0.2 mGy (20 mrad)
(B) 1.5 mGy (150 mrad)
(C) 3 mGy (300 mrad)
(D) 10 mGy (1 rad)
(E) 40 mGy (4 rad)

(i) Head CT scan
(ii) Skull radiograph (lateral)
(iii) Lumbosacral spine (lateral)
(iv) Chest radiograph (PA)
(v) Abdomen (AP)

19. Match the following fetal radiation doses with the relevant x-ray examinations.

(A) < 0.01 mGy (< 1 mrad)
(B) 1 mGy (100 mrad)
(C) 15 mGy (1.5 rad)
(D) 100 mGy (10 rad)

(i) 10 minutes abdominal fluoroscopy (AP)
(ii) Chest radiograph (AP)
(iii) CT scan of the abdomen/pelvis
(iv) Abdomen radiograph (AP)

20. Patient doses from CT scans have all the following features EXCEPT

(A) skin dose of about 40 mGy (4 rad) for a head scan
(B) skin dose of about 20 mGy (2 rad) for a body scan
(C) skin to central axis dose ratio of 1:1 for head scans
(D) skin to central axis dose ratio of 2:1 for body scans
(E) the same risk for a single 10 mm section as for a single 1 mm section

21. Match the following average United States annual radiation exposures to their sources.

(A) < 0.01 mSv (< 1 mrem)
(B) 0.5 mSv (50 mrem)
(C) 2 mSv (200 mrem)
(D) 5 mSv (500 mrem)

(i) Medical exposure (x-rays and NM)
(ii) Domestic radon
(iii) Regulatory limit for the public
(iv) Nuclear power generation

22. True (T) or False (F). Current average annual doses in the U.S. are approximately

(A) 3 mSv (300 mrem) from natural background
(B) 0.1 mSv (10 mrem) from domestic TVs and computer VDUs
(C) 0.3 mSv (30 mrem) from cosmic background
(D) 0.4 mSv (40 mrem) from internal radionuclides such as ^{40}K
(E) 1 mSv (100 mrem) from Chernobyl fallout

23. The mean radiation dose to the lungs is highest from

(A) a standard chest x-ray
(B) occupational exposure for x-ray technologist (1 year)
(C) exposure to domestic radon (1 year)
(D) cosmic radiation (1 year)

24. The genetically significant dose (GSD) from radiology is

(A) the number of genetic defects caused by x-rays
(B) used to estimate an individual's risk
(C) an index of potential genetic damage
(D) rapidly increasing each year
(E) 25 mSv (2.5 rem) per year in the United States

25. An operator standing 1 meter from a patient undergoing a head CT scan will most likely receive a dose that is

(A) 0.1% of the patient skin dose
(B) about 0.04 mGy (4 mrad)
(C) able to blacken a 600 speed screen/film
(D) below the annual dose limit for workers
(E) all of the above

26. True (T) or False (F). For x-ray shielding

(A) half-value layer (HVL) is independent of x-ray energy
(B) 1 cm of Pb and 1 cm of concrete are equally effective
(C) it is essential to use Pb or other high Z materials
(D) doubling the distance from a source $\equiv$ 2 HVLs shielding
(E) 2 tenth-value layers (TVLs) are better than 6 HVLs
(F) 1 TVL is better than 4 HVLs

27. Match the following terms and definitions as they relate to room shielding needs.

(A) Workload
(B) Use factor
(C) Occupancy factor

(i) Total weekly intensity of a radiation source
(ii) Fraction of time a source points in a given direction
(iii) Fraction of time any given area is occupied

28. Radiation shielding for diagnostic x-ray rooms is normally required to be

(A) less than a TVL
(B) about 1.6 mm (1/16 in.) Pb or equivalent attenuation
(C) in compliance with NRC requirements
(D) greater in the ceiling than in the walls
(E) all of the above

29. Match the following measuring devices with the application.

(A) Film dosimeter
(B) Ionization chamber
(C) Geiger-Müller tube
(D) NaI well counter
(E) Dose calibrator

(i) ^{99m}Tc contamination on hands
(ii) Identification of radioactive contamination
(iii) Personnel dosimetry
(iv) X-ray tube output
(v) Measuring activity before patient administration

30. Personnel film badges are

(A) most sensitive to 25 keV photons
(B) used to measure doses below 0.02 mSv
(C) generally insensitive to heat
(D) not dependent on the photon energy
(E) all of the above

Answers and Explanations

1–C. At the low doses normally encountered in diagnostic radiology, the only significant effect will be the production of ionization.

2–A. Bone marrow cells, which are continually proliferating, are the most radiosensitive.

3–D. At LD$_{50/60}$, 50% of the exposed population is killed within 60 days.

4. A–iii; B–iv; C–i; D–ii.

5. A–2 Gy (200 rad); B–1 Gy (100 rad); C–6 Gy (600 rad); D–5 Gy (500 rad).

6–A. Stochastic (random) effects, including carcinogenesis and genetic damage, are the most significant risks encountered in diagnostic radiology.

7. A–ii; patients treated with radiation had subsequent increased incidence of leukemia; **B–iii;** women undergoing chest fluoroscopy for tuberculosis had elevated breast doses and subsequent increased incidence of breast cancer; **C–i;** ingested ^{226}Ra was taken up by the bone resulting in an increased incidence of osteosarcoma.

8–E. All of the statements are true.

9. A–True; data for solid tumors shows no departure from linearity, whereas leukemia may be fitted by a linear or linear–quadratic curve; **B–True;** the dosimetry system developed in 1986 (DS86) replaced the previous dosimetry of 1965 (TD65); **C–True;** this is the principal reason for the upward revision of radiation risks; **D–False;** lung cancer has been observed in uranium miners exposed to radon, but not at domestic exposure levels; **E–False;** current radiation protection philosophy assumes there is "no threshold."

10. A–iii; B–ii; C–i; D–iv; E–v.

11–C. The entrance skin dose in fluoroscopy is typically 30 to 50 mGy/min (3 to 5 rad/min); for an AP projection, the attenuation by soft tissue would likely result in a threefold reduction in dose to the fetus.

12. A–iv; B–ii; C–v; D–iii; E–i.

13–B. NCRP assumes a linear dose response curve with no threshold dose for induction of detrimental effects.

14–E. Only the radiation received from *occupational exposure* is included for regulatory purposes.

15–E. None of the statements are correct. A fetus is treated as a member of the public, and current regulations would therefore limit the fetal dose to 5 mSv (500 mrem).

16–D. About 20 "non-agreement" states are regulated directly by the NRC. The "agreement" states must have regulations for nuclear materials that are as stringent as those of the NRC.

17. A–iii; exposure in mR; **B–v;** dose–area product in mGy-cm^2; **C–iv;** absorbed dose in mGy; **D–ii;** integral dose (energy imparted) in mJ; **E–i;** effective dose equivalent in mSv.

18. A–iv; chest x-ray = 0.2 mGy (20 mrad); **B–ii;** lateral skull x-ray = 1.5 mGy (150 mrad); **C–v;** AP abdomen x-ray = 3 mGy (300 mrad); **D–iii;** lateral lumbosacral spine x-ray = 10 mGy (1 rad); **E–i;** head CT scan = 40 mGy (4 rad); all doses are entrance skin doses.

19. A–ii; in a chest x-ray, only scatter radiation reaches the fetus and the entrance skin dose is only 0.15 mGy (15 mrad); **B–iv; C–iii;** CT body doses range between 10 and 20 mGy (1 and 2 rad); **D–i;** the entrance skin dose is about 300 mGy since the dose rate is typically 30 mGy/min ($\equiv$ 3 rad/min) and the fetal dose is one third this value.

20–E. The risk will be approximately proportional to the energy imparted which is 10 times greater for a 10 mm thick slice.

21. A–iv; B–i; there are about 300 million diagnostic procedures performed in the United States every year, and the population average dose is approximately 0.5 mSv (50 mrem); **C–ii;** this is an average value for the U.S. with significant regional variations; **D–iii;** current value with the ICRP recommending a reduction to 1 mSv.

22. A–True; B–False; any x-ray output from TVs and VDUs is very low energy and easily absorbed by the screen; **C–True;** note that people living in Leadville, CO, at an elevation of 3000 m, receive an additional 0.7 mSv (70 mrem) per year; **D–True; E–False;** in North America, fallout from Chernobyl detectable in 1986 but doses were negligible.

23–C. The average *effective dose equivalent* from 1 year of exposure to domestic radon is 2 mSv (200 mrem), and the mean lung dose will be much higher than this.

24–C. GSD is a measure of the gonadal dose modified by the relative child expectancy of irradiated individuals. The GSD in the U.S. from diagnostic radiology is about 0.25 mSv (25 mrem) per year.

25–E. All of the statements are true. Skin dose to patient will be about 40 mGy (4 rad) and the scatter will be about 0.1%.

26. A–False; attenuation is generally strongly dependent on photon energy; **B–False;** the Pb is much more effective because it has a higher atomic number and density; **C–False;** the only factor that matters is how much of the incident radiation gets through the barrier, with high Z materials used because they are more convenient; **D–True;** both reduce intensity by a factor of four; **E–True;** attenuation from 2 TVLs $\equiv$ $(10)^2$ = 100, whereas 6 HVLs $\equiv$ $(2)^6$ = 64; **F–False;** 4 HVLs $\equiv$ $(2)^4$ = 16, which is better than a tenfold attenuation from one TVL.

27. A–i; B–ii; C–iii.

28–B. Most diagnostic x-ray rooms require 1.6 mm Pb (1/16 in.). Note that the NRC regulates nuclear material, not diagnostic x-ray rooms.

29. A–iii; most personnel dosimetry is performed using film dosimeters; **B–iv;** ionization chambers are very accurate for exposure measurements but do not have high sensitivity; **C–i;** GM tubes are very sensitive and convenient to use; **D–ii;** the use of a well counter with pulse height analysis will permit the photon energy of the contamination to be determined; **E–v;** dose calibrators must be used to measure the amount of activity being administered to patients.

30–A. The film badge is most sensitive to photons with an energy just above the K-edge of silver (i.e., 25 keV).

10

Ultrasound

I. Ultrasound Physics

A. Ultrasound waves

–**Sound waves** are a mechanical disturbance that propagate through a medium.

–**Wavelength (λ)** is the distance between successive wave crests.

–**Frequency (f)** is the number of oscillations per second measured in hertz. **Hertz (Hz)** is 1 cycle per second.

–The **period** is the time between oscillations, or $1/f$.

–For sound waves, the relation between velocity (v), measured in m/s, frequency, and wavelength is $v = f \times \lambda$ (m/s).

–Audible sound has frequencies ranging from 15 Hz to 20,000 Hz.

–Ultrasound frequencies are higher than that of audible sound, and are greater than 20 kHz.

–**Diagnostic ultrasound** uses **transducers** with frequencies ranging from 1 to 20 MHz (1 MHz = 10^6 Hz).

–Ultrasound waves are transmitted through tissue as **longitudinal waves** of alternating compression and rarification.

–Ultrasound waves may be **reflected, refracted, scattered,** or **absorbed**.

B. Velocity

–The **velocity** of sound is dependent on the nature of the medium through which it is traveling and is (approximately) **independent of frequency**.

–Because velocity is constant, increases in frequency result in decreases in wavelength and vice versa $(v = f \times \lambda)$.

–Velocity is inversely proportional to compressibility. The less compressible the medium, the greater the velocity.

–Sound travels fastest in solids and slowest in gases.

–The **average velocity** of sound in soft tissue is **1540 m/s,** with much higher values in bone and metal and much lower values in lung and air.

–Table 10-1 lists ultrasound velocities for various media.

Table 10-1. Ultrasound Properties

Material	Velocity (m/s)	Attenuation coefficient (dB/cm at 1 MHz)	Acoustic impedance $(kg/m^2/s \times 10^6)$
Air	330	12.0	0.0004
Fat	1450	0.63	1.38
Water	1540	0.0022	1.54
Kidney	1560	1.0	1.62
Blood	1570	0.18	1.61
Muscle	1585	3.3	1.70
Eye lens	1620	2.0	1.84
Bone	3300	20.0	7.8
Metals	> 4000	< 0.02	>30.0

C. Acoustic impedance

–The **acoustic impedance (Z)** of a material is the product of the density (ρ), measured in kg/m^3, and the velocity of sound in the medium, measured in m/s: $\mathbf{Z = \rho \times v}$ $(kg/m^2/s)$.

–The acoustic impedance unit is called the **Rayl** $(kg/m^2/s)$.

–Acoustic impedance is independent of frequency in the diagnostic range.

–Air and lung media have low values, and bone and metal have high values of acoustic impedance.

–Table 10-1 lists acoustic impedance values for various media with most tissues having values of about 1.6×10^6 $kg/m^2/s$ (Rayls).

–Acoustic impedance determines the amount of energy reflected at an interface.

D. Sound intensity

–The **amplitude** of a wave is the **size** of the wave displacement or pressure.

–Larger amplitudes of vibration produce denser compression bands and, hence, higher intensities of sound.

–Ultrasound beam **intensity (I)** is a measure of the energy associated with the beam and is proportional to the square of the amplitude.

–Ultrasonic intensities are normally expressed in terms of **milliwatts per unit area (mW/cm²)**.

–The intensity of a beam may be averaged over the transducer area and over long time periods (many pulses) as a crude measure of ultrasound beam strength.

–The intensity at a single point during a single pulse is known as the **spatial peak pulse average intensity (I_{sppa})**.

–The intensity at a single point averaged over a long time period (many pulses) is the **spatial peak temporal average intensity (I_{spta})**.

–I_{sppa} and I_{spta} are important parameters when considering the possibility of inducing bioeffects.

E. Decibels

–**Relative sound intensity** is measured on a logarithmic scale and may be expressed in bels (B) or **decibels (dB),** where 1 B = 10 dB.

–Relative intensity in decibels is equal to $\mathbf{10 \times \log_{10}(I/I_o)}$, where I_o is the original intensity and I is the measured intensity.

–Negative decibel values correspond to signal attenuation, and positive values correspond to signal amplification.

–Intensity reduced to 50% is -3 dB, to 10% is -10 dB, to 1% is -20 dB, and to 0.1% is -30 dB.

–A change of +3 dB corresponds to a twofold increase in intensity, +10 dB to a 10-fold increase, +20 dB to a 100-fold increase, and so on.

II. Interaction of Ultrasound and Matter

A. Attenuation

–**Attenuation** is a composite effect of loss by scatter and absorption.

–Attenuation generally **increases with frequency**.

–Due to its high frequency, ultrasound is attenuated more readily than audible sound.

–The attenuation of ultrasound in a homogeneous tissue is exponential.

  –In soft tissues, there is a nearly linear relation between the frequency and attenuation of ultrasound.

–At an ultrasound frequency of 1 MHz, attenuation in soft tissue is approximately 1 dB/cm.

  –At 5 MHz, attenuation in soft tissue is approximately 5 dB/cm, and at 10 MHz, attenuation is approximately 10 dB/cm.

  –For water and bone media, attenuation increases approximately as frequency squared.

–The absorbed sound wave energy is converted into **heat**.

–Little absorption and almost no scatter or reflection occur in fluids.

–Table 10-1 lists ultrasound attenuation coefficients for a range of media.

B. Reflection angle

–A portion of the ultrasound beam is reflected at tissue interfaces as shown in Figure 10-1. The sound reflected back toward the source is called an **echo** and is used to generate the ultrasound image.

–The percentage of ultrasound intensity reflected depends, in part, on the **angle of incidence** of the beam.

–Angles of incidence and reflection are equal as shown in Figure 10-1, similar to the reflection of light.

–As the angle of incidence increases, reflected sound is less likely to reach the transducer.

  –No reflection is generally detected by the transducer if the beam strikes the patient surface at angles greater than approximately 3 degrees from the perpendicular to the interface.

–**Specular reflections** occur from large, smooth surfaces.

–**Nonspecular reflections** are diffuse scatter from "rough" surfaces where the irregular contours are bigger than the ultrasound wavelength.

–Specular reflections are the major contributors to ultrasound images.

C. Reflection intensity

–The percentage (intensity) of ultrasound reflected also depends on the **acoustic impedance** of the tissues.

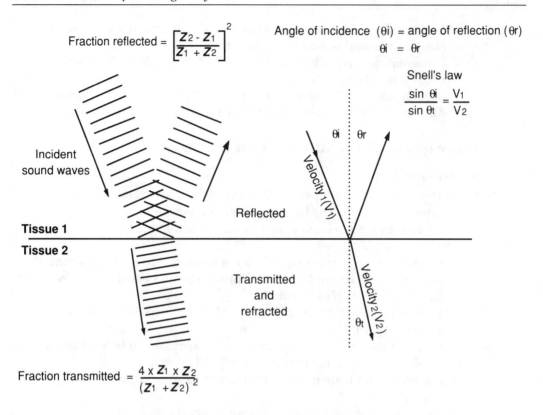

$$\text{Fraction reflected} = \left[\frac{Z_2 - Z_1}{Z_1 + Z_2}\right]^2$$

Angle of incidence (θi) = angle of reflection (θr)

$$\theta i = \theta r$$

Snell's law

$$\frac{\sin \theta i}{\sin \theta t} = \frac{V_1}{V_2}$$

Incident sound waves

Reflected

Tissue 1

Tissue 2

Transmitted and refracted

$$\text{Fraction transmitted} = \frac{4 \times Z_1 \times Z_2}{(Z_1 + Z_2)^2}$$

Figure 10-1. Reflection and refraction of sound waves.

- At normal incidence (90 degrees), the fractional amount of ultrasound intensity **reflected** is $[(Z_2 - Z_1)/(Z_2 + Z_1)]^2$ (see Figure 10-1).
- Because the amount transmitted and the amount reflected must always equal 1, the amount **transmitted** is $(4Z_1 \times Z_2)/(Z_1 + Z_2)^2$.
  - From chest wall ($Z = 1.7$) to lung ($Z = 0.0004$), the intensity reflected is 99.9% and transmitted is 0.1%.
  - From kidney ($Z = 1.62$) to fat ($Z = 1.38$), the intensity reflected is 0.64% and transmitted is 99.36%.
- Table 10-2 lists values of reflected intensities for a range of interfaces encountered in diagnostic ultrasound.

Table 10-2. Percentage of Energy Reflected from an Ultrasound Beam Perpendicular to the Tissue Interface

	Muscle (%)	**Liver (%)**	**Blood (%)**	**Bone (%)**
Fat	1.1	0.8	0.6	49
Muscle	—	0.02	0.1	41
Liver	0.02	—	0.02	42
Blood	0.1	0.02	—	43

D. Tissue reflections

–Air/tissue interfaces reflect virtually all of the incident ultrasound beam.

–Gel is applied between the transducer and skin to displace the air and minimize large reflections that would interfere with ultrasound transmission into the patient.

–Bone/tissue interfaces also reflect substantial fractions of the incident intensity.

–Imaging through air or bone is generally not possible.

–The lack of transmissions beyond these interfaces results in an area void of echoes called **shadowing**.

–In imaging the abdomen, the strongest echoes are likely to arise from gas bubbles.

–Organs such as the kidney, pancreas, spleen, and liver are comprised of subregions that contain many scattering sites, which results in a speckled texture on ultrasound images.

–Organs that contain fluids such as the bladder, cysts, and blood vessels have no internal structure and almost no echoes (i.e., show black).

E. Refraction

–**Refraction** is the change in direction of an ultrasound beam when passing from one medium to another as shown in Figure 10-1.

–When ultrasound passes from one medium to another, the frequency remains the same but the wavelength changes to accommodate the new velocity of sound in the second medium.

–The wavelength of sound shortens when the velocity is reduced.

–Refraction is described by **Snell's law**: $\sin\theta_i/\sin\theta_t = v_1/v_2$, where θ_i is the angle of incidence, θ_t is the transmitted angle, v_1 is the velocity in medium 1, and v_2 is the velocity in medium 2.

III. Transducers

A. Introduction

–A **transducer** is a device that can convert one form of energy into another.

–**Piezoelectric transducers** convert electrical energy into ultrasonic energy. Piezoelectric means **pressure electricity**.

–High-frequency voltage oscillations are produced by a **pulse generator** and sent to the ultrasound transducer by a **transmitter**.

–The electrical energy causes the crystal to momentarily change shape.

 –This change in shape of the crystal increases and decreases the pressure in front of the transducer, thus producing ultrasound waves.

 –The returning ultrasound echoes are converted back into electrical energy signals using either the same or another transducer.

–Return voltage signals are transferred from the receiver to a computer to create an ultrasound image.

–Transducer crystals do not conduct electricity.

–The piezoelectric effect of a transducer is destroyed if heated above its curie temperature limit.

–Most transducers are made of natural crystal quartz or a synthetic ceramic such as lead-zirconate-titanate (PZT).

B. Transducer frequency

–The thickness and acoustic velocity of a piezoelectric crystal determine the resonant frequency of the transducer.

–**Resonant frequency** is the natural frequency of oscillation.

–Transducer crystals are normally manufactured so that their thickness (t) is equal to one-half of the wavelength (λ) of the ultrasound produced by the transducer ($t = \lambda/2$).

–Changing the thickness of the crystal changes the frequency but not the ultrasound amplitude or velocity.

  –For example, if a crystal has a thickness of 1 mm and the velocity of sound is 4000 m/s, then the resonant frequency is $f = v/\lambda = v/(2 \times t)$, or 2 MHz.

–High-frequency transducers are thin, and low-frequency transducers are thicker.

C. Transducer design

–The **Q factor** is related to the frequency response of the crystal.

–The Q factor determines the purity of sound and the length of time a sound persists, or **ring down time**.

–**High Q transducers** produce a relatively pure frequency spectrum; low Q transducers produce a wider range of frequencies.

–The Q factor is determined by the ratio of the operating frequency to the bandwidth at full width half maximum (FWHM).

–Short pulses correspond to reduced Q values and vice versa.

–Most transducers are designed to have short pulses with low Q values.

–Blocks of damping material, usually tungsten/rubber in an epoxy resin, are placed behind transducers to reduce vibration (ring down time) and shorten pulses.

–A **matching layer** of material is placed on the front surface of the transducer to improve the efficiency of energy transmission into the patient.

  –The matching layer material has an impedance in between that of the transducer and tissue.

  –The matching layer thickness is one fourth the wavelength of sound in that material and is referred to as **quarter wave matching.**

–Figure 10-2 shows the components of a typical transducer.

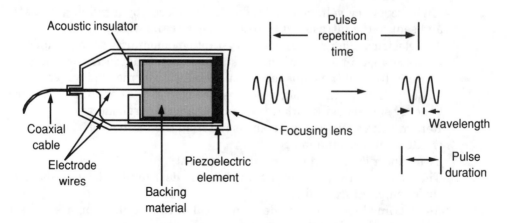

Figure 10-2. Components of an ultrasound transducer and a typical ultrasound beam.

D. Ultrasound fields

–The near (parallel) field of the ultrasound beam is known as the **Fresnel zone** (Figure 10-3).

–The far (diverging) field is known as the **Fraunhofer zone**.

–Beam intensity falls off in both zones because of attenuation, and in the far zone because of beam divergence.

–Ultrasound imaging normally uses the Fresnel zone but not the Fraunhofer zone in which resolution is poor.

–The length of the Fresnel zone is $d^2/4\lambda$, where d is the diameter of the transducer and λ is the wavelength.

–The Fresnel zone increases with transducer size and frequency (lower wavelengths).

–Table 10-3 lists Fresnel zone dimensions for a 10-mm diameter transducer at different frequencies.

–Low-frequency transducers have better tissue penetration.

–**Side lobes** are small beams of greatly reduced intensity that are emitted at angles to the primary beam (see Figure 10-3) and that may cause image artifacts.

E. Focused transducers

–Focused transducers reduce beam width, which improves lateral resolution. Focused transducers also concentrate beam intensity, thereby

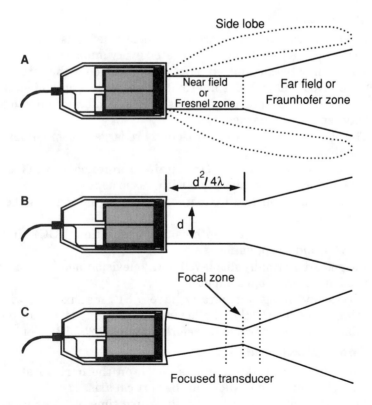

Figure 10-3. Transducer zones and focus.

Table 10-3. Wavelength and Fresnel Zone Length in Soft Tissue for a 10-mm Diameter Transducer

Frequency (MHz)	Wavelength (mm)	Fresnel Zone (mm)
0.5	3.0	8.3
1.0	1.5	17
2.0	0.75	33
5.0	0.3	83
10.0	0.15	170

increasing penetration and echo intensities and improving image quality (see Figure 10-3).
- Most diagnostic transducers are focused, which is achieved using a curved piezoelectric crystal or acoustic lens.
- The **focal zone** is the region over which the beam is focused.
- The **focal length** is the distance from the transducer to the center of the focal zone.
- The **depth of focus** is the distance over which the beam is in reasonable focus.
- A small-diameter transducer has a shorter focal zone and spreads more rapidly in the far zone.

IV. Ultrasound Displays

A. Introduction
- Most ultrasound beams are emitted in brief pulses with a duration of about 1 μs and are typically repeated every millisecond.
- The span between emitted pulses allows time for the returning echoes to be received and provides information about the depth of an interface.
- The strength of returning echoes provides information about differences between the two tissues.
- The objects imaged with ultrasound are large in comparison to the wavelength being used.
- Ultrasound scanners use **time gain compensation (TGC)** to compensate for increased attenuation with tissue depth.
  - This is accomplished by increasing the signal gain as the echo return time increases.
  - TGC is also known as depth gain compensation (DGC), time varied gain (TVG), and swept gain.
- Images are normally displayed on a television monitor and may be digitized and stored in a computer.
- Ultrasound images generally have a 512 matrix size, with each pixel being 8 bits deep (1 Byte), allowing 256 (2^8) gray levels to be displayed.
  - Each ultrasound frame therefore contains 0.25 MByte of information.

B. A-Mode ultrasound
- **A-mode** (amplitude) displays depth on the horizontal axis and echo intensity (pulse amplitude) on the vertical axis.
- For soft tissue ($v = 1540$ m/s), a return time of 13 μs corresponds to a depth of 1 cm (round trip of 2 cm).

–A-mode systems have no memory, and a permanent record is obtained by photographing the CRT monitor.

–Little use is made of the spike amplitude.

–A-mode may be used in ophthalmology or when accurate distance measurements are required.

–A-mode only provides information along the line of sight and has been superseded by M-mode (motion mode) and two-dimensional B-mode (brightness mode) imaging.

C. M-Mode ultrasound

–**M-mode or T-M mode** (time-motion mode) displays time on the horizontal axis and depth on the vertical axis.

–The spikes of A-mode are converted into dots, and brightness replaces amplitude.

–Sequential ultrasound pulses are displayed adjacent to each other, allowing the change in position of interfaces to be seen.

–A camera records the entire (horizontal) sweep to produce an image.

–M-mode thus displays **time-dependent motion**.

–Longer times may be recorded with strip chart recorders.

–M-mode is valuable for studying rapid movement, such as cardiac valve motion.

D. B-Mode ultrasound

–**B-mode** displays a static image of a section of tissue.

–The gray scale is used to display the intensity of an echo from a given region.

–The transducer functions as both transmitter and receiver.

–The transducer sweeps the beam back and forth through the patient's body, acquiring single lines of data that display echo intensity as a function of location.

–The sweeping motion may be mechanical, that is, a single transducer is wobbled back and forth or a multielement transducer is continually rotated.

–Phased arrays consist of multiple small transducers that are sequentially activated to image a plane (Figure 10-4).

–Phased arrays electronically steer the beam.

–Linear phased arrays have parallel elements. Curvilinear phased arrays diverge and allow a wider field of view (FOV).

–A single image frame is created by adding together individual lines.

–**Line density** is the number of vertical lines per FOV.

–The frame rates for **real time imaging** are 15 to 40 frames per second, which permits motion to be followed.

–Increased line density results in improved lateral resolution but decreased frame rate.

E. Pulse repetition frequency

–**Pulse rate** or **pulse repetition frequency (PRF)** refers to the number of separate packets of sound that are sent out every second.

–Each sonic pulse is short (2 to 3 wavelengths, or a duration of about 1 μs); between pulses, the transducer acts as a receiver.

–Common PRFs are approximately 1 kHz, or 1000 pulses/s.

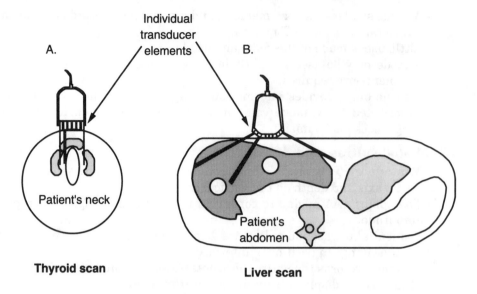

Figure 10-4. Typical clinical transducers. **A,** Linear phased array transducer. **B,** A curvilinear phased array transducer.

–High pulse rates limit the penetration depth (range) that may be detected because of the time required for the signal to return.

–A low PRF limits the line density and frame rate, which impacts the ability to follow motion.

–For example, a 20-cm deep object requires 260 μs for a round trip.

–The maximum number of lines is then $1/(260 \times 10^{-6})$, or 3846.

–With 3846 total lines, it is possible to have 113 lines per image and 34 frames/s, or 225 lines per image and 15 frames/s, and so on.

V. Clinical Ultrasound

A. Clinical transducers

–Transducers used for abdominal imaging are generally in the 2.5- to 5-MHz range.

–Specialized high-resolution and shallow penetration probes (8 to 20 MHz) have been developed for studying the eye.

–In infants, 3.5- to 7-MHz transducers are used for echoencephalography.

–B-mode, M-mode, and Doppler systems are used to study the cardiovascular system.

–Special systems include **endovaginal** transducers for imaging the pelvic region and fetus, **endorectal** transducers for imaging the prostate, **transesophageal** transducers for imaging the heart, and **intravascular** probes for imaging inside blood vessels.

–Phased array transducers, which may be operated at high frame rates, are also better suited for Doppler imaging in which one image line must be sampled many times.

–Table 10-4 lists types of ultrasound transducers and their clinical applications.

Table 10-4. Clinical Transducers

Transducer Type	Frequency	Body Regions	Resolution Axial	Resolution Lateral	Comments
Sector scanner or curvilinear array	3 MHz (2 MHz for obese patients)	Abdomen	Moderate	Moderate	Good depth penetration (grainy images at 2 MHz)
Linear array	5–10 MHz	Thyroid; testicles; carotids; breast; legs	Excellent	Very good	Poor depth penetration (used for superficial organs)
Curvilinear array	5 MHz	Pediatric abdomen; large thyroid; large breast	Very good	Good	Used for large superficial organs
Vaginal	7.5 MHz	Ovaries; uterus	Excellent	Very good	Limited range; may be accompanied by transabdominal study
Endorectal	5–7 MHz	Prostate; rectal wall	Very good to excellent	Very good	Limited range

B. Resolution

–**Axial resolution** is the ability to separate two objects lying along the axis of the beam and is determined by the **pulse length**.

–Axial resolution is limited to half the pulse length and is, therefore, dependent on pulse frequency and duration.

–With a typical wavelength of 0.3 mm and three waves per pulse, the axial resolution is approximately 0.5 mm.

–Axial resolution deteriorates with increasing pulse length, decreasing frequency, and increasing wavelength.

–The use of damped transducers (low Q) produces short pulses that improve axial resolution.

–**Lateral resolution** is the ability to resolve two adjacent objects and is determined by the width of the beam and line density.

–Lateral resolution is best in the Fresnel zone where ultrasound waves are parallel.

–A focused transducer produces a narrower beam at the focal zone and, therefore, has better lateral resolution than an unfocused transducer of the same size (see Figure 10-3).

–Lateral resolution is generally a few millimeters.

C. Artifacts

–Reverberations occurring in the patient's body degrade image quality.

–**Reverberation** echoes are the result of multiple reflections occurring from two adjacent interfaces.

–The number of reverberations is limited by the power of the beam and sensitivity of the detector.

–**Image noise** is the result of random signals produced in the electronic preamplifier of the transducer.

–Noise reject controls can be adjusted to filter out weak echoes, but this also eliminates weak signals.

–**Refraction,** defined by Snell's law, generally causes artifacts, spatial distortion, and loss of resolution in the resultant image.

D. Ultrasound bioeffects

–At high power levels, ultrasound can cause **cavitation,** which is the creation and collapse of microscopic bubbles.

–Viscous stress can occur, resulting in small-scale fluid motions called microstreaming.

–**Tissue heating** occurs as a result of energy absorption and is the basis of using ultrasound for hyperthermia treatments.

–At low MHz frequencies, there have been no independently confirmed, significant biological effects in mammalian tissues at intensities below approximately 100 mW/cm^2 for unfocused beams or below 1 W/cm^2 for focused beams.

E. Ultrasound safety

–The American Institute of Ultrasound in Medicine has established a Bioeffects Committee to review ultrasound safety.

–Typical values of I_{spta} for pulse ultrasound are 1 to 10 mW/cm^2.

–More than half of pregnant women in the United States undergo ultrasonic examinations with no real evidence of detrimental effects.

–Diagnostic ultrasound is widely held to be biologically safe and current data suggest that the benefit to patients outweighs the risks, if any, when diagnostic ultrasound is used in appropriate clinical situations.

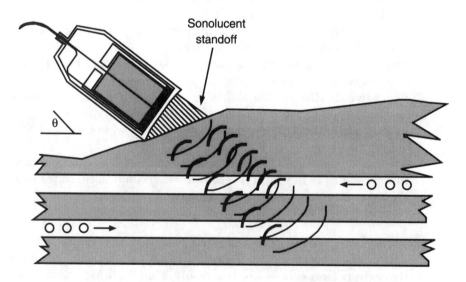

Change in frequency (f) = 2 x transducer frequency x $\dfrac{\text{(Velocity of blood)}}{\text{(Velocity of sound in tissue)}}$ x cos θ

Figure 10-5. Doppler ultrasound.

VI. Doppler Ultrasound

A. Introduction

–The **Doppler** effect refers to the change in frequency that results from a moving sample or ultrasound source (Figure 10-5).

  –Objects moving toward the detector appear to have a higher frequency and shorter wavelength.

  –Objects moving away from the detector appear to have a lower frequency and longer wavelength.

  –If the object is moving perpendicular to the ultrasound beam, there is no change in frequency or wavelength.

–Doppler ultrasound is used primarily to identify and evaluate blood flow in vessels.

–Velocity and waveform information can be used to evaluate stenoses, resistance, and vessel patency (Figure 10-6).

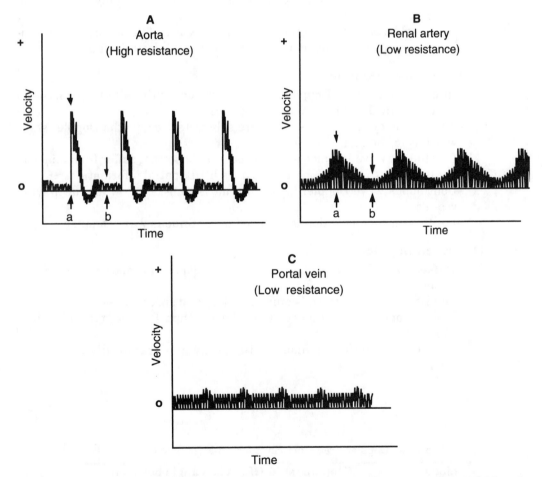

Figure 10-6. A Doppler waveform is a tracing that shows the relation between velocity (determined from the Doppler shift frequency) and time and is unique to the flow pattern in the vessel. **A,** A high-resistance arterial vessel demonstrates a rapid fall in velocity following systole. **B,** A low-resistance artery shows flow during diastole as well. **C,** Veins typically have a low velocity and low resistance. The maximum amplitude (*a*) represents peak velocity. The slowest forward flow measured in diastole is *b*. The resistive index is (*a* – *b*)/*a,* and the higher the resistance to blood flow, the higher the resistive index. Negative velocity represents flow away from the transducer.

B. Doppler physics

–High Q transducers are desirable for Doppler because they produce a narrower range of ultrasound frequencies.

–Doppler systems tend to run at lower frequencies than B-mode systems because resolution is not as important and there is a need to minimize attenuation (blood is a weak scatterer).

–The shift in frequency is $2f(v/c)\cos\theta$, where f is the ultrasound frequency, c is the velocity of sound, v is the speed of the moving object, and θ is the angle between the ultrasound beam and the moving object.

–Table 10-5 lists typical values of Doppler ultrasound frequency shift for moving blood.

–**Aliasing artifacts** can occur in pulsed Doppler, resulting in errors in estimating velocity.

–The use of lower frequencies allows higher velocities to be measured without aliasing.

–The range and distribution of flow velocities can be displayed as a spectrum (see Figure 10-6).

–**Spectral broadening** is the result of a mixture of velocities in the sample and produces a shaded area below the peak velocity value.

C. Continuous Doppler

–In continuous wave Doppler, one transducer continually transmits and another transducer continuously receives.

–The frequency of the two signals are subtracted to give the Doppler shift, which is in the audio range.

–Continuous wave Doppler is inexpensive and does not suffer from aliasing, but lacks depth resolution and provides little spatial information.

–Continuous wave Doppler is good for measuring fast flow and deep lying vessels.

–Depth gain compensation is not used in continuous wave Doppler.

D. Pulsed Doppler

–**Pulsed Doppler** allows both velocity and depth information (ranging) to be obtained.

–The Doppler information is only provided for a specific area.

–Pulsed Doppler uses a longer pulse length than B-mode, typically up to 15 mm long.

–Doppler information is displayed audially and graphically as a waveform.

Table 10-5. Doppler Frequency Shift for a 3-MHz Beam

Blood velocity (cm/s)	Doppler shift (Hz) when angle between transducer and flow direction is:		
	0°	30°	60°
5	190	170	100
10	390	340	190
20	780	670	390

–**Duplex scanning** involves displaying Doppler data on real time (B-mode) images and allows velocity and position information to be obtained simultaneously.

–Figure 10-6 shows examples of Doppler waveforms for a range of normal blood vessels.

E. Color Doppler

–**Color Doppler** is a hybrid that combines anatomic information obtained using a B-mode system with flow information obtained using pulsed Doppler analysis.

–Pulse length in color Doppler is typically 2 mm.

–Colors (blue and red) are assigned dependent on motion toward or away from the transducer.

–Information is provided over a large area and superimposed on a gray scale image.

–Color Doppler can detect flow in vessels too small to see by imaging alone.

–Spectral analysis may also be obtained using commercial color Doppler systems.

–Modern instruments incorporate both color Doppler and spectral Doppler.

Review Test

1. True (T) or False (F). Sound waves

(A) have the same velocity in all media
(B) are the low frequency of the electromagnetic spectrum
(C) can ionize atoms
(D) cannot travel in a vacuum
(E) transfer energy to tissue via side lobes
(F) are longitudinal waves
(G) are audible for frequencies between 15 Hz and 20 kHz

2. The velocity of an ultrasound beam is always

(A) constant for all solids
(B) proportional to frequency cubed
(C) equal to the velocity of the molecules of the medium
(D) equal to frequency times wavelength

3. Match the ultrasound propagation velocity with the material.

(A) Air
(B) Fat
(C) Soft tissue
(D) Bone
(E) Metal

(i) 1540 m/s
(ii) 330 m/s
(iii) 1450 m/s
(iv) 3300 m/s
(v) 6000 m/s

4. Acoustic impedance (Z) is primarily dependent on tissue

(A) density (ρ)
(B) attenuation (dB/cm)
(C) thickness
(D) temperature
(E) color

5. Match the attenuation factor (%) with the relative echo intensity.

(A) 50%
(B) 10%
(C) 5%
(D) 1%
(E) 0.1%

(i) -30 dB
(ii) -20 dB
(iii) -10 dB
(iv) -13 dB
(v) -3 dB

6. Match the following relative acoustic impedances (Z) in Rayls with the appropriate tissues.

(A) 0.0004
(B) 1.38
(C) 1.54
(D) 1.84
(E) 7.8

(i) Bone
(ii) Fat
(iii) Air
(iv) Water
(v) Eye lens

7. The wavelength (λ) of a 1 MHz sound beam is NOT

(A) the same in all solid media
(B) 0.3 mm in air
(C) 1.54 mm in soft tissue
(D) 4.1 mm in bone
(E) velocity divided by frequency

8. An ultrasound beam traveling through tissue CANNOT normally be

(A) absorbed
(B) amplified
(C) scattered
(D) reflected
(E) refracted

9. The most important factor determining the fraction of ultrasound energy reflected at a large interface is the

(A) depth of the interface
(B) transducer diameter
(C) transducer output intensity
(D) difference in acoustical impedances at the interface
(E) scan mode (A, B, M)

10. The fraction of a normally incident ultrasound beam transmitted at an interface of Z_1 and Z_2 is

(A) $1 - [(Z_2 - Z_1)/(Z_1 + Z_2)]^2$
(B) $1 - 4Z_1Z_2/(Z_1 + Z_2)^2$
(C) $(Z_1Z_2)^{1/2}(Z_1 + Z_2)$
(D) given by Snell's law
(E) none of the above

11. Reflections occur from all of the following EXCEPT

(A) smooth surfaces
(B) kidney interior
(C) fat–kidney interfaces
(D) bladder wall
(E) bladder contents

12. Snell's law describes the relation between the

(A) angle of incidence and angle of transmission
(B) dispersion angle and wavelength in the Fraunhofer zone
(C) angle of incidence and angle of reflection
(D) focusing angle and transducer curvature
(E) none of the above

13. The resonant frequency of an ultrasound transducer is determined primarily by the

(A) crystal thickness
(B) refraction law (Snell's law)
(C) Q factor
(D) applied voltage
(E) velocity of light

14. Higher frequency transducers have

(A) large thicknesses
(B) no need for gel coupling
(C) higher attenuation in tissue
(D) higher velocities in tissue
(E) inferior axial resolution

15. The Q factor of a transducer is all the following EXCEPT

(A) the maximum intensity produced by the transducer
(B) a measure of the purity of the frequency
(C) high for Doppler ultrasound
(D) low for short pulse lengths
(E) ratio of the operating frequency to the bandwidth

16. A high Q transducer has a small

(A) focal zone
(B) Fresnel zone
(C) bandwidth
(D) diameter
(E) none of the above

17. The damping material behind the crystal transducer reduces the

(A) pulse frequency
(B) ring down time
(C) echo amplitude
(D) lateral resolution
(E) none of the above

18. An ultrasound beam with a short pulse length is most likely to result in an improved

(A) axial resolution
(B) lateral resolution
(C) echo intensity
(D) tissue penetration
(E) pulse repetition frequency

19. Time gain compensation (TGC) corrects for which of the following?

(A) Attenuation at gel skin interface
(B) Frequency change of moving objects
(C) Intensity decrease with tissue penetration
(D) Transducer damping material
(E) Image fading on cathode ray tube

20. In B-mode ultrasound, the pulse repetition frequency

(A) is typically 1000 Hz
(B) influences the frame rate
(C) influences the number of lines per frame
(D) determines the maximum penetration depth
(E) all of the above

21. In B-mode ultrasound, the choice of frequency is most likely to result in a trade off between patient penetration and

(A) contrast
(B) pulse repetition frequency
(C) noise
(D) lateral resolution
(E) axial resolution

22. Ultrasound signals are converted from digital data to a video monitor display using a

(A) log amplifier
(B) photomultiplier tube
(C) photocathode
(D) scan converter
(E) none of the above

23. Match the following ultrasound probes with the best single descriptor.

(A) Endorectal
(B) Phased array
(C) Annular array

(i) Is electronically steered
(ii) Can be steered horizontally and vertically
(iii) High frequency (limited range)

24. True (T) or False (F). Clinical ultrasound beams normally have

(A) intensities of 10 W/cm^2
(B) focal lengths of 3 mm
(C) negligible divergence in the Fraunhofer zone
(D) large numbers of discrete photons
(E) cavitation effects
(F) chromosome aberration effects

25. Match the following transducers with the most appropriate resolution performance.

(A) 2 MHz phased array real time
(B) 5 MHz linear array real time
(C) 10 MHz pulsed sector real time
(D) 3 MHz continuous wave doppler

(i) Superior axial resolution
(ii) Moderate axial resolution
(iii) Inferior axial resolution
(iv) No measure of resolution applicable

26. Ultrasound lateral resolution is affected by

(A) the number of scan lines
(B) focusing
(C) transducer diameter
(D) all of the above

27. True (T) or False (F). Ultrasound shadowing artifacts may be caused by reduced sound intensity behind

(A) any strong attenuator
(B) bone
(C) air
(D) water
(E) kidney–fat interface

28. All of the following may cause significant ultrasound artifacts EXCEPT

(A) reverberation
(B) side lobes
(C) non-specular reflections
(D) refraction

29. The frequency of the doppler shift depends on all of the following EXCEPT

(A) speed of ultrasound beam
(B) frequency
(C) angle between ultrasound beam and moving object
(D) depth of moving object
(E) speed of moving object

30. True (T) or False (F). In doppler studies

(A) changes in frequency are measured
(B) a low Q factor is desirable
(C) frequency shift is dependent on incident angle
(D) continuous doppler uses two transducers

Answers and Explanations

1. A–False; in air, the speed of sound is 330 m/sec but in tissue this increases to 1540 m/sec; **B–False;** ultrasound is not electromagnetic radiation; **C–False;** photons or charged particles can ionize atoms; **D–True;** there is no "medium" to propagate the wave motion; **E–True;** side lobes are emitted by most transducers; **F–True;** the displacement is along the direction of travel whereas electromagnetic waves are transverse since the displacement is perpendicular to the direction of the wave motion; **G–True;** the audible range for humans is 15 Hz to 20,000 Hz.

2–D. The velocity (v) of any wave is always equal to the product of the frequency (f) and wavelength (λ) [i.e., $v = f \times \lambda$].

3. A–ii; B–iii; C–i; D–iv; E–v.

4–A. Acoustic impedance is dependent on tissue density and is obtained using the equation $Z = \rho \times v$, where ρ is the tissue density and v is the velocity of sound in the tissue.

5. A–v; B–iii; C–iv; D–ii; E–i.

6. A–iii; B–ii; C–iv; D–v; E–i; acoustic impedance is the product of the density and velocity of sound.

7–A. Wavelength generally changes with medium since frequency will be the same, but velocity depends on the medium.

8–B. There is no mechanism for amplifying ultrasound beams in patients. Echoes from tissue interfaces, however, may be amplified by the system electronics.

9–D. The difference in acoustic impedance between the two tissues (Z_1, Z_2) determines the fraction (F) of incident energy reflected. For normal incidence, $F = (Z_2 - Z_1)^2/(Z_1 + Z_2)^2$.

10–A. Transmitted fraction is (1 – reflected fraction), and the reflected fraction is $(Z_1 - Z_2)^2/(Z_1 + Z_2)^2$.

11–E. There are no reflections from fluids in the bladder. Specular reflections occur from interfaces that are smooth relative to the ultrasound wavelength.

12–A. Snell's law describes the angle of refraction that occurs when an ultrasound beam passes from one medium to another.

13–A. Crystal thickness (t) is half the wavelength (λ) and therefore determines the frequency.

14–C. The attenuation in tissue is about 1 dB/cm at 1 MHz and increases approximately linearly with frequency.

15–A. Q has nothing to do with the intensity produced by the transducer, but with the range of frequencies generated.

16–C. The bandwidth is very narrow and the ultrasound pulse is relatively pure.

17–B. The ring down time is reduced and very short pulses of only two or three wavelengths are generated.

18–A. Axial resolution is generally equal to one half the pulse length.

19–C. TGC corrects for normal attenuation in tissue (~1 dB/cm @ 1 MHz).

20–E. All of the statements are true.

21–E. As frequency increases, the wavelength is reduced, which improves resolution but reduces patient penetration.

22–D. Scan converters convert the digital image data into a video signal that is displayed on a TV monitor.

23. A–iii; B–i; C–ii.

24. A–False; 1 to 10 mW/cm^2 are typical diagnostic intensities; **B–False;** short focal lengths would be 4 to 6 cm; **C–False;** the

Fraunhofer (far) zone is where beam divergence occurs and cannot reliably be used for imaging; **D–False;** x-ray beams have photons, which are "discrete"; **E–False;** high beam intensities are required to produce cavitation effects; **F–False;** ionizing radiation can induce chromosome breaks.

25. A–iii; lowest frequency has the longest wavelength and will thus have the longest pulse length and produce the worst axial resolution; **B–ii; C–i; D–iv;** with continuous wave doppler, there is no spatial information provided and hence spatial resolution cannot be quantified.

26–D. All of the factors listed may affect lateral resolution.

27. A–True; B–True; C–True; D–False; E–False; for the artifact to occur, there has to be a large loss of transmitted signal intensity caused by either attenuation or reflection.

28–C. Non-specular reflection will result in the beam being scattered in all directions and is unlikely to be the direct cause of image artifacts.

29–D. The depth of the moving object is immaterial.

30. A–True; B–False; pure frequencies are needed, which requires high Q values; **C–True;** the smaller the angle, the higher the frequency shift, and at 90 degrees there is no observed frequency shift at all; **D–True;** one transducer to transmit the ultrasound and the second to receive the echoes.

11

Magnetic Resonance (MR)

I. Basic Physics

A. Magnetic nuclei

- —As a result of their nuclear spin and charge distribution, protons and neutrons have a magnetic field called a **magnetic dipole**.
  - —Although neutrons have no net charge, they do have a charge distribution.
- —**Magnetic moment** is a vector that represents the strength and orientation of a magnetic dipole.
- —Nuclei with an even number of protons and neutrons have no net magnetic moment.
  - —The protons and neutrons pair up with their magnetic moments aligned in opposite directions and cancel each other.
- —Nuclei with an odd number of protons or neutrons have a net magnetic moment and behave like a bar magnet.
  - —These nuclei are candidates for magnetic resonance as listed in Table 11-1.
- —The hydrogen nucleus has the largest magnetic moment, and its abundance in the body makes it the basis of most clinical MR imaging (MRI).

B. Tissue magnetization

- —There are more than 10^{20} hydrogen protons in each cubic centimeter (cm^3) of tissue.
- —These protons are normally randomly oriented and, therefore, have no net magnetic moment (**magnetization vector**).
- —In a magnetic field, hydrogen nuclei (protons) may be orientated either **spin up** (i.e., aligned along the field) or **spin down** (i.e., aligned opposite to the field).
  - —Spin-down alignment has slightly more energy.
  - —A small excess of protons go into the spin-up alignment.
  - —The magnetic fields of the remaining spin-up and spin-down nuclei cancel.

Table 11-1. Nuclei Used for Magnetic Resonance

Nucleus	Clinical Uses	Natural Abundance (%)	Relative Sensitivity*
^{1}H	MRI, MRS	99.985	1.00
^{2}H	MRS	0.015	1.45×10^{-6}
^{19}F	MRI, MRS	100	0.833
^{23}Na	MRI, MRS	100	0.093
^{31}P	MRS	100	0.066

*Includes differences in natural abundance and innate sensitivity per nucleus.
MRI = magnetic resonance imaging; MRS = magnetic resonance spectroscopy.

—Any tissue placed in a large magnetic field therefore has a net **magnetization vector** of unpaired hydrogen protons aligned in the direction of the external field.
—Only the excess nuclei in the lower energy (spin up) state generate the MR signal.
  —This excess is approximately 3 per million proton nuclei at a magnetic field strength of 1 tesla (T).
—MR signals are weak and considerable technical ingenuity is required to maximize signal-to-noise ratios (SNRs).

C. Larmor frequency

—When magnetic moments are placed into a magnetic field, a torque causes the moments to perform a precession motion similar to a spinning top.
—The **Larmor frequency** (f_L) is the precession frequency (MHz) of nuclei in a magnetic field (B). $f_L = \gamma/2\pi \times B$. The gyromagnetic ration (γ) is a constant for any nucleus.
—Replacing the Larmor frequency (f_L) with the angular frequency (ω), where $\omega = 2\pi \times f_L$, allows the Larmor equation to be expressed as $\omega = \gamma \times B$.
—Protons have a Larmor frequency of 21 MHz at 0.5 tesla (T), 42 MHz at 1 T, and 63 MHz at 1.5 T.
—For comparison, ^{19}F has a Larmor frequency of 40 MHz at 1 T, and ^{23}Na has a Larmor frequency of 11 MHz at 1 T.

D. Resonance

—**Resonance** occurs when the net magnetization vector is perturbed from its equilibrium orientation.
—Electromagnetic radiation applied at the Larmor frequency (f_L) and perpendicular to the external magnetic field (z-axis) causes the magnetization vector to rotate out of alignment with the field toward the x-y plane.
  —This electromagnetic radiation is in the radio frequency (RF) part of the electromagnetic spectrum.
—The component of the net magnetization vector parallel to the magnetic field is called the **longitudinal magnetization**.
—The component perpendicular to the magnetic field is called the **transverse magnetization**.
—The rotation angle (flip angle) depends on the strength of the applied RF field and the total time that it is switched on (**pulse duration**).

–A **180-degree RF pulse** reorients the magnetization vector in a direction opposite to the external magnetic field.

–A **90-degree RF pulse** reorients the magnetization vector into the plane perpendicular to the external magnetic field.

–A 90-degree RF pulse takes half as long as a 180-degree RF pulse.

E. Free induction decay

–After a 90-degree RF pulse, each spin is aligned and the magnetization vector precesses at the Larmor frequency about the external magnetic field.

–This rotation gives rise to the **free induction decay (FID)** signal.

–FID signals can be detected as an oscillating voltage, at the Larmor frequency (f_L), in a receiver coil placed around the sample.

–The FID signal is weak because of the small number of nuclei that contribute to the signal (approximately 3 per 10^6) and the small size of the nuclear magnetic moments.

–The receiver coil may be the same as the RF transmitter coil.

–FID signals are detected, digitized, and, through use of reconstruction algorithms, used to generate MR images.

F. T1 relaxation

–Protons placed into a strong magnetic field produce a net magnetization (M) parallel to the magnetic field axis.

–This magnetization grows exponentially from the initial value of zero to the equilibrium value of M with a time constant T1.

–At time equal to T1, 63% of the signal has returned and at $3 \times$ T1, 95% has returned.

–Equilibrium at full magnetization M occurs after a time interval of $5 \times$ T1.

–If the field is switched off, magnetization M decays exponentially with the same time constant T1 (i.e., as $e^{-t/T1}$), where t is the elapsed time.

–T1 relaxation is called **longitudinal** or **spin-lattice relaxation**.

–Figure 11-1*A* shows the T1 relaxation curve for two different tissues.

–For most tissues, T1 times are a few hundred milliseconds (Table 11-2).

–T1 is long in small molecules like water and in large molecules like proteins.

–T1 is short in fats and in intermediate-sized molecules.

–Contrast agents such as gadolinium-DTPA can cause T1 shortening.

–In general, T1 increases with increasing magnetic field strength.

G. T2 relaxation

–After a 90-degree pulse, the magnetization vector rotates at the Larmor frequency in a plane perpendicular to the external magnetic field.

–The FID signal produced is proportional to the magnetization vector, which decays exponentially.

–In perfectly uniform magnetic fields, the decay rate constant is T2, and the induced FID signal decays as $e^{-t/T2}$.

–At a time equal to T2, the signal has decayed to 37% of its maximum.

–At $3 \times$ T2, the signal has decayed to 5%, and at approximately $5 \times$ T2, the signal has almost completely decayed.

–Figure 11-1*B* shows the T2 decay curves for two different tissues.

–T2 relaxation is called **transverse** or **spin–spin relaxation**.

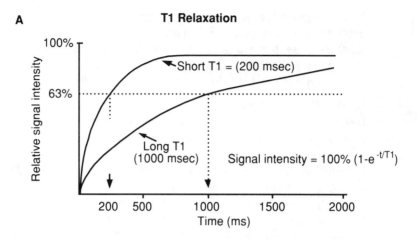

A   **T1 Relaxation**

Short T1 = (200 msec)

Long T1
(1000 msec)

Signal intensity = $100\% \ (1\text{-}e^{-t/T1})$

Relative signal intensity

Time (ms)

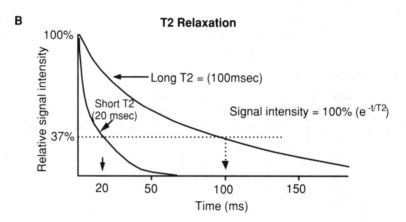

B   **T2 Relaxation**

Long T2 = (100msec)

Short T2
(20 msec)

Signal intensity = $100\% \ (e^{-t/T2})$

Relative signal intensity

Time (ms)

Figure 11-1. T1 and T2 relaxation times. **A,** The T1 relaxation is represented as return to equilibrium of the longitudinal component of magnetization. At time T1, the signal has grown to 63% of its maximum value. **B,** The T2 relaxation is represented as a decrease in the transverse component of magnetization due to dephasing. At time T2, the signal has decayed to 37% of its maximum.

       –For most tissues, T2 times are typically tens of milliseconds (see Table 11-2).

       –T2 increases with increasing molecular size and decreased molecular mobility.

       –Liquids generally have long T2 times, whereas large molecules and solids generally have short T2 times.

       –T2 has little apparent dependence on the magnetic field strength.

H. T2*

       –Normal magnets have magnetic field inhomogeneities of a few parts per million (ppm) or a few μT in fields of 1 T.

       –Decay in transverse magnetization caused by **spin dephasing** is a result of inhomogeneities in the main magnetic field.

       –Spins that are in slightly higher fields rotate slightly faster and vice versa, resulting in dephasing of the spins.

       –This dephasing results in a decrease in magnetization vector intensity.

Table 11-2. T1 and T2 Relaxation Times

Tissue	T1 (ms) at Field Strength of:		T2 (ms)
	0.5 T	1.5 T	
Fat (adipose)	200	260	80
Liver	320	490	45
Kidney	500	650	60
White matter	530	780	90
Spleen	540	780	60
Muscle	550	870	50
Grey matter	650	920	100
Cerebrospinal fluid	2000	2400	180

–The observed FID signal falls exponentially with a decay rate constant $T2^*$ (i.e., $e^{-t/T2^*}$).

–$T2^*$ is a few milliseconds and is much shorter than T2.

–Dephasing due to $T2^*$ may be overcome by generating echoes, whereas signal loss due to true T2 relaxation is irreversible.

–Materials such as paramagnetic and ferromagnetic contrast agents disrupt the local magnetic field homogeneity and shorten $T2^*$.

–For all tissues, $\mathbf{T2^* \leq T2 \leq T1}$.

II. Magnetic Resonance Instrumentation

A. Magnets

–Powerful magnets capable of generating strong, stable, spatially uniform magnetic fields are essential for MRI.

–Magnetic fields are measured in tesla (T), where 1 T = 10,000 gauss (G).

–The Earth's magnetic field is weak (50 μT, or 0.5 G).

–To perform MRI, the magnetic field must have a high homogeneity of approximately 1 ppm.

  –**Shim coils** superimpose small corrective field differences on the main field to improve the magnetic field uniformity.

–The large whole-body magnets used in MRI scanners may be **resistive, permanent,** or **superconducting**.

  –Permanent magnets have low operating costs and small fringe fields, but are heavy and can only generate fields up to approximately 0.35 T.

  –Resistive magnets can generate magnetic fields up to approximately 0.5 T.

  –Resistive magnets can be turned on and off, but consume a large amount of power and need cooling because of the heat generated.

–As MRI field strength increases, so does the T1 relaxation time, SNR, image artifacts, and RF energy deposition in the patient.

B. Superconducting magnets

–The best MR images are achieved at field strengths higher than those of resistive and permanent magnets.

  –Field strengths of 2 T or higher can be generated by superconducting magnets.

–**Superconductivity** is the ability of certain materials to conduct electrical current without any resistance.

–Superconductors use a wire-wrapped cylinder (i.e., a solenoid) to generate the magnetic field.

–Superconducting magnets are generally kept cool using liquid helium (4.2°K) surrounded by liquid nitrogen (77°K).

  –A constant electric current creates the magnetic field, which is on at all times.

–If the temperature of the magnet rises, the system loses its superconducting properties and the resultant power dissipation causes the magnet to **quench**.

–Figure 11-2 is a cutaway view of a superconducting MR imaging system.

C. Gradient coils

–Magnetic gradients are used to code the spatial location of the MR signal and are essential for generating MR images.

–MRI systems have magnetic field gradients in the z, x, and y orientations.

  –When activated, these gradients superimpose a small field gradient on the main magnetic field.

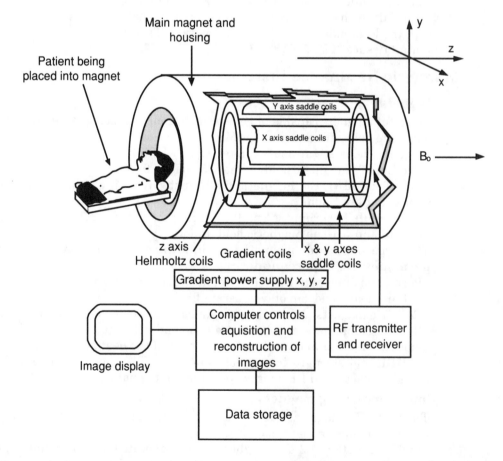

Figure 11-2. Superconducting magnetic resonance system showing the main magnetic field (Bo) produced by the superconducting magnet, which is cooled by helium and nitrogen. Three paired coils apply the gradients. An RF coil transmits and receives the RF signal.

—With gradients superimposed on the main magnetic field, each magnetic field value corresponds to a slightly different Larmor frequency, which alters the precession frequency of nuclei in this specific region.

—Combinations of the three sets of gradients allow the gradient field to be oriented in any direction.

—Gradient strengths range from 1 to 10 mT/m (0.1 to 1 G/cm).

—Axial gradients (z) are produced using **Helmholtz coils**.

—Figure 11-3 shows a pair of Helmholtz coils being used to produce a gradient along the z-axis for section selection.

—Gradients in the perpendicular plane are normally produced by **saddle coils**.

—Gradients may need to be switched on and off rapidly (within less than 500 μs).

—Gradients generate small, rapidly decaying eddy currents in other coils or metal structures nearby; these currents impair scanner performance and may create image artifacts.

D. Radio frequency coils

—RF is electromagnetic radiation with frequencies in the range of approximately 1 MHz to 10 GHz.

—Transmitter coils are used to generate RF pulses. The same or separate coils are used as receivers to detect FID signals from the patient.

—RF coils maximize the **SNR** of the weak FID signals.

  —Small coils generally increase the SNR but restrict the region or volume being imaged.

  —The SNR may also be improved by using special coils designed for particular anatomic regions.

—Surface coils are simple loops placed directly on the region of interest.

  —**Surface coils** have increased sensitivity, but the detected signal intensity falls off rapidly with distance from the coil.

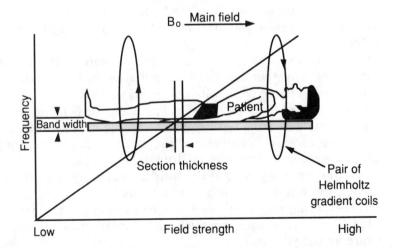

Figure 11-3. Section selection along the z-axis using a pair of Helmholtz gradient coils which superimpose a magnetic field on the main field. The resultant variation in Larmor frequency along the gradient allows a section of tissue perpendicular to the gradient to be selected.

Table 11-3. Limiting Fields Close to Magnets

Field Limit (mT)	Object
0.5 (5 G)	Pacemakers, cathode ray tubes
1 (10 G)	Credit cards, watches
2 (20 G)	Floppy disks
5 (50 G)	Power supplies

–RF coils include **quadrature coils** and **phased array coils,** which generally improve SNR performance and may also increase the field of view (FOV).

E. Shielding

–The **magnetic flux lines** from the main magnetic field can extend out to a large distance from the magnet.

–The peripheral magnetic field is called the **fringe field,** and can affect magnetically sensitive devices (Table 11-3).

–Large metallic objects (e.g., elevators and ferromagnetic structures) can disrupt the uniformity of the main magnetic field and degrade MR image quality.

–**Magnetic shielding** usually consists of steel plates placed around the MR magnet.

–MRI units also require **RF shielding** to prevent powerful RF signals from escaping and interfering with electronic equipment.

 –The RF shielding is a **faraday cage,** which consists of copper wire mesh or plates surrounding the MR imager or room.

 –RF shielding is also essential in limiting outside interference from sources such as radio broadcasts.

F. Magnetic resonance hazards

–Detrimental biological effects from exposure to static magnetic fields are not evident below 10 T. Static fields, however, have been known to augment the T-wave amplitude on electrocardiograms.

–One of the greatest potential hazards around a magnet is the **missile effect**.

 –Ferromagnetic objects such as pens, scissors, screwdrivers, oxygen cylinders, and other metallic devices may be pulled into the magnet.

–Pacemakers may be deactivated by magnetic fields.

–Because of the torque produced by the magnetic field, hazards also exist for patients who have ferromagnetic devices implanted in their bodies, including cerebral aneurysm clips, cochlear implants, shrapnel, implanted electrodes, and internal drug infusion pumps.

–The **time-varying magnetic fields** created by the gradients are of greater concern than static magnetic fields.

 –Time-varying magnetic fields induce currents in the patient and can induce mild cutaneous sensations, involuntary muscle contractions, and cardiac arrhythmias.

 –Looped wires on the patient's skin can heat up and cause burns.

 –Time-varying magnetic fields can also produce magnetophosphenes (light flashes).

Table 11-4. Food and Drug Administration Guidelines for Magnetic Field and RF Power Levels Below Level of Concern

Parameter	Limit	Comment
Static fields	2 T*	Several 4 T whole-body systems are in use
Rate of change of magnetic field	dB /dt < 3 T/s*	Prevents peripheral nerve stimulation
Average limit for RF specific absorption rate	< 0.4 W/kg < 3.2 W/kg < 8 W/kg	Whole body Head Any gram of tissue
Core body temperature rise	< 1°C	< 38°C in head < 39°C in body < 40°C in extremities (local heating)

*In general, use above these levels requires additional evidence of safety.

G. Magnetic resonance safety

- —There are no hazards beyond the 0.5 mT (5 G) fringe field of an MR magnet.
    - —General access is restricted in areas having magnetic fields above 0.5 mT (5 G).
    - —Warning signs must be posted in areas having magnetic fields above 1.5 mT (15 G).
- —The measure of **dose** of RF fields is the **specific absorption rate (SAR)** in watts per kilogram (W/kg) and is a measure of power absorbed per unit of mass, or tissue.
    - —Absorption of RF power can increase tissue temperature. Limits are imposed on the average and maximum power deposition rates in any gram of tissue, and on the rise in tissue temperature.
- —Food and Drug Administration (FDA) guidelines for magnet and RF power levels are listed in Table 11-4.
- —The noise level in MR systems ranges from 65 to 95 dB, and there have been anecdotal reports of hearing loss.

III. Magnetic Resonance Imaging

A. Magnetic resonance signal localization

- —Signal localization for image construction is based on adding a magnetic field gradient onto the main (constant) magnetic field.
- —Along the gradient, a unique magnetic field strength corresponds to each location.
- —Each specific field strength (location) corresponds to a specific Larmor frequency in the detected signal.
- —A frequency analysis of the MR signal permits the origin of each signal to be determined.
- —To identify the location of the MR signal, frequency analysis of FID signals is performed using Fourier techniques.
- —Image reconstruction is performed digitally by computers using two-dimensional Fourier transform reconstruction algorithms.

B. Two-dimensional image formation

- —Pulse sequences are repeated n times using a repetition time interval of TR to obtain phase-encoding.

–The number of **phase-encoding steps** (n) determines the number of pixels in the y-direction, with n typically ranging from 128 to 256.

–The number of pixels in the x-direction is related to the **frequency-encoding gradient** and is typically 256.

–For a constant FOV, increasing the number of pixels in the x-direction increases resolution and reduces signal strength.

–The total time to complete an imaging sequence is $N_{ex} \times n \times TR$, where n is the number of phase-encoding steps, TR is the repetition time, and N_{ex} is the number of acquisitions taken.

  –For a typical sequence of TR = 500 ms, N_{ex} = 2, and n = 128, imaging time is 128 seconds (approximately 2 minutes).

–Multiple images are usually obtained during an acquisition by exciting several sections during each TR interval in an interleaved fashion.

C. **Magnetic resonance pulse sequences**

–Diverse **pulse sequences** are used to generate signal intensities from a given region.

–Pulse sequences are the **strength, order, duration,** and **repetition of RF pulses** and **magnetic gradients** used to generate an image.

–The most commonly used pulse sequences in clinical imaging are **spin echo (SE), inversion recovery (IR),** and **gradient recalled echo (GRE).**

–The pulse sequence chosen determines the type of contrast observed in the resultant MR image.

  –Image contrast is markedly influenced by tissue differences in T1, T2, and proton density.

D. **Spin echo**

–**SE** pulse sequences commence with 90-degree pulses to rotate the magnetization vector into the transverse plane where the magnetization rapidly dephases (T2* effects).

–**Spin rephasing** is achieved by using a 180-degree RF pulse at a time TE/2 that generates a SE at time **TE (echo time).**

–The intensity of the SE at time TE is reduced by a factor of $e^{-TE/T2}$ due to T2 effects.

–The 180-degree pulse can be repeated to generate **multiple echoes** with progressively longer TE values.

–The sequence is repeated with a **repetition time (TR),** which is the time interval between successive 90-degree pulses.

–For TR values less than $5 \times T1$, the tissue magnetization vector is unable to fully recover after a 90-degree pulse.

  –An equilibrium tissue magnetization vector size is generally reached after a few successive 90-degree pulses; the size of this magnetization is reduced in intensity for longer T1 values.

–Figure 11-4A shows the specific components of a spin echo pulse sequence.

E. **Spin echo weighting**

–SE sequences can be modified to emphasize T1 differences (T1 weighting), T2 differences (T2 weighting), or proton density differences.

–T1-weighted images are obtained with a short TR (less than 600 ms) to emphasize T1 differences and a short TE (less than 20 ms) to minimize T2 differences.

A Spin echo

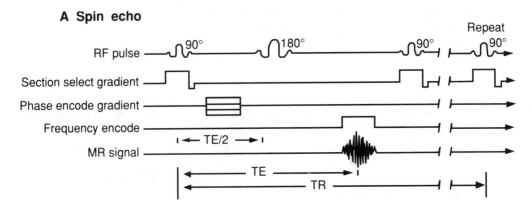

B Inversion recovery

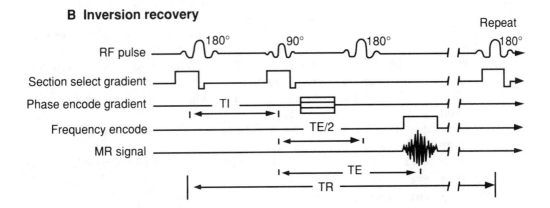

Figure 11-4. Spin echo and inversion recovery pulse sequences.

–Short T1 tissues have a high signal intensity because of their complete relaxation.

–T2-weighted images are obtained with a long TR (more than 2000 ms) to minimize T1 differences, because all tissues exhibit full relaxation, and a long TE (more than 90 ms) to emphasize T2 differences.

–For long TEs, tissues with long T2s appear bright, and tissues with short T2s appear dark.

–Proton density weighted images are obtained with a long TR (more than 2000 ms) to minimize T1 differences and a short TE (less than 20 ms) to minimize T2 differences.

–Table 11-5 summarizes the influence of TE and TR times on the type of contrast obtained in MR images.

F. Fast spin echo

–**Fast spin echo (FSE)** techniques resemble multiecho SE sequences but change the phase-encoding gradients for each echo.

–In FSE, the number of repeat pulses separated by time TR is greatly reduced with a corresponding reduction in imaging time.

–FSE shortens acquisition time by applying multiple phase-encoding steps and 180-degree echoes after every 90-degree pulse.

Table 11-5. Effects of TE and TR Parameters on Spin Echo Images

	Short TE	Long TE
Short TR	T1 weighted	Mixed
Long TR	Proton density	T2 weighted

–T1-weighted images acquired in this way have more T2 weighting than conventional SE images.

–Compared to conventional SE imaging, FSE techniques decrease the number of interleaved slices that can be obtained because there is a greater fraction of the TR interval used to obtain MR signals.

G. Inversion recovery

–**Inversion recovery (IR)** uses 180-degree pulses to invert the magnetization vector.

–The longitudinal magnetization vector recovers with a time constant T1, and complete recovery occurs after a time of $5 \times$ T1.

–The 180-degree pulse is followed by a 90-degree (readout) pulse after time TI (inversion time) to flip the relaxed spins into the transverse plane.

–A second 180-degree pulse at time TE/2 produces an echo at time TE, which is the detected signal intensity.

–The size of the signal obtained with the readout pulse is strongly dependent on the value of T1 and TI.

–IR emphasizes T1 differences, and tissues with short T1 values produce high-intensity signals.

–Figure 11-4*B* shows the specific components of an inversion recovery pulse sequence.

H. Gradient recalled echoes

–Gradient recalled echo techniques make use of short TRs, short TEs, and low flip angles.

  –This combination permits fast acquisition times and permits three-dimensional imaging within reasonable times.

  –Sequences may use TRs of only 5 ms, and 256 acquisitions can be acquired in 1.3 seconds.

–GRE imaging relies on reversing the polarity of the magnetic field gradients instead of 180-degree refocusing of RF pulses to generate echoes.

  –This is accomplished by reversing the polarity of the magnetic gradient to rephase the spins and generate an echo FID signal.

–Short TE values emphasize T1 differences between tissues.

–Examples of fast imaging include fast low-angle shot (FLASH), fast imaging with steady state precession (FISP), and gradient recalled acquisition in the steady state (GRASS).

  –Parameters can be adjusted to emphasize blood flow and, therefore, angiographic images can be constructed.

I. Three-dimensional imaging

–Three-dimensional Fourier transform (3DFT) imaging techniques are possible to image relatively small volumes such as knees.

–In three-dimensional imaging, two sets of orthogonal phase-encoding gradients are used in addition to the frequency encoding gradient.

–A nonselective RF pulse simultaneously excites the entire sample volume.

–A 3DFT is applied along all three axes for image reconstruction.

–After the volume data are reconstructed, two-dimensional images in any selected plane can be constructed.

–Three-dimensional imaging times are $N_{ex} \times n_1 \times n_2 \times TR$, where n_1 is the number of phase-encoding steps in one plane and n_2 is the number in the orthogonal plane.

–Disadvantages of 3DFT techniques include longer acquisition times and susceptibility to motion artifacts.

–Advantages of 3DFT include the high resolution in all three orientations and the availability of contiguous sections.

IV. Image Quality

A. Magnetic resonance images

–MR images typically have matrix sizes of 128×256, 192×256, 256×256, or 256×512 pixels.

–Each pixel needs 12 to 16 bits to code the pixel intensity level, which is achieved using 2 Bytes.

–MR images have image contents ranging from 0.06 to 0.25 MB.

–The MR imaging parameters selected determine the trade-offs that influence contrast, noise, resolution, and acquisition time.

–Regular quality control (QC) measurements should be taken to ensure that the MR system is functioning optimally.

–QC tests may measure section thickness, resolution, SNR, field uniformity, gradient linearity, spatial distortion, and image contrast.

B. Image contrast

–Contrast in MR images depends on the type of MR imaging pulse sequence used and on tissue characteristics such as differences in T1 and T2 relaxation times.

–Tissues with short T1 values appear bright on T1-weighted images.

–Tissues with long T2 values appear bright on T2-weighted images.

–Proton density weighted images demonstrate little intrinsic contrast because of the small variations (approximately 10%) in proton density for most tissues.

–Flow can also affect image contrast and is the basis for MR angiography (MRA).

–Image contrast may be modified by the administration of contrast agents such as gadolinium-DTPA.

C. Signal-to-noise ratio

–The inherent contrast of MR is high because of the large differences in the relaxation properties of different tissues.

–The **SNR** affects the acquired image quality.

–The SNR is increased by increasing slice thickness, decreasing matrix size, and reducing RF bandwidth.

–High magnetic fields also increase the SNR.

–SNR increases as the square root of the number of image acquisitions $\sqrt{N_{ex}}$.

–The trade-off for increased SNR and the resultant improved image quality is an increase in imaging time.

D. Resolution

–The spatial resolution achieved on MR systems is determined by the FOV and matrix size, which is typically 128^2 to 256^2.

–Pixel size equals the FOV divided by the matrix size and is approximately 1 mm for head images and 1.4 mm for body images.

–MR resolution is approximately one half to one fourth of that achieved by computed tomography and is usually no better than approximately 0.3 line pairs per millimeter.

–Higher resolution may be achieved by using stronger gradients and more phase-encoding steps.

–The trade-offs for improved resolution include loss of signal intensity and increases in image acquisition time.

E. Magnetic resonance artifacts

–Artifacts are areas of high or low signal intensity or distortion in the image that can simulate or mask anatomic structures or pathologic conditions such as when truncation artifacts in the spinal cord simulate a syrinx.

–To minimize or overcome MR artifacts, their origin must be understood.

–It is important to be able to differentiate MR artifacts from both normal anatomy and pathologic condition.

F. Chemical shift artifacts

–Chemical shift artifacts are caused by the slight difference in resonance frequency of protons in water and in fat.

–Molecular structure and local magnetic environment differences cause protons in fat and water to have slightly different resonance frequencies.

–This difference is noticeable at fat/water interfaces with high magnetic field strength and results in misregistration of the signal from the two proton groups.

–Chemical shift artifacts can result in light and dark bands at the edges of the kidney or the margins of vertebral bodies.

G. Miscellaneous artifacts

–**Patient motion** is common because of the long image acquisition times.

–Patient motion results in **ghost images** that normally appear in the phase-encode direction due to mismapping of measured signals.

–Respiratory gating or phase reordering may be used to minimize motion artifacts in body imaging.

–Flowing blood and cerebrospinal fluid also result in MR image artifacts.

–Inhomogeneities in the main magnetic field have a significant impact on GRE and other fast imaging techniques.

–**Aliasing** or **wrap around** artifact occurs when the FOV is smaller than the structure, and imaged objects outside the FOV are mapped to the opposite side of the image.

–Aliasing is generally caused by nonlinearities in field gradients or undersampling of the acquired image data.

–There are many other sources of MR artifacts, including **truncation, zipper,** and **central point**.

V. Magnetic Resonance Contrast Agents

A. Introduction

–Contrast agents may result in image enhancement in anatomic regions that are perfused by these agents.

–**Paramagnetism, superparamagnetism,** and **ferromagnetism** all act as sources of local magnetic field inhomogeneity.

–These types of materials produce **spin relaxation** and may be used as contrast agents.

–Contrast agents that reduce T1 more than T2 produce hyperintensity on T1-weighted images and are called **positive contrast agents**.

–Contrast agents that reduce T2 more than T1 produce hypointensity on T2-weighted images and are called **negative contrast agents**.

B. Diamagnetism

–**Magnetic susceptibility** is the extent to which matter becomes magnetized when placed in an external magnetic field (B).

–The local (internal) magnetic field is $B \times (1 + \chi)$, where χ is the susceptibility.

–**Diamagnetic** materials result in small decreases in magnetization relative to the external field and, therefore, have small **negative values of susceptibility**.

–Most tissues are diamagnetic with a negative χ in the range 10^{-4} to 10^{-6}.

–At tissue interfaces, especially between air and bone, changes in magnetic susceptibility result in changes in the local field, which may result in imaging artifacts.

C. Paramagnetism

–Paramagnetism is caused by the presence of **unpaired atomic electrons** or molecular electrons.

–When paramagnetic atoms are placed in an external magnetic field, the local (internal) magnetic field is increased.

–Paramagnetic materials thus have **positive values of susceptibility,** which are typically approximately 10^{-3}.

–Paramagnetism has a much larger effect than diamagnetism and results in an enhancement of the local (internal) field.

–Paramagnetism occurs with chelates of metals such as Cr, Fe, Mn, Co, Cu, Gd, and Dy, as well as with molecular oxygen.

D. Ferromagnetism

–Ferromagnetism is a property of a **large group of atoms**, whereas diamagnetism and paramagnetism are properties of individual atoms or molecules.

–The group of atoms in ferromagnetic substances is called a **domain**.

–Ferromagnetic substances such as iron, nickel, and cobalt have unpaired electrons that are strongly coupled, resulting in large local fields and **high positive susceptibilities**.

–Ferromagnetic materials generally consist of large numbers of domains whose relative orientations depend on the external magnetic fields.

–Ferromagnets may have residual magnetization even after the external field is removed.

E. Superparamagnetism

–Small particles of Fe_3O_4, less than approximately 350 Å and thus consisting of a **single domain,** are termed superparamagnetic.

–When placed in an external magnetic field, superparamagnetic particles develop a strong internal magnetization.

–Superparamagnetism differs from ferromagnetism in that superparamagnets have a single domain, no magnetic memory, and a moderate degree of induced magnetism.

–Superparamagnetic crystals of iron oxide are used for imaging the liver and reticuloendothelial system.

F. Contrast agents

–**Gadolinium-DTPA** is an example of a **paramagnetic contrast agent**.

–Gadolinium has **seven unpaired electrons** with magnetic moments approximately 1000 times stronger than the proton magnetic moment.

–Gadolinium acts as a relaxation agent of nearby protons and reduces T1 significantly and T2 slightly. The overall effect is highly dependent on the concentration of gadolinium.

–Contrast agents under investigation include complexes of transition elements and rare earth elements such as iron and manganese.

–Contrast agents are useful for evaluating blood–brain barrier breakdown and renal lesions.

VI. Advanced Magnetic Resonance Techniques

A. Flow effects

–Flowing blood changes position between excitation by the RF pulses and signal reception, resulting in signal void on SE images.

–The opposite phenomenon is known as **entry slice enhancement,** which occurs when unsaturated protons enter the first section and generate a greater signal intensity than stationary, partially saturated tissues.

–Depending on the sequences used, signal is affected by the direction, speed, and pattern of blood flow.

–In GRE imaging, the presence of unsaturated protons produces high signal from moving fluid.

–The degree of enhancement depends on the TR, slice thickness, and flow velocity.

B. Magnetic resonance angiography

–Noninvasive MRA is quickly being established in the clinical setting.

–MRA techniques include time of flight and phase contrast.

–**Time of flight** techniques rely on bright signal from unsaturated protons in flowing blood entering the imaging section.

–**Phase contrast** techniques use bipolar gradients to produce phase changes in moving blood.

  –The surrounding tissues, which are stationary, exhibit no net phase change.

–The phase change is related to the time between bipolar gradients and flow velocity, which provides a correlation between signal intensity and blood flow velocity.

–MRA images are produced by projecting the stack of sections onto a single two-dimensional image because display of tortuous blood vessels is inadequate on thin-section images.

–MRA is useful in patients who cannot tolerate iodinated contrast agents.

C. Echo planar imaging

–**Echo planar imaging (EPI)** uses rapidly switching gradients to refocus echoes.

–Frequency-encode gradients that rapidly change polarities are paired with an applied phase-encode gradient.

–EPI can generate MR images in 50 ms but with limited resolution (64^2 or 128^2 matrix) and poor signal-to-noise ratio.

–Special gradients with values of 20 to 40 mT/m (2 to 4 G/cm) are required to perform EPI.

D. Magnetization transfer

–**Magnetization transfer contrast (MTC)** techniques modulate image contrast by saturating a pool of protons in macromolecules and their associated bound water.

–Narrow band RF pulses, shifted slightly away from the water resonance frequency, are used to selectively excite the protons in macromolecules.

–Some of this magnetization is transferred from the macromolecules to water. These water molecules, which have a modified signal intensity, are then imaged using conventional MR pulse sequences.

–MTC is useful in reducing background signal in MRA and may also have applications in breast imaging.

E. Fat suppression

–Fat suppression techniques are used to eliminate unwanted signals from fat in breast and brain imaging.

–Fat suppression techniques work best on high field systems with good uniformity.

–Fat suppression may be accomplished using variations of the chemical shift selection pulse sequences.

F. Magnetic resonance spectroscopy

–**MR spectroscopy (MRS)** makes use of the slight difference in resonance frequency of protons or other nuclei bound in different molecular structures.

–^{1}H and ^{31}P are the nuclei most often used for spectroscopy.

–Phosphorus spectroscopy can be used to evaluate cellular metabolism by identifying the relative concentration of inorganic phosphate, phosphocreatine, and adenosine triphosphate.

–MRS requires a stronger and more uniform field than conventional hydrogen imaging.

–A typical minimum voxel size used in MRS studies is approximately 1 cm^3 for ^1H and 8 cm^3 for ^{31}P.

–MRS is a research tool and has not yet been introduced into routine clinical practice.

G. Functional imaging

–**Functional imaging** relies on local physiologic changes in the brain associated with activation of visual, motor, auditory, or other brain system.

–Cerebral stimulation of specific regions of the brain increases local venous blood oxygenation. This enhances the detected MR signal intensity from regions with increased blood flow.

–Functional images are obtained from the difference of images obtained before and during the cerebral stimulation.

–Functional imaging maps the areas of cerebral stimulation with better temporal and spatial resolution than positron emission tomography.

–Functional imaging is best performed at high field strengths (2 T or higher) using EPI.

–Functional imaging is likely to become a powerful research tool in brain research.

Review Test

1. True (T) or False (F). The following nuclei have been used in biomedical MR.

(A) ^{18}F
(B) ^{19}F
(C) ^{23}Na
(D) ^{31}P
(E) ^{32}P
(F) ^{40}K

2. The Larmor frequency is the

(A) pulse repetition frequency
(B) nuclear precession frequency
(C) phase encoding frequency
(D) spatial encoding frequency
(E) none of the above

3. The gyromagnetic ratio depends on the

(A) magnetic field strength
(B) flip angle
(C) type of nucleus
(D) RF pulse duration
(E) longitudinal relaxation

4. True (T) or False (F). For most tissues

(A) T1 is of the order of a few seconds
(B) T2 is of the order of tens of ms
(C) T2 < T2*
(D) T2 is relatively independent of field strength
(E) T1 increases as field strength increases
(F) T1 and T2 often increase with malignancy

5. Cortical bone in MR has

(A) long T1
(B) short T2
(C) no detectable free induction decay (FID) signal
(D) proton nuclei
(E) all of the above

6. Following a 90-degree RF pulse

(A) spins dephase with a time constant T1
(B) after a time T2, an echo occurs
(C) magnetization is parallel to the external field
(D) FID signal can be observed at time T1
(E) in time $5 \times$ T1 the initial magnetization has recovered

7. Match the following approximate magnetic field strength with the appropriate source.

(A) 50 μT
(B) 0.3 T
(C) 1 T
(D) 4 T

(i) Typical superconducting magnet
(ii) Highest field strength whole body MRI
(iii) Earth's magnetic field
(iv) Typical permanent magnet

8. The superconducting magnets used in MR normally have

(A) no magnetic field inhomogeneities
(B) water cooling to dissipate heat production
(C) coils with alternating electric currents (AC)
(D) magnetic fields perpendicular to the bore axis
(E) none of the above

9. Gradient fields in MRI are used most commonly to

(A) maintain uniform magnetic fields
(B) localize sources of MRI signals
(C) shorten T1 values
(D) increase the signals from larger body depths
(E) all of the above

10. MR "shimming" is used to

(A) minimize the noise in RF coils
(B) correct for magnetic field inhomogeneities
(C) reduce the noise level in MRI systems
(D) minimize the possibility of quenches
(E) none of the above

11. Which of the following is acceptable for MRI at 1.5 T?

(A) Chochlear implants
(B) Pacemakers
(C) Ferromagnetic aneurysm clips
(D) Claustrophobic patients
(E) None of the above

12. All of the following items may be adversely affected by stray magnetic fields from an MRI system EXCEPT

(A) cardiac pacemakers
(B) image intensifiers
(C) optical disks
(D) computer displays
(E) floppy disks

13. Match the most appropriate MRI imaging method with the listed characteristics.

(A) Spin echo imaging
(B) Gradient echo imaging
(C) 2DFT imaging
(D) 3DFT imaging

(i) 1 phase encoding gradient is used
(ii) 2 phase encoding gradients are used
(iii) Flip angles less than 90 degrees used
(iv) Echo is generated by a 180-degree RF pulse

14. In inversion recovery sequences, the TI value is the time

(A) of the complete scan
(B) to the interval echo
(C) between successive 90-degree pulses
(D) between successive 180-degree pulses
(E) between a 180-degree and subsequent 90-degree pulse

15. In spin echo imaging, the FID signal normally is measured after

(A) the initial 180-degree pulse
(B) a time TE
(C) time $5 \times T1$
(D) time T2
(E) an interval TR

16. Match the following spin echo sequences.

(A) T1 weighted
(B) T2 weighted
(C) Proton density
(D) T1 and T2 weighted

(i) TR = 500 ms, TE = 20 ms
(ii) TR = 500 ms, TE = 90 ms
(iii) TR = 2000 ms, TE = 90 ms
(iv) TR = 2000 ms, TE = 20 ms

17. Increased signal intensity in MRI CANNOT arise as a result of

(A) short T1
(B) long T2
(C) flow effects
(D) flip angles larger than 90 degrees
(E) dephasing effects

18. Slow-flowing blood on conventional spin echo MRI sequences will normally appear

(A) bright on the initial section
(B) bright on all sections
(C) dark on the initial section
(D) dark on all sections

19. MRI signal-to-noise ratio (SNR) can be improved by

(A) switching from a body to a head coil
(B) increasing the number of acquisitions
(C) increasing the static magnetic field strength
(D) increasing the section thickness
(E) all of the above

20. Chemical shift artifacts are caused by differences in the

(A) T1 relaxation time
(B) T2 relaxation time
(C) spin density
(D) Larmor frequency
(E) atomic number

21. All the following are artifacts in MRI EXCEPT

(A) chemical shift
(B) flow
(C) motion
(D) beam hardening
(E) aliasing

22. Contrast in MRI may be due to all the following differences EXCEPT

(A) presence of flow
(B) proton density
(C) T1 relaxation times
(D) atomic number
(E) T2 relaxation times

23. Match the following magnetic susceptibility values with the appropriate effect.

(A) − 10^{-5}
(B) + 10^{-3}
(C) > + 1

(i) Ferromagnetism
(ii) Diamagnetism
(iii) Paramagnetism

24. Superparamagnetic materials

(A) are small particles (< 350 Å)
(B) only have single domains
(C) develop strong internal magnetism in an external field
(D) are related to ferromagnetic materials
(E) all of the above

25. Proton relaxation by Gd-DTPA is due mainly to the effect of the

(A) Gd nucleus
(B) DTPA
(C) unpaired Gd electrons
(D) Gd K-edge energy
(E) none of the above

26. The paramagnetic contrast agent used in MRI increases tissue

(A) resonance frequency
(B) T2
(C) T1
(D) diffusion
(E) spin relaxation

27. Common magnetic resonance angiography (MRA) techniques are based on

(A) phase contrast
(B) phase encoding
(C) T1 contrast
(D) time-to-inversion
(E) none of the above

28. Echo planar imaging generally requires all of the following EXCEPT

(A) gradient-recalled echoes
(B) gradients between 20 and 40 mT/m
(C) rapid gradient switching
(D) high magnetic fields (> 0.3 T)
(E) rapid sequence of 64 or 128 180-degree RF pulses

29. True (T) or False (F). MR spectroscopy can

(A) use ^{32}P
(B) measure phosphorus metabolites
(C) create images of each chemical form of phosphorus
(D) obtain spectra from volumes as small as 0.1 mm^3
(E) detect phosphocreatinine using ^{31}P

30. Functional imaging using magnetic resonance shows

(A) brain activation sites
(B) increased venous oxygenation
(C) superior temporal resolution to PET
(D) superior spatial resolution to PET
(E) all of the above

Answers and Explanations

1. A–False; ^{18}F is a positron emitter used in positron emission tomography; **B–True;** ^{19}F has been used mainly for imaging; **C–True;** ^{23}Na has been used to generate images of Na distribution in the head; **D–True;** ^{31}P is used mainly in spectroscopy; **E–False;** ^{32}P is a pure beta emitter used in biological research; **F–False;** ^{40}K is a naturally occurring radioactive material found in humans.

2–B. Magnetic nuclei precess at the Larmor frequency when placed into a magnetic field.

3–C. The nucleus determines the gyromagnetic ratio (equal to 42 MHz/tesla for protons).

4. A–False; T1 is of the order of hundreds of ms; **B–True; C–False;** T2* includes the effects of T2, and therefore cannot be longer than T2; **D–True; E–True;** T1 values increase by about 50% when the field increases from 0.5 T to 1.5 T; **F–True;** due to increased water content.

5–E. All of the statements are true. Bone results in no *detectable* signal because the very short T2 associated with all solids means the FID dephases very rapidly. T1s for solids are generally very long.

6–E. After the 90-degree pulse, the spins dephase with a time constant T2*, initial magnetization is recovered with time constant of T1, and the initial value is restored after about $5 \times$ T1.

7. A–iii; 50 µT (0.5 gauss) is the strength of the earth's magnetic field; **B–iv; C–i;** most superconducting magnets used in commercial scanners are in the range of 0.5 to 1.5 T; **D–ii;** a small number of 4 T whole-body systems are currently being used for research.

8–E. None of the statements are true.

9–B. Gradients define the MR image plane and are used for frequency and phase encoding to determine the spatial origin of the detected signals.

10–B. Shimming is used to reduce field inhomogeneities to a few parts per million.

11–E. None are acceptable for MRI scans. Claustrophobic patients may be scanned on some "open" low field systems, but superconducting magnets are required to achieve 1.5 T.

12–C. Optical disks do not contain magnetic media and are not affected by magnetic fields.

13. A–iv; B–iii; C–i; D–ii.

14–E. An inversion recovery sequence starts with a 180-degree inversion pulse followed by a 90-degree readout pulse after time TI.

15–B. A phase-refocusing 180-degree pulse is applied at time TE/2, which results in the FID echo at time TE.

16. A–i; B–iii; C–iv; D–ii.

17–E. Dephasing effects reduce signal intensities (they may increase contrast, but not signal intensity).

18–A. The initial section appears bright due to the entry section phenomenon.

19–E. All of the methods listed will improve the SNR ratio.

20–D. Chemical shifts arise from the differing Larmor frequencies of nuclei in differing chemical structures, such as protons in water and fat molecules.

21–D. Beam-hardening artifacts occur in CT, not MRI.

22–D. Atomic number (Z) does not give rise to image contrast in MR, but does give rise to image contrast in x-ray imaging.

23. A–ii; B–iii; C–i.

24–E. All the listed items are generally true.

25–C. The seven unpaired electrons in Gd result in the relaxation of adjacent nuclei.

26–E. The large magnetic moments of contrast agents such as Gd increase relaxation rates (shorten T1 and T2).

27–A. Phase contrast and time-of-flight are the two common methods used in MRA.

28–E. No MRI sequences require such a rapid set of RF pulses.

29. A–False; ^{32}P is radioactive and used in biochemical research; ^{31}P is used in MR; **B–True; C–True;** images may be created of the spatial distribution of selected phosphorus metabolites, but the resolution will be poor because of low signal intensities; **D–False;** the smallest practical volumes for spectroscopy are of the order of 1 cc; **E–True;** this is a phosphorus metabolite.

30–E. All of the listed statements are generally true of functional MR imaging, which is becoming an important neurologic research tool.

12

Breast Imaging

I. Mammography

A. Breast cancer

–Breast cancer accounts for 32% of cancer incidence and 18% of cancer deaths in women in the United States.
  –The incidence is increasing, with 182,000 new cases and 46,000 breast cancer deaths in 1993.
  –Approximately 9% of women in the United States ultimately develop breast cancer.
–Figure 12-1 shows breast cancer incidence and mortality rates.
–Early detection with screening mammography significantly reduces breast cancer mortality rates for women older than age 50.
–Screening asymptomatic women between the ages of 40 and 50 is controversial.
–The American College of Radiology (ACR) recommends a baseline mammogram by age 40, biannual examinations between ages 40 and 50, and yearly examinations after age 50.
–As many as 10% of breast cancers are not detected by mammography.

B. Imaging requirements

–Detection of breast cancer requires specialized imaging equipment and diagnostic expertise.
  –This imaging equipment must be shown to be functioning properly by means of a dedicated quality control (QC) program.
–Radiographic recognition of breast cancer depends on detection of subtle architectural distortion, masses near normal breast tissue density, skin thickening, and microcalcifications.
  –**Microcalcifications** are specks of calcium hydroxyapatite $[Ca_5(PO_4)_3OH]$, which may have diameters as small as 0.1 mm.
–Screening mammography normally includes a **craniocaudal** and a **mediolateral oblique** view of each breast.
  –Diagnostic mammographic examinations may include additional views and magnification to resolve ambiguous findings.

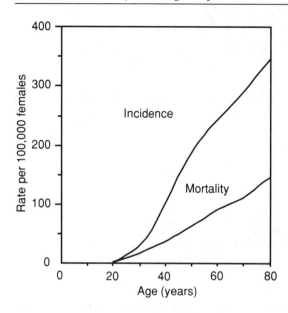

Figure 12-1. Breast cancer incidence and mortality.

C. Modern mammography

–Screen/film mammography is technically demanding and requires radiographs with excellent resolution, contrast, and film density.

  –The small differences in attenuation between normal and malignant tissue result in low subject contrast and make cancer detection difficult.

  –Detection of microcalcifications is difficult because their small dimensions also result in low subject contrast.

–Table 12-1 summarizes the key physical properties of the major breast tissues and pathologic conditions.

–Dedicated mammography equipment is essential for quality and low-dose screen/film imaging.

–Modern mammography equipment employs small focal spots, low kVp techniques, breast compression devices, and low ratio grids, and is configured for optimal patient positioning.

  –Low kVps are used to maximize the relative contribution of the photoelectric effect, thereby increasing subject contrast and minimizing scatter.

  –Special screens, films, and dedicated film processing are also important in mammography.

–Specific technical x-ray requirements are listed in Table 12-2.

Table 12-1. Properties of Breast Tissue

Tissue Type	Density (g/cm³)	Linear Attenuation Coefficient at 20 keV (cm⁻¹)
Adipose	0.93	0.45
Fibroglandular	1.035	0.80
Carcinoma	1.045	0.85
Skin	1.09	0.80
Calcification	2.2	12.5

Table 12-2. Typical Specifications for a Dedicated Mammography Unit

Parameter	Specification
Power rating	3–10 kW
X-ray tube output (at breast entrance)	0.5–0.8 R/s at 28 kVp
High voltage waveform	Three-phase or high-frequency
kVp selection	24–35 kVp (1-kVp steps)
mAs selection	2–600 mAs
Target material	Molybdenum ($Z = 42$)
Window material	Beryllium ($Z = 4$)
Added filtration	30–60 μm molybdenum
Half-value layer	0.30–0.37 mm aluminum at 28 kVp
Nominal focal spot size	0.3 mm
Magnification focal spot	0.1–0.15 mm

D. Mammography accreditation

–The ACR developed an accreditation program in 1990 to improve the quality of screen/film mammography.

–Accreditation is based on the five steps listed in Table 12-3.

–Accredited physicians are required to interpret a minimum of 10 mammograms per week.

–Annual tests to be performed on all dedicated mammography equipment are listed in Table 12-4.

–Centers meeting these ACR standards receive a certificate of accreditation.

–As of October 1994, the Food and Drug Administration (FDA) required all of the estimated 10,000 mammography facilities operating in the United States to be formally certified.

–The FDA standards are no less stringent than those of the ACR accreditation program.

II. Screen/Film Techniques

A. X-ray tube

–In visualizing breast tissue, the x-ray energy level that optimizes subject contrast is approximately **20 keV**.

–Higher energy x-rays decrease subject contrast.

–Lower energy photons have inadequate breast penetration and substantially increase the patient radiation dose.

–Both **molybdenum** and **rhodium** are used as target materials in the anode because they produce characteristic x-ray radiation at optimal energy levels.

Table 12-3. American College of Radiology Accreditation Requirements

Site survey questionnaire completed
Assessment of image quality using a phantom
Dosimeter assessment of mean glandular dose
    [3 mGy (300 mrad) per view, maximum]
Assessment of clinical images by independent radiologists
Assessment of quality control program

Table 12-4. Mammography Quality Control Tests To Be Performed Annually by a Certified Medical Physicist

Unit assembly and cassette performance
Collimation
Focal spot size
Peak voltage accuracy and reproducibility
Beam quality (half-value layer)
Automatic exposure control performance
Uniformity of screen speeds
Entrance skin exposure and mean glandular dose
Image quality (mammography phantom)
Artifact evaluation

—**Molybdenum** has characteristic x-rays of 17.9 and 19.5 keV.
—**Rhodium** has characteristic x-rays of 20.2 and 22.7 keV.
—For these characteristic x-rays to be produced, the x-ray tube peak voltage must be higher than these values, that is, typically 25 to 30 kVp.
—The slightly higher energy x-rays from rhodium provide better penetration of thicker or denser breasts.
—Typical x-ray tube currents are 80 to 100 milliamperes (mA).
—Exposure times are usually about 1 second, but may be as long as 4 seconds for dense, thick breasts.
—Three-phase or high-frequency generators are used to minimize voltage fluctuations and reduce exposure times.
—Figure 12-2 shows the x-ray spectra from a molybdenum target.

B. **X-ray output**

—The **heel effect** (higher x-ray intensity on the cathode side) is used to increase the intensity of radiation near the chest wall where greater penetration is needed.
—This is accomplished by placing the cathode side of the tube toward the patient.

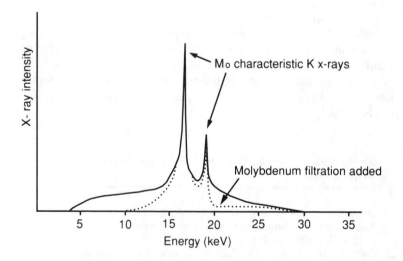

Figure 12-2. X-ray spectra from a molybdenum target at 30 kVp showing the effect of adding a molybdenum filter.

—A beryllium ($Z = 4$) x-ray tube window is used to minimize x-ray beam attenuation.

—Molybdenum filters (30 μm thick) remove most bremsstrahlung radiation above the molybdenum K-edge energy level.

  —Removal of this high-energy bremsstrahlung radiation improves subject contrast.

—The molybdenum also filters out the very low energy x-rays that would only contribute to patient dose.

—For rhodium anodes ($Z = 45$; K-edge = 23.2 keV), a rhodium filter is used to remove the high-energy bremsstrahlung radiation.

—The correct x-ray tube output is obtained using phototiming with special **automatic exposure control** systems designed to operate correctly at low x-ray energy levels.

C. Compression

—Optimal mammography requires the use of breast compression, which is achieved using radiotranslucent paddles that have an x-ray transmission of about 80% at 30 kVp.

—Compression generally results in **greater sharpness, less scatter,** and **reduced patient dose**.

—Spot compression, or dual focus compression, may be used to achieve maximum compression in a limited region of interest.

—Compression reduces the thickness of the breast and allows low peak voltages to be used, thereby improving subject contrast.

  —Compressed breasts are normally 3 to 8 cm thick.

  —Compression spreads the breast tissue out, making pathologic conditions easier to detect.

—Compression brings the breast closer to the image plane, minimizes image magnification, and reduces focal spot blur (geometric unsharpness).

—Compression also reduces exposure times, thus minimizing patient motion blur and film reciprocity law breakdowns associated with long exposure times.

—The principal drawback of compression is patient discomfort.

D. Grids

—Scatter to primary ratios in mammography range from 0.6 to 1.0.

  —Although these ratios are low compared to general radiology, they can noticeably reduce image contrast.

—Grids are commonly used to **maximize image quality** by reducing scatter.

—Scatter increases with breast thickness and peak voltage.

—Mammography is normally performed using a moving grid (Bucky or reciprocating grid).

  —Typical values for grid line densities range from 30 to 60 lines per centimeter.

  —Typical grid ratios are 4:1 or 5:1 for moving grids.

—Grids decrease scatter but increase patient dose up to threefold.

E. Screen/film combinations

—Rare earth intensifying screens, such as terbium-activated gadolinium oxysulfide (Gd_2O_2S:Tb), are used in mammography.

–Screens may incorporate light absorbers to limit screen diffusion and improve resolution.

–The photon absorption efficiency in mammography screens may be as high as 50% due to the use of low energy x-ray photons.

–Single emulsion films are normally used to reduce receptor blur by eliminating crossover and parallax effects.

–The film is placed between the x-ray source and screen to reduce blur because the x-rays are mainly absorbed at the front of the screen.

–A typical screen/film combination in mammography requires 5 to 10 mR at the screen to generate a reasonable film density.

–Mammography films generally have high gradients (approximately 3), resulting in low film latitude.

　–Limited latitude, however, is normally not a problem when there is adequate breast compression.

–Figure 12-3 shows the characteristic curve of several typical mammography screen/film combinations.

F. Film processing

–Mammography films have relatively thick single emulsions, which makes them much more sensitive to **processor artifacts**.

–Optimal film processing is critical to ensure high image quality, and dedicated mammography processors are recommended.

–Special processors with extended cycle times of 3 minutes and higher developer temperatures may be used.

　–The extended development time optimizes development of the latent image, resulting in increased film speed and contrast.

–Optimal film processing requires careful QC, which results in improved image quality and reduced patient dose.

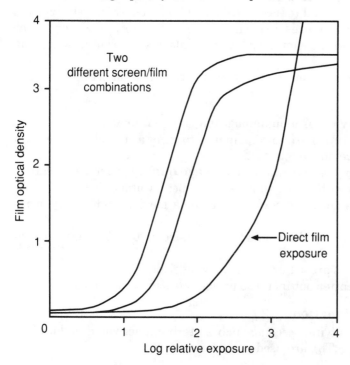

Figure 12-3. Characteristic curves for two screen/film combinations, compared with direct-exposure film.

—For optimal image contrast, the mean optical density of mammograms should be in the range of 1.2 to 1.8.

III. Image Features and Dosimetry

A. Magnification mammography

—Magnification mammography improves visualization of mass margins and fine calcifications. The amount of breast coverage in a single magnification radiograph is reduced.

—**Small focal spots** (0.1 or 0.15 mm in diameter) are essential to minimize geometric unsharpness.

  —Use of a small focal spot requires longer exposure times, which may result in increased patient motion and blur.

  —Magnification with small focal spot sizes, however, increases resolution and signal-to-noise ratios.

—Magnification is achieved by moving the breast away from the film using a 15- to 30-cm standoff.

  —Source to image receptor distance is normally constant, resulting in images magnified 1.5 to 2 times.

  —The presence of an air gap reduces the amount of scatter reaching the film and eliminates the need for a grid.

B. Viewing mammograms

—For optimal viewing of the images, bright viewboxes with luminance values of approximately 3000 candelas per square meter (cd/m^2) (900 foot-lamberts) should be used, whereas most viewboxes are approximately 1500 cd/m^2 (450 foot-lamberts).

—Viewing rooms should be darkened, and hot lights should be available.

—Extraneous light decreases contrast perception.

  —Regions beyond the mammogram border should be covered to improve low contrast visibility.

—A magnifying glass should be used to view microcalcifications.

C. Image quality

—The limiting spatial resolution of state-of-the-art mammographic screen/film combinations is 15 to 22 line pairs per millimeter (lp/mm).

—**Quantum mottle** and **film granularity** are major sources of noise in screen/film mammography.

—Grids may improve the contrast by a factor of 2, but also increase the radiation dose by a factor of 2 to 3.

—Low kVp techniques increase contrast but also increase patient dose.

—Magnification imaging with a small focal spot improves the achievable spatial resolution.

—The screen/film cassettes must be meticulously cleaned and carefully handled to minimize artifacts and maintain high image quality.

D. Breast dose

—The glandular tissue in the breast is sensitive to cancer induction by radiation.

—The **mean glandular dose (MGD)** is the preferred measure of dose in mammography and is determined using a special phantom.

–The MGD may be estimated from the measured entrance skin exposure, the x-ray beam peak voltage, and the half-value layer.

–The MGD also depends on breast composition. A 50% glandular tissue and 50% adipose tissue composition is generally assumed for dosimetry purposes.

–Use of a grid normally doubles the MGD value.

–The ACR recommends that the MGD for a 4.5-cm thick breast should be less than 1 mGy (100 mrad) for screen/film, less than 3 mGy (300 mrad) for screen/film with a grid, and less than 4 mGy (400 mrad) for xeromammography.

–Doses should be determined annually by a certified medical physicist.

–Typical MGD values for breast imaging are shown in Table 12-5.

E. Radiation risks

–The principal risk after radiation exposure is the induction of breast cancer in the glandular tissue.

–Epidemiological studies of high-dose radiation-induced breast cancer include studies of atomic bomb survivors, tuberculosis patients who underwent extended fluoroscopy, and radiation therapy patients.

–Most radiation-induced breast cancers result from MGD doses in the range 1 to 20 Gy (100 to 2000 rad) with little data from doses below 0.5 Gy (50 rad).

–Radiation risks for women undergoing mammography are based on extrapolations of risk estimates made at high doses.

–Based on current risk estimates, exposing 1 million 45-year-old women to an MGD of 1 mGy (100 mrad) may result in two excess breast cancer deaths.

F. Risk versus benefits

–For a screening examination with an MGD of 2.5 mGy (250 mrad), the theoretical radiation-induced breast cancer fatalities in 1 million examined women is about five.

  –This mammogram radiation risk is equivalent to the risk of dying in an accident when traveling 5000 miles by airplane or 450 miles by car.

–In this population of 1 million women, 1500 cases of breast cancer surface clinically in 1 year.

–Without a screening program, the breast cancer fatality rate is about 50%.

–A screening program might be expected to reduce the fatality rate by about 40%, or save about 300 lives.

–The benefit to risk associated with mammography screening is, therefore, high.

Table 12-5. Mean Glandular Dose per View*

Receptor	Average	Range
Screen/film (no grid)	0.77 mGy	0.12–2.48 mGy
	77 mrad	12–248 mrad
Screen/film (grid)	1.28 mGy	0.15–7.45 mGy
	128 mrad	15–745 mrad
Xeroradiography	2.90 mGy	0.56–8.90 mGy
	290 mrad	56–890 mrad

*For facilities applying for American College of Radiology accreditation in 1992.

IV. Alternative Breast Imaging Modalities

A. Xeromammography

–Xeroradiography uses selenium-coated aluminum plates.
  –**Selenium** is an x-ray–sensitive photoconductive material with a K-edge of 12.7 keV.
–Detectors have a selenium thickness of 150 or 320 μm.
–X-ray tubes used with xeroradiography have tungsten anodes, aluminum filtration (1 to 2 mm), and operate at about 45 kVp.
–Before exposure, the selenium plate is charged with a surface potential of about 1000 V.
–X-rays absorbed by the selenium liberate electrons and ions, which reduce the initial charge on the plates.
–After exposure, the plates hold a latent image of the x-ray exposure pattern with high exposures corresponding to low charge and low exposures corresponding to high charge.
–Special processing equipment, using liquid or powder toners, is required to visualize the latent image on an exposed plate.
–Inside the processor, the plate is sprayed with an ionized toner, which consists of particles about 1 μm in size.
–The toner forms an image by being preferentially deposited in the high or low voltage regions of the plate.
–This pattern of toner deposition is then transferred to plastic-coated paper.

B. Xeroradiography versus screen/film

–Characteristic image quality aspects of xeromammography are **wide latitude** and **edge enhancement** in the resultant image.
–A high kVp permits visualization of thick, dense breasts and silicon implants, which cannot be imaged at the low kVp used in screen/film mammography.
–Compared with screen/film mammography, xeroradiography has a lower **large area** contrast, which is the corollary of a wide latitude.
–Xeromammography has typical mean glandular doses in the range of 2 to 4 mGy (200 to 400 mrad), which is higher than those for screen/film.
–In 1990, Xerox discontinued manufacture of xeroradiography equipment, and its clinical use is being phased out.

C. Ultrasound and breast imaging

–High-resolution and high-frequency transducers (7.5 or 10 MHz) are used for ultrasound imaging of the breast.
–Ultrasound can improve diagnostic accuracy and decrease the need for surgical biopsy in women who have suspicious findings at screen/film mammography.
–The main clinical role of ultrasound is to **differentiate cysts from solid masses**.
  –Ultrasound may also be used to evaluate palpable masses not seen on mammograms and for biopsy guidance.
–Ultrasound is ineffective for routine screening of asymptomatic patients.

D. Magnetic resonance and breast imaging

—Magnetic resonance imaging (MRI) may supplement conventional imaging methods in the diagnosis of breast disease.

—Special breast coils are used to perform three-dimensional imaging of the breast with a typical volume matrix of $128 \times 256 \times 256$ pixels.

—Fat suppression techniques may be used to generate T1-weighted images.

—Breast MRI normally uses gadolinium-DTPA contrast (0.1 mmol/kg).

   —Contrast-enhanced MR has a high sensitivity and is better able to identify tumor margins.

—The improved sensitivity of MRI may be used to determine whether patients with presumed solitary nodules actually have multifocal disease.

—Lack of contrast enhancement from fat and scar tissue may also be used to identify mammographically suspicious lesions.

—Benign lesions such as fibroadenomas are often difficult to distinguish from malignancies.

—MR is useful in evaluating breast implants for tears and leaks.

—MR can distinguish silicone from enhancing tumor.

—MRI-guided biopsies cannot be performed with current commercial MR scanners.

E. Stereotaxic localization

—Stereotaxic localization has been developed to perform **core needle biopsies**.

   —Benefits of core needle biopsies over open biopsies include a short procedure time (30 minutes), minimal local anesthetic, reduced cost and risk, and no residual scarring of breast tissue.

—Sterotaxic localizations are best achieved using digital imaging systems, which eliminate time-consuming film processing.

—The limitations of core needle biopsy devices include their high cost and the limited field of view of real-time images, which are typically 5 by 5 cm.

F. Miscellaneous

—**Computed radiography** has been used for screening mammography, but the low resolution (5 lp/mm) is a major limitation for visualization of microcalcifications.

—High-resolution digital x-ray detectors are being developed for use in mammography and are undergoing clinical trials.

—**Light diaphanography** involves shining light through the breast and detecting its transmission using special cameras.

—Clinical diaphanography screening results have been poor.

—A major problem of diaphanography is the significant amount of scatter compared with light absorption.

—Differential absorption effects appear to be caused by increases in vascularity, which results in nonspecific findings.

—**Thermography** involves imaging the infrared radiation emitted by tissues; the amount emitted depends on body temperature.

   —Carcinomas near the breast surface may thus show up as hot spots when compared to the contralateral breast.

—The ACR deems thermography to be ineffective for detecting breast cancer, and its use for this purpose is not recommended.

Review Test

1. Modern mammography equipment uses

(A) three-phase or high-frequency generators
(B) small focal spots (0.1–0.3 mm)
(C) automatic exposure control
(D) built-in compression paddles
(E) all of the above

2. Conventional screen/film radiographic techniques, in comparison with mammography

(A) use the same kVp
(B) have lower half-value layers
(C) use longer exposure times
(D) require the same exposures
(E) none of the above

3. True (T) or False (F). Dedicated film/screen mammography equipment usually uses

(A) tungsten anodes
(B) SID of 100 cm
(C) 0.5 mm added Al filtration
(D) the same x-ray tubes as xeromammography
(E) focal spots of 0.3 mm
(F) short exposure times (< 10 ms)

4. The low kVp used in screen/film mammography reduces

(A) subject contrast
(B) dose
(C) microcalcification visibility
(D) scatter
(E) film processing time

5. True (T) or False (F). The molybdenum filters used in mammography

(A) are usually 30 μm thick
(B) preferentially attenuate x-ray energies > 20 keV
(C) preferentially absorb Mo characteristic x-rays
(D) have a higher atomic number than Al filters
(E) are generally used for xeroradiography

6. Breast compression in mammography

(A) improves image contrast
(B) eliminates the need for a grid
(C) requires the use of a wide-latitude film
(D) increases radiation dose
(E) permits the use of higher kVps

7. Mammography screen/film cassettes are likely to have

(A) carbon fiber or plastic cassette fronts
(B) single emulsion film
(C) high gradient films
(D) a single intensifying screen
(E) all of the above

8. Grids in screen/film mammography

(A) improve contrast
(B) increase the radiation dose
(C) have grid ratios of about 5:1
(D) all of the above

9. Contrast in screen/film mammography is best improved by using

(A) tungsten targets
(B) breast compression
(C) a high kVp
(D) no grid
(E) wide-latitude film

10. Optimal viewing of screen/film mammograms requires

(A) a bright viewbox (~3000 cd/m^2)
(B) availability of a hotlight
(C) use of a magnifying glass
(D) a darkened room
(E) all of the above

11. Geometric unsharpness

(A) is unimportant in mammography
(B) is minimized with a large focal spot size
(C) is reduced by a small SID
(D) increases with magnification
(E) none of the above

12. Magnification radiography using current imaging equipment

(A) reduces the entrance skin exposure
(B) improves definition of fine detail
(C) requires large focal spots > 0.3 mm
(D) reduces film density
(E) requires moving the film further from the tube

13. Breast doses in mammography are most likely to be reduced by *increasing* the

(A) x-ray tube kVp
(B) x-ray tube mA
(C) focal spot size
(D) grid ratio
(E) number of views taken

14. Answer True (T) or False (F). The American College of Radiology recommends that the mean glandular dose for an average 4.5 cm breast should be less than

(A) 4 mGy (400 mrad) for xeroradiography
(B) 3 mGy (300 mrad) for film/screen + grid
(C) 1 mGy (100 mrad) for film/screen + no grid
(D) 10 mGy (1 rad) for a chest CT scan
(E) 3 mGy (300 mrad) for a mammogram taken using a conventional x-ray unit

15. The mean glandular dose of screen/film mammography is

(A) higher than of xeromammography
(B) > 3 mGy with a grid
(C) reduced with a grid
(D) without any radiation risk
(E) none of the above

16. The radiation risk of a screening mammogram for a 45-year-old woman is

(A) about 1 in 200,000
(B) from the induction of breast cancer
(C) much lower than the potential benefit
(D) associated with a long latent period
(E) all of the above

17. Benefits of xeromammography include

(A) equipment availability
(B) edge enhancement
(C) lower dose
(D) high large-area contrast
(E) all of the above

18. Xeromammography requires all the following EXCEPT

(A) toner for processing
(B) about 45 kVp
(C) small focal spots
(D) selenium-coated plates
(E) 30 μm Mo filters

19. Tubes used in xeromammography have

(A) Mo targets
(B) Be filters
(C) 0.5 kW power ratings
(D) 1 mm focal spots
(E) none of the above

20. The primary use of ultrasound in breast imaging is

(A) routine screening of asymptomatic women
(B) visualization of microcalcifications
(C) differentiation of benign from malignant masses
(D) staging of malignant disease
(E) none of the above

21. Breast imaging using MR may use

(A) fat suppression techniques
(B) Gd-DPTA contrast
(C) special breast coils
(D) three-dimensional imaging techniques
(E) all of the above

22. The clinical use of MR breast imaging may include all of the following EXCEPT identification of

(A) tumor margins
(B) multifocal disease
(C) microcalcification clusters
(D) scar tissue
(E) tumors in patients with silicone implants

23. Benefits of stereotaxic localization for core needle biopsies compared to surgical biopsies include all the following EXCEPT

(A) short procedure time (30 minutes)
(B) absence of ionizing radiation
(C) minimal local anesthetic
(D) reduced cost
(E) reduced scarring

24. The major limitation of computed radiography (CR) for breast imaging is its inferior

(A) x-ray detection efficiency
(B) display contrast
(C) noise characteristic
(D) dose performance
(E) limiting spatial resolution

25. The use of thermography to detect breast cancer

(A) uses ionizing radiation
(B) makes use of TLD detectors
(C) is most effective near the chest wall
(D) is deemed by the ACR to be ineffective
(E) none of the above

Answers and Explanations

1–E. All of the parts mentioned are used.

2–E. None are true.

3. A–False; molybdenum targets are used; **B–False;** typical SIDs are 50 cm to 65 cm, with exposure times becoming too long when larger distances are used; **C–False;** 30 μm Mo is the usual filter; **D–False;** xeroradiography uses tungsten targets, aluminum filtration, and ~45 kVp; **E–True;** 0.3 mm for normal mammography and 0.15 mm for magnification mammography; **F–False;** exposure times tend to be long due to the limited x-ray tube exposure outputs.

4–D. As the photon energy is reduced, the photoelectric effect becomes more important, and Compton scatter is reduced.

5. A–True; B–True; the Mo K-edge is 20 keV, so photoelectric absorption will be very high for photons with energy levels just above this value; **C–False;** Mo filters are relatively transparent to Mo-characteristic x-rays because their energy levels are *just below* the K-edge; **D–True;** Z for Al is 13; Z for Mo is 42; **E–False;** Al filters are used in xeroradiography where x-ray voltages are typically about 45 kVp.

6–A. Compression generally improves image contrast.

7–E. All the listed items are features associated with screen/film mammography.

8–D. All of the listed statements are true.

9–B. Compression reduces the breast thickness and improves contrast by reducing scatter.

10–E. All of the listed elements are required.

11–D. Geometric unsharpness increases with magnification and requires smaller focal spots.

12–B. Magnification improves detail visibility and is achieved by moving the breast closer to the x-ray tube.

13–A. Increasing the kVp will make the beam more penetrating, thus reducing the radiation dose. It will also, however, reduce the resultant image contrast, which in turn lessens the potential benefit of the examination.

14. A–True; B–True; C–True; D–False; the ACR says nothing about CT examinations where the typical mean glandular dose would be about 20 mGy; **E–False;** the ACR requires *dedicated* screen/film mammography units.

15–E. None of the statements are true.

16–E. All of the statements are true.

17–B. Edge enhancement is unique to xeroradiography.

18–E. Filtration in xeroradiography is normally 1 mm or 2 mm Al. Mo filters are used in screen/film mammography.

19–E. None are true.

20–E. None of the uses listed is the primary use. The primary role of ultrasound in breast imaging is the differentiation of cysts from solid masses.

21–E. All of the listed features are common in MR breast imaging.

22–C. MR does not visualize microcalcifications.

23–B. Radiographs are obtained to correctly localize the needle.

24–E. The limiting spatial resolution of CR is 5 line pairs/mm which is much worse than that of screen/film (~20 line pairs/mm).

25–D. Thermography, the imaging of infrared radiation that is emitted by all bodies, is ineffective for detecting breast cancer.

13

Statistics

I. Statistical Definitions and Distributions

A. Population statistics

–**Fatality rate** is the death rate in a diseased group.
–**Mortality rate** is the number of deaths in a particular time period for a specific population.
–**Incidence** is the number of people who develop a particular condition within a specific time period.
–**Prevalence** is the number of people in a population at risk who have a particular condition at a specific time.

B. Data distribution

–**Mean** is the arithmetic average of a group of data.
–**Median** is a measure of the central tendency and is the value that separates the data in half and defines the fiftieth percentile.
–**Mode** is the most common data point.
–**Range** is the difference between the highest and lowest values and is a measure of dispersion of the data distribution.
–**Standard deviation** (defined as σ for a population) is used to describe the spread or distribution of a data set and is the square root of the average of the square of all the sample deviations.
–**Variance** is the standard deviation squared (σ^2).
–**Bias** is the presence of systematic error.
–**Precision** is the reproducibility of a result but does not imply accuracy.
–**Accuracy** refers to how close a measured value is to the true value.
–Figure 13-1 shows a dart player whose results illustrate these terms.

C. Gaussian (normal) distribution

–**Gaussian curves** are **bell shaped** and represent a normal probability distribution.
–They are symmetrical around a central mean value (m) with a standard deviation (σ).
–All Gaussian curves have the same mean, median, and mode value (Figure 13-2).

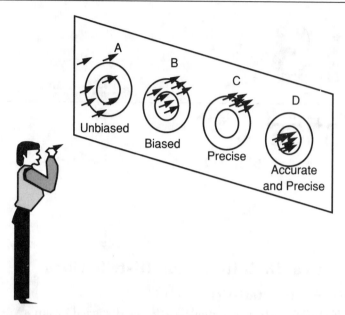

Figure 13-1. Board **A** shows an unbiased distribution, which is imprecise and inaccurate. Board **B** is biased, imprecise, and inaccurate. Board **C** is precise, but inaccurate. Board **D** is accurate and precise.

—By definition, 68% of the data fall within 1 σ of the mean ($m \pm \sigma$); 95% of the data fall within 2 σ of the mean ($m \pm 2\sigma$); 99% of the data fall within 3 σ of the mean ($m \pm 3\sigma$).

—A Gaussian curve has the equation $Y = \sqrt{(1/2\pi)} \times e^{-X^2/2}$, where Y is the probability density of the value X.

—The standard **normal curve** is a special case, where $m = 0$ and $\sigma = 1$.

D. Poisson distribution

—**Poisson distribution** is used to model the probability distribution of uncommon events such as radioactive decay.

—For a given observation, the number of counts obtained in t seconds vary about some average value m.

—Repeat experiments of counts observed in t seconds generate a Poisson distribution in which the average is m counts.

—The probability of observing exactly n counts in this time interval is $(e^{-m}) \times (m^n)/n!$, where $n!$ (pronounced n factorial) is the product of $n \times (n-1) \times (n-2)...(2) \times (1)$.

—The **variance** of a Poisson distribution is equal to the mean.

—The **standard deviation** is the square root of the variance ($\sqrt{m}$).

—The Poisson distribution is not symmetrical for low values of m.

—The Poisson distribution approaches a Gaussian distribution for values of m greater than about 10.

II. Test Results

A. Definitions

—**True positives (TPs)** are positive test results in patients who have the disease.

—**False positives (FPs)** are positive test results in patients who do not have the disease.

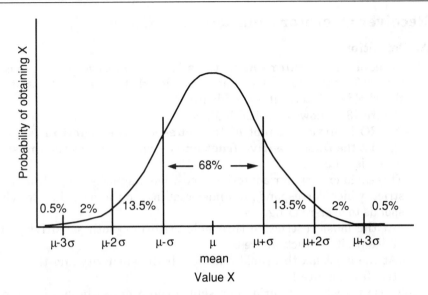

Figure 13-2. Gaussian probability distribution (normal curve). The percentage values correspond to the areas between the specified limits.

–**True negatives (TNs)** are negative test results in patients who do not have the disease.

–**False negatives (FNs)** are negative test results in patients who have the disease.

–Table 13-1 is a truth table that may be applied to any diagnostic test.

B. Test outcomes

–**Sensitivity** is the ability to detect disease and is TP/(TP + FN), also known as the **true-positive fraction**.

–A **sensitive test** has a low false-negative rate.

–**Specificity** is the ability to identify the absence of disease and is TN/(TN + FP), also known as the **true-negative fraction**.

–A **specific test** has a low false-positive rate.

–**Accuracy** is the fraction of correct diagnosis and is (TP + TN)/(TP + FP + TN + FN).

–**Positive predictive value** is the probability of having the disease given a positive test and is TP/(TP + FP).

–**Negative predictive value** is the probability of not having the disease given a negative test and is TN/(TN + FN).

–**Prevalence** of the disease is (TP + FN)/(TP + FP + TN + FN).

Table 13-1. Truth Table for Any Diagnostic Test

		Diagnostic Test Result	
		Positive	**Negative**
Patient	Disease present	True positive (TP)	False negative (FN)
Status	Disease absent	False positive (FP)	True negative (TN)

III. Receiver Operator Characteristic Curve

A. Definition

–A **receiver operator characteristic (ROC) curve** is used to compare the performance (sensitivity and specificity) of diagnostic tests at various thresholds of interpreter confidence.

–Figure 13-3 shows a typical ROC curve.

–An ROC curve is a plot of the **true-positive fraction** (sensitivity) against the **false-positive fraction** (1 – specificity) as the threshold criterion is relaxed.

–Threshold criteria for accepting a positive diagnosis range from the most strict, which corresponds to under-reading, to the most lax, which corresponds to over-reading.

   –At the most restrictive threshold criterion, both sensitivity and the false-positive fraction are 0.

   –At the most lax threshold criterion, both sensitivity and the false-positive fraction are 1.

–These threshold criteria represent a compromise between the need to increase sensitivity and minimize the false-positive fraction.

B. Area under the ROC curve

–As the threshold criterion is relaxed, both the sensitivity and the false-positive fraction increase from 0 to 1.

–The area under an ROC curve is a measure of overall imaging performance and is commonly called A_z.

–The maximum area under the curve is 1.0.

–For random guessing, the ROC curve is a straight line through the points (0,0) and (1,1), and the area under the curve is 0.5.

–As the imaging performance improves, the ROC curve moves toward the upper left-hand corner, and the area under the ROC curve increases.

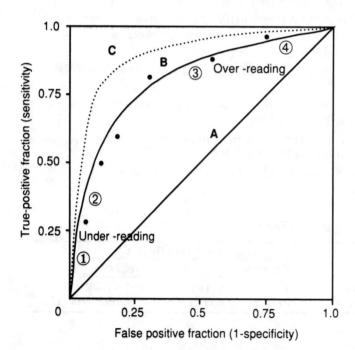

Figure 13-3. ROC curves. Curve **A** represents the results of random guessing and has no predictive value. Curve **B** represents a typical result, and curve **C** represents an improved performance. *1* represents an area of high specificity where the interpreter is certain the test is normal. *2* represents under-reading by the interpreter with specificity remaining high. *3* has increased sensitivity caused by over-reading. *4* is the point of greatest sensitivity where all results are called positive.

C. Significance of ROC analysis

–ROC analysis is generally considered the best way to compare two imaging modalities.

–For any imaging modality, the ROC curve generally moves to the upper left-hand corner as the signal-to-noise ratio increases.

–One logistical difficulty of ROC analysis is determination of the clinical truth, which is needed to compute sensitivity and specificity.

IV. Tests of Statistical Significance

A. t-Test

–The **t-test** is an example of a parametric test in which it is assumed that measurements are normally distributed.

–The t-test is used to compare the mean of two small groups (less than 30) or to compare the mean of a small group with a known normal value.

–If the mean measurements made for two populations differ by a value M, then the t-statistic is M/SE, where SE is the standard error.

–For a paired t-test, the SE is $\sigma/\sqrt{N}$, where σ is the standard deviation of the paired differences and N is the number of measurements.

–The t-statistic values are compared with values provided in tables to determine the p value and are dependent on the "degrees of freedom" (one less than the number of independent observations in the sample).

–The p value is a measure of statistical significance and represents the probability that a given result occurred as a result of chance.

–A p value of 0.05 means that there is a 5% probability that the result occurred by chance.

B. t-Test example

–As an example, consider two screen/film combinations, A and B, used in mammography.

–A study is performed to determine whether film B improves the detectability of microcalcifications.

–Six readers count the number of microcalcifications seen in each film taken of the same patient, as summarized in Table 13-2.

–The mean difference between the two films is 3.5, with a standard deviation of 1.87 as given in column 4 of Table 13-2.

–Is this difference statistically significant or could such a difference arise by chance alone?

Table 13-2. Number of Microcalcifications Counted by Six Observers on Two Films (A and B) of the Same Patient

Reader (i)	N_{Ai}	N_{Bi}	$\Delta N_i = N_{Bi} - N_{Ai}$
1	8	12	4
2	6	12	6
3	9	14	5
4	10	12	2
5	8	11	3
6	9	10	1
Mean difference ($\pm \sigma$) between films A and B			3.50 ($\pm$ 1.87)

Table 13-3. Values of the t-Statistic for Selected Probabilities and Degrees of Freedom

Degrees of Freedom	Probability (p)		
	0.05	0.01	0.001
1	12.71	63.66	636.62
2	4.30	9.93	31.60
5	2.57	4.03	6.87
10	2.23	3.17	4.59
30	2.04	2.75	3.65

–For six readings, the SE is $1.87/\sqrt{6}$ or 0.76. The t-statistic is thus 3.5/0.76 or 4.61.

–Table 13-3 lists values of the t-statistic for different p values and degrees of freedom.

–The number of degrees of freedom is $(N - 1)$ for N readers.

–With six readers, there are 5 degrees of freedom and the t-statistic value is 4.03 ($p = 0.01$) and 6.87 ($p = 0.001$).

–Thus, the probability of getting a t-statistic greater than 4.03 purely by chance is only 0.01 (1%), and the value (4.61) obtained in this study is greater than 4.03 and, therefore, significant at the $p = 0.01$ level.

–This t-statistic value is not significant at the $p = 0.001$ level because it is less than the required value of 6.87.

–In this example, film B is significantly better than film A, with the chance of this improvement arising solely by chance being less than 1%.

C. Chi-square test

–The chi-square test is a common measure of statistical significance. It is used to determine if the categorical information from two groups is equivalent or independent. This is a nonparametric test, and there are no underlying assumptions about the distribution of the data.

–The chi-square statistic is given by

$$\chi^2 = \Sigma_i \ \frac{(O_i - E_i)^2}{E_i}$$

where O_i is the observed value and E_i is the expected value.

–The computed values of the chi-square statistic are compared in statistical tables similar to that shown in Table 13-3.

–Chi-square is used to determine statistical significance by calculating the departure from randomness of a pattern.

–If a pattern is nonrandom and there is a strong association between variables, then a statistically significant χ^2 value results.

Review Test

1. The incidence of a disease in a given population is the

(A) percentage of new cases per year
(B) number of new cases per year
(C) total number of patients with disease
(D) same as the prevalence
(E) all of the above

2. For a Gaussian distribution, the mean is always equal to the

(A) full width half maximum
(B) variance
(C) mode
(D) standard deviation
(E) none of the above

3. All of the following are true for Poisson distributions EXCEPT

(A) they are used to describe radioactive decay
(B) they are used to describe quantum mottle
(C) the variance is equal to the mean
(D) the symmetrical for means < 10
(E) the approximate to a Gaussian for means > 10

4. If the mean number of radioactive transformations in one second is 100, the chance of getting less than 70 counts is

(A) 32%
(B) 5%
(C) 1%
(D) 0.5%
(E) require more information

5. Sensitivity is given by the

(A) number of true positives
(B) ratio of true positives to all patients with disease
(C) ratio of true positives to all patients
(D) patients with disease minus the false positives
(E) none of the above

6. Specificity is given by the

(A) true negative fraction
(B) 1 – false positive fraction
(C) true negatives/(true negatives + false positives)
(D) all of the above

7. A receiver operator characteristic (ROC) curve may be used to measure diagnostic imaging

(A) performance
(B) accuracy
(C) specificity
(D) sensitivity
(E) all of the above

8. The area under the ROC curve is

(A) a measure of performance
(B) unlikely to be less than 0.5
(C) 0.5 for random guesses
(D) 1.0 for a perfect diagnostic tool
(E) all of the above

9. Six consecutive measurements made on two radioactive sources differ by 100 ± 1 counts; the t-test statistic

(A) is given by the mean divided by the standard error
(B) should be checked in a table for 5 degrees of freedom
(C) will show a significant difference in the means
(D) all of the above

10. The chi-square test

(A) is a parametric test
(B) assumes measurements are normally distributed
(C) sums differences between observed and expected values
(D) sums squares of the observed to expected ratios
(E) none of the above

Answers and Explanations

1–B. Incidence is the number of new cases during some specific time interval. Prevalence is the total number of existing cases.

2–C. For a Gaussian curve, the mean, median, and mode are all equal.

3–D. A Poisson distribution is not symmetrical at low mean values (< 10), but is approximately symmetrical for large means (> 10).

4–D. 0.5%. The standard deviation is $\sqrt{100}$ or 10; thus only 1% of all measurements lie beyond $100 \pm 3\sigma$, or below 70 and above 130; only half of these will be below 70.

5–B. Sensitivity is TP/(TP + FN) or the true positive fraction.

6–D. All of the statements are true.

7–A. Performance is obtained from the area under the ROC curve. (Note that both sensitivity and specificity change with threshold criterion.)

8–E. All of the statements are true.

9–D. All of the statements are true, and the two samples are almost certain to be statistically different.

10–E. None of the definitions are true. The chi-square statistic is the sum of $(O - E)^2/E$ values, where O is the observed value, and E is the expected value.

PRACTICE EXAMINATIONS

Examination Guide

Education is what survives when what has been learnt has been forgotten.

—BF Skinner

Following are two mock examinations, each consisting of 120 questions and answers. These questions cover all the material summarized in this book. The examinations provided should be taken without consulting textbooks and should take no longer than 3 hours to complete. Taking mock examinations under realistic test conditions serves several useful purposes, including:

A. Practice for the real examination. Taking these practice examinations will enable you to learn whether you are taking too long to read and answer questions. It is also an excellent opportunity for you to develop a strategy for dealing with difficult questions, such as guessing *after* eliminating all "wrong" answers or by temporarily skipping difficult questions and returning to complete them at a later time.

B. Highlighting areas of weakness. Once the examinations have been completed, you should have a very good idea of your areas of weakness. Weaknesses should be corrected by consulting the appropriate chapter in this review book or, if greater depth is required, by reading an appropriate textbook.

C. Building confidence. Successful completion of the mock examinations demonstrates that the material has been satisfactorily covered, which may help to ease any pre-examination nervousness.

It is recommended that you first read the appropriate material in selected textbooks to ensure sufficient knowledge of the subject. You should then review the material in each chapter of this book and answer the appended questions. Having completed these steps, you should be ready to take these mock examinations. The following is a list of guidelines for successfully completing examinations.

1. Read and follow all examination instructions.
2. Read each question *carefully*.
3. Do not assume information; focus on key words (e.g., almost, never, most, not).
4. Eliminate obviously incorrect answers and focus on remaining answers.
5. Do not spend more than 2 minutes on any question.
6. Check the time every 30 minutes.
7. Should time permit, reread the questions and verify your answers.
8. Answer *all* questions, even if you have to guess; you have nothing to lose and everything to gain.

PRACTICE EXAMINATION A

A1. Which of the following is expressed in non-SI units?

(A) Meter
(B) Roentgen
(C) Kilogram
(D) Second
(E) Becquerel
(F) Sievert

A2. Match the quantity with the units in which it is measured.

(A) Absorbed dose
(B) Power
(C) Exposure
(D) Activity
(E) Dose equivalent

(i) Becquerel
(ii) Watt
(iii) C/kg
(iv) Gray
(v) Sievert

A3. Match the atomic number with the correct element.

(A) 29
(B) 42
(C) 50
(D) 74

(i) Tin
(ii) Tungsten
(iii) Copper
(iv) Molybdenum

A4. Outer-shell electrons differ from K-shell electrons by their

(A) rest mass energy
(B) charge
(C) magnetic moment
(D) binding energy
(E) none of the above

A5. Match the following particles and masses.

(A) Electron
(B) Alpha particle
(C) Neutrino
(D) Proton

(i) 4 AMU
(ii) 1 AMU
(iii) (1/1836) AMU
(iv) Zero mass

A6. Match the wavelength with the type of wave.

(A) 10^{-10} meters
(B) 7 meters
(C) 0.001 meters
(D) 5×10^{-7} meters

(i) Visible light
(ii) Diagnostic x-rays
(iii) Ultrasound
(iv) MRI signal (1 tesla)

A7. Ionizing radiations include all of the following EXCEPT

(A) photons
(B) electrons
(C) neutrons
(D) alpha particles
(E) pulsed ultrasound waves

A8. True (T) or False (F). In the following transformations

(A) beta minus decay, Z increases by 1
(B) beta minus decay, A increases by 1
(C) beta plus decay, Z increases by 1
(D) isomeric transitions, A and Z remain constant
(E) alpha decay, Z decreases by 2

A9. Match the particle with the description.

(A) Nucleus of a hydrogen atom
(B) Emitted during electron capture
(C) Created during pair production
(D) Source of electric currents
(E) Produced during decay of ^{222}Rn (radon)

(i) Proton
(ii) Neutrino
(iii) Positron
(iv) Alpha particle
(v) Electron

A10. An activity of 10 mCi corresponds to

(A) 3.7 kBq
(B) 370 kBq
(C) 3.7 MBq
(D) 370 MBq
(E) 3.7 GBq

A11. Full-wave, compared with half-wave rectification

(A) requires no diodes in the rectification circuit
(B) reduces the voltage ripple
(C) delivers the same radiation output in half the time
(D) increases the effective energy of the beam
(E) reduces the heel effect

A12. 50 keV electrons striking tungsten CANNOT lose energy by

(A) K-shell characteristic x-ray production
(B) L-shell characteristic x-ray production
(C) Bremsstrahlung x-ray production
(D) excitation and ionization of outer-shell electrons

A13. The cloud of electrons surrounding an x-ray tube filament is called

(A) a space charge
(B) a diode
(C) a grid
(D) an impurity
(E) none of the above

A14. Tungsten (Z = 74) is used for the target of most x-ray tubes rather than lower Z materials because

(A) shorter wavelength x-rays are produced
(B) the intensity of the resulting x-ray beam is high
(C) there is no characteristic radiation from tungsten
(D) x-rays from tungsten are emitted toward the patient
(E) the heel effect is minimized with tungsten targets

A15. An x-ray beam produced by monoenergetic 90 keV electrons strikes a tungsten target. Match the statements below.

(A) Electron beam energy converted to heat
(B) Electron beam energy converted to x-rays
(C) Total x-ray and heat energy
(D) X-rays accounted for by characteristic x-rays

(i) 1%
(ii) 10%
(iii) 100%
(iv) 99%

A16. A focal-spot rating is defined as the product of the maximum kV and mA for an exposure time of

(A) 0.01 s
(B) 0.1 s
(C) 1 s
(D) no exposure time needs to be specified

A17. The x-ray tube mAs mainly controls image

(A) density
(B) resolution
(C) speed
(D) magnification

A18. The heel effect results in the greatest x-ray beam intensity

(A) at the anode edge
(B) at the cathode edge
(C) in the middle of the field
(D) transmitted through the collimator
(E) transmitted through the x-ray tube housing

A19. Pair production interactions

(A) have no threshold
(B) occur in the electric field of the nucleus
(C) produce 1.022 MeV annihilation radiation
(D) are important in radiology
(E) all of the above

A20. After photoelectric interactions, the following emission CANNOT occur.

(A) Photoelectrons
(B) Scattered photons
(C) Characteristic x-rays
(D) Auger electrons

A21. True (T) or False (F). Concerning the photoelectric effect and Compton scatter in water

(A) photons may undergo two successive photoelectric effects
(B) Compton scatter has a threshold energy of 1.022 MeV
(C) at diagnostic x-ray energies, the photoelectric effect increases with photon energy
(D) the photoelectric and Compton effects are equal at 25 keV

A22. The energy of the scattered photon in Compton processes primarily depends on the

(A) atomic number
(B) density
(C) electron density
(D) molecular structure
(E) scattering angle

A23. In the following situations, which interaction predominates: photoelectric effect; Compton scatter; coherent scatter?

(A) 28 kVp in soft tissue
(B) 60 kVp in bone
(C) 100 kVp in soft tissue
(D) 100 kVp in iodine contrast
(E) 100 kVp in LaOBr intensifying screen

A24. If the linear attenuation is 0.1 cm^{-1}, and the density is 2 g/cm^3, then the mass attenuation coefficient is

(A) 0.2 cm^2/g
(B) 0.05 cm^2/g
(C) 0.05 g/cm^2
(D) 20 g/cm^2
(E) cannot be determined

A25. Increasing aluminum filtration will generally lead to increased

(A) subject contrast
(B) x-ray output
(C) tube heat loading
(D) entrance skin exposure
(E) phototimed film densities

A26. X-ray beam quality is

(A) directly proportional to the tube current (mA)
(B) reduced by additional x-ray beam filtration
(C) measured in mm of aluminum
(D) used to convert dose (Gy) to dose equivalent (Sv)
(E) independent of the applied kV and waveform

A27. Subject contrast depends on

(A) kVp
(B) tube current (mA)
(C) type of film
(D) development time and temperature
(E) film density

A28. Which of the following is the non-SI unit of dose equivalent?

(A) Roentgen
(B) Rad
(C) Rem
(D) RBE
(E) None of the above

A29. The quality factor (QF) is used to

(A) convert rem to sievert
(B) convert absorbed dose to dose equivalent
(C) determine the linear energy transfer (LET)
(D) determine the relative biological effectiveness
(E) all of the above

A30. Match the tissue with the appropriate f-factor (rad/R) for an 80 kVp diagnostic x-ray beam.

(A) Fat
(B) Muscle
(C) Bone

(i) 0.9
(ii) 3.0
(iii) 0.6

A31. Match the SI unit with the corresponding non-SI unit.

(A) Gray
(B) Becquerel
(C) Sievert
(D) Coulomb/kg
(E) Joule

(i) Rem
(ii) Rad
(iii) Curie
(iv) Erg
(v) Roentgen

A32. How will an increase in developer temperature generally affect the resultant film density?

(A) Increase density
(B) No change
(C) Reduce density
(D) Cannot be determined

A33. Match the following examinations with the appropriate type of film.

(A) High gradient
(B) Wide latitude
(C) Fast

(i) Chest x-ray examination
(ii) Abdomen examination
(iii) Mammography examination

A34. Films with high contrast CANNOT have

(A) low fog
(B) low noise
(C) wide latitude
(D) high speed
(E) high resolution

A35. Match each instrument to the measurement procedure, using each option only once.

(A) Survey for radionuclide contamination
(B) X-ray tube output
(C) Personnel monitoring
(D) Xeroradiograph

(i) Geiger-Müller (GM) meter
(ii) Thermoluminescent dosimeter (TLD)
(iii) Ionization chamber survey meter
(iv) Charged selenium plate

A36. The ratio of the x-ray exposures without a screen to the corresponding exposure with a screen is called the

(A) resolving power
(B) intensification factor
(C) exposure ratio
(D) Bucky ratio
(E) conversion ratio

A37. Matching the K-edge of the intensifying screen with the energy of incident x-rays improves the

(A) conversion efficiency
(B) spatial resolution
(C) subject contrast
(D) image contrast
(E) none of the above

A38. True (T) or False (F). Regarding screen/film combinations

(A) LaOBr emits mainly blue light
(B) Gd_2O_2S emits mainly green light
(C) $CaWO_4$ emits mainly blue light
(D) ortho film is sensitive to green light
(E) most radiographic films are sensitive to red light

A39. What determines grid efficiency of removal of scattered radiation?

(A) Grid ratio
(B) Focus distance
(C) Gap distance
(D) Strip height
(E) None of the above

A40. The ability of an imaging system to reproduce fine detail in the image is best characterized by the system

(A) x-ray absorption efficiency
(B) spatial frequency
(C) modulation transfer function
(D) quantum mottle
(E) magnification

A41. For a film with a gradient of 2.0, a 3-cm nodule in the lung will reduce film density by about

(A) < 0.01
(B) 0.1
(C) 0.6
(D) > 2.0

A42. Focal spot size affects image quality by modifying

(A) resolution in contact radiography
(B) resolution in magnification radiography
(C) patient entrance skin exposure
(D) image noise
(E) film latitude

A43. Film image contrast may be reduced by

(A) increasing developer temperature
(B) lowering kVp
(C) using a grid
(D) reducing beam filtration
(E) none of the above

A44. Doubling screen thickness is likely to increase the

(A) exposure time
(B) patient dose
(C) fraction of x-ray photons absorbed
(D) film processing time
(E) image noise

A45. Match the following grid ratios with the most likely application.

(A) Magnification mammography
(B) Barium study
(C) Screen/film mammography
(D) Portable abdomen

(i) 4:1
(ii) 6:1
(iii) 12:1
(iv) None

A46. Which of the following does NOT affect image noise for a given film density?

(A) Intensifying screen conversion efficiency
(B) Film processor temperature
(C) Film speed
(D) Screen thickness

A47. Match the technique change with its most likely effect on a phototimed radiographic image.

(A) Increase kVp but same mA
(B) Lower mA with the same kVp
(C) Increase the grid ratio
(D) Use a larger focal spot size

(i) Increased motion blur
(ii) Improved contrast
(iii) Reduced spatial resolution
(iv) Reduced contrast

A48. Compared to screen/film, computed radiography has

(A) the potential to reduce patient doses
(B) reduced spatial resolution
(C) image processing capabilities
(D) the ability to store data digitally
(E) all of the above

A49. Match the fluorescent phosphor with imaging modality.

(A) NaI
(B) CsI
(C) $La_2O_2S:Tb$

(i) Screen/film radiography
(ii) Fluoroscopy
(iii) Nuclear medicine

A50. The photocathode of an image intensifier converts

(A) electrons to light
(B) x-rays to light
(C) x-rays to electrons
(D) electrons to x-rays
(E) none of the above

A51. All of the following degrade image quality in image intensifiers EXCEPT

(A) vertically oriented CsI crystals
(B) pincushion distortion
(C) vignetting
(D) misaligned electronic focussing lens
(E) x-rays impinging on the *output* phosphor

A52. Fluoroscopic entrance skin exposures are normally

(A) equal to a few R/min
(B) not allowed to exceed 10 R/min
(C) dependent on the kV used
(D) dependent on the II size
(E) all of the above

A53. A noisy fluoroscopic image is most likely to be improved by increasing the

(A) focal spot size
(B) x-ray beam filtration
(C) grid ratio
(D) exposure level
(E) monitor gain

A54. To perform cine studies, a fluoroscopic system would require addition of all the following EXCEPT

(A) x-ray tube voltages 150 kVp
(B) grid controlled x-ray tube
(C) synchronization circuit
(D) cine camera
(E) optical distributor

A55. What is the pixel size if a 256^2 matrix is used to image a 25 cm-wide field?

(A) 0.5 mm
(B) 1 mm
(C) 2 mm
(D) None of the above

A56. Basic computation in a computer is performed by the

(A) random access memory (RAM)
(B) read only memory (ROM)
(C) central processing unit (CPU)
(D) small computer system interface (SCSI)
(E) none of the above

A57. True (T) or False (F). Regarding computer memory

(A) RAM is used for permanent memory
(B) buffer memory is used for temporary storage
(C) floppy disks hold more information than hard disks
(D) magnetic tapes have access times of less than 1 msec
(E) optical jukeboxes can have a storage capacity of over 10^{12} Bytes

A58. An efficient picture archive and communication system (PACS) should reduce all of the following EXCEPT

(A) use of film
(B) lost images
(C) use of view boxes
(D) radiology capital costs
(E) film library clerks

A59. Match the imaging modality with the appropriate limiting spatial resolution.

(A) Digital subtraction angiography
(B) Magnetic resonance imaging
(C) Computed tomography
(D) Nuclear medicine
(E) Computed radiography

(i) 3 line pairs/mm
(ii) 2 line pairs/mm
(iii) 0.7 line pairs/mm
(iv) 0.3 line pairs/mm
(v) < 0.1 line pairs/mm

A60. The Hounsfield unit (HU) assigned to a pixel in a clinical CT image may be significantly affected by all of the following tissue factors EXCEPT

(A) density
(B) electron density
(C) atomic number
(D) homogeneity
(E) temperature

A61. Increasing the CT image matrix from 256^2 to 512^2, at a fixed kV and mAs, may be expected to increase the

(A) patient throughput
(B) x-ray tube loading
(C) patient dose
(D) limiting spatial resolution
(E) film printing time

A62. Increasing the kV *alone* in CT scanning reduces

(A) anode loading
(B) subject contrast
(C) partial volume effects
(D) reconstruction time
(E) all of the above

A63. Which of the following artifacts does not appear in CT images?

(A) Motion artifacts
(B) Phase-encoding artifacts
(C) Streak artifacts
(D) Ring artifacts
(E) Beam-hardening artifacts

A64. The limiting spatial resolution in CT is affected by all of the following EXCEPT

(A) field of view
(B) detector aperture size
(C) mA
(D) matrix size
(E) focal spot size

A65. Increasing the width of the CT image display window will reduce

(A) displayed contrast
(B) quantum mottle
(C) section thickness
(D) field of view
(E) none of the above

A66. CT beam-hardening artifacts

(A) reduce CT numbers in the image center
(B) are independent of x-ray beam filtration
(C) reduce all CT numbers
(D) do not occur on 4th generation scanners
(E) none of the above

A67. Give "ballpark" values for each of the following levels of radioactivity.

(A) Detection limit using a Geiger meter
(B) Administered for thyroid uptake assessment
(C) Administered for nuclear medicine (NM) imaging procedure
(D) Technetium-99m generator
(E) Cobalt-60 radiotherapy source
(F) Released during the Chernobyl disaster

A68. Technetium generators

(A) are eluted with sterile water
(B) last for 67 hours
(C) have ^{99}Tc as the parent radionuclide
(D) can be eluted on a daily basis
(E) can be disposed of in the regular garbage after use

A69. The NaI crystals routinely used in gamma cameras

(A) are between 6 and 12 mm thick
(B) have high photoelectric absorption at 140 keV
(C) convert about 5% of absorbed energy into light
(D) result in an intrinsic resolution of 3 mm FWHM
(E) all of the above

A70. Increasing the distance between the patient and a parallel hole collimator results in

(A) reduced resolution
(B) reduced field of view
(C) increased patient dose
(D) image distortion
(E) all of the above

A71. Using radionuclides with a higher photon energy generally increases

(A) detector efficiency
(B) septal penetration
(C) amplifier gain setting
(D) image magnification
(E) resolution

A72. Which of the following nuclear medicine studies require a computer?

(A) Lung scan
(B) Liver scan
(C) MUGA study
(D) Thyroid uptake
(E) All of the above

A73. All of the following factors will affect the organ dose for a radioisotope study EXCEPT the

(A) organ size
(B) organ shape
(C) uptake of isotope
(D) clearance of isotope
(E) gamma camera imaging time

A74. True (T) or False (F). When estimating the *therapeutic* thyroid dose following administration of ^{131}I, the following data are essential.

(A) Activity administered to the patient
(B) Γ factor for ^{131}I (Gy/Bq at 1 meter)
(C) Fractional uptake by the thyroid
(D) Thyroid mass
(E) Biological clearance of activity from thyroid

A75. Radiopharmaceuticals can suffer from all of the following impurities EXCEPT

(A) radionuclide
(B) crystal
(C) chemical
(D) biological
(E) all of the above

A76. In SPECT imaging

(A) resolution is generally superior to CT
(B) imaging times are typically < 2 minutes
(C) annihilation radiation is detected in coincidence
(D) multiple views must be obtained
(E) scatter and attenuation corrections are never needed

A77. Positron emission tomography (PET) scanners generally make use of all of the following EXCEPT

(A) short-lived radionuclides such as ^{15}O
(B) cyclotrons
(C) directly detected positrons
(D) filtered-back projection reconstruction algorithms
(E) solid-state detectors

A78. Following an acute whole body exposure of 1 Gray (100 rad), the following is likely to be observed.

(A) Erythema
(B) Diarrhea
(C) Reduced lymphocyte count
(D) Permanent sterility
(E) Death within 60 days

A79. Exposure to x-rays

(A) during the first 10 days postconception can result in embryo death
(B) between 20 days and 40 days postconception can cause fetal deformations
(C) during the second trimester can cause growth retardation
(D) during the third trimester increases childhood cancers
(E) all of the above

A80. Match the skin dose with the radiographic examination.

(A) 30 mGy (3 rad)
(B) 0.1 mGy (10 mrad)
(C) 3 mGy (300 mrad)

(i) Chest x-ray (PA)
(ii) Abdominal x-ray
(iii) 1 minute of fluoroscopy

A81. After a single-view lateral lumbar spine x-ray examination (600 speed screen/film combination), a woman discovers she is pregnant. The radiation dose to the fetus is likely to

(A) be sufficient that the woman will require an abortion
(B) exceed 100 mGy (10 rad)
(C) exceed 10 mGy (1 rad)
(D) be less than 10 mGy (< 1 rad)
(E) be difficult to assess

A82. The ALARA concept requires that design of an x-ray facility should ensure that

(A) doses be kept as low as reasonably achievable
(B) all unnecessary x-rays should be avoided
(C) account be taken of social and economic factors
(D) doses received by patients be minimized
(E) all of the above

A83. Lead aprons for radiographers

(A) should be worn at the radiographic control panel
(B) have a higher lead equivalence than for nuclear medicine technologists
(C) are generally 0.50 mm in lead equivalence
(D) reduce the thyroid dose
(E) reduce exposure from radon

A84. Leaded glasses are required

(A) to have an attenuation equivalent of 5 mm lead
(B) for all radiographic exposures
(C) for all fluoroscopic exposures
(D) none of the above

A85. True (T) or False (F). ^{222}Rn (radon)

(A) is a product of ^{226}Ra
(B) concentrates in poorly ventilated basements
(C) can cause lung cancer
(D) is a pure beta emitter
(E) has a half-life of greater than 1 year

A86. Increasing the ultrasound frequency from 1 MHz to 10 MHz usually reduces the

(A) material acoustical impedance
(B) beam penetration
(C) material viscosity
(D) lateral resolution
(E) beam velocity

A87. An ultrasound beam intensity attenuated by 3 dB is how much lower than the original signal?

(A) 3%
(B) 30%
(C) 50%
(D) 97%
(E) Depends on the ultrasound velocity

A88. Signal attenuation in ultrasound is

(A) normally measured in decibels
(B) very high in the lung
(C) proportional to frequency
(D) about 1 dB/cm at 1 MHz in soft tissue
(E) all of the above

A89. Refraction of an ultrasound beam refers to the

(A) change of beam frequency
(B) multiple reflections at two interfaces
(C) loss of signal intensity
(D) change in direction of the beam at an interface
(E) all of the above

A90. The Q factor of an ultrasound transducer describes the

(A) crystal resonance frequency
(B) Fresnel zone length
(C) frequency response of the crystal
(D) FWHM value of the beam intensity
(E) power penetration into patient

A91. True (T) or False (F). The following generally improve the transmission of ultrasound into the patient.

(A) Quarter-wave matching layer
(B) Time gain compensation (TGC)
(C) Gel applied to the transducer
(D) Scan converter

A92. Time gain compensation (TGC) compensates for tissue attenuation by increasing the

(A) transducer output
(B) echo intensity
(C) focal zone length
(D) echo velocity
(E) all of the above

A93. Clinical ultrasound beams may have all the following EXCEPT

(A) frequencies of several MHz
(B) velocities of 1540 m/s in tissue
(C) wavelengths of about 0.5 mm
(D) pulse repetition frequencies (PRF) of 100 kHz
(E) pulses contain only a few wavelengths

A94. Increasing the ultrasound pulse length will generally reduce the

(A) axial resolution
(B) amount of power deposited in the patient
(C) acoustical impedance
(D) transducer Q factor
(E) lateral resolution

A95. A Doppler ultrasound examination can use

(A) specular reflections to characterize tissue
(B) pulsed ultrasound to eliminate aliasing
(C) continuous ultrasound to measure flow
(D) echo amplitude to measure impedance
(E) time to measure interface depth

A96. True (T) or False (F).

(A) All naturally occurring nuclei have a magnetic moment
(B) Protons in magnetic fields precess at the Larmor frequency
(C) Protons aligned parallel to the field have higher energy than those aligned antiparallel
(D) Most protons in a region contribute to the MR signal

A97. The Larmor equation in MR involves all of the following EXCEPT

(A) magnetic field strength
(B) gyromagnetic ratio for nucleus of interest
(C) nuclear precession frequency
(D) spin–spin relaxation rate

A98. Following a 90-degree RF pulse, spins in a uniform magnetic field will likely lose their phase coherence in a time comparable to

(A) T1
(B) T2
(C) TE
(D) TI
(E) TR

A99. True (T) or False (F). For commercial whole body MR magnets

(A) resistive magnets need coolant to dissipate heat
(B) resistive magnets have a maximum strength of 2 T
(C) permanent magnets have small fringe fields
(D) permanent magnets are generally very heavy
(E) superconducting magnets have uniformities approaching 1 part per million (ppm)
(F) superconducting magnets have field strengths up to 4 T

A100. The RF coils used in proton MR imaging do NOT

(A) resonate at about 42 MHz at 1 T
(B) emit RF pulses of short duration
(C) detect RF signals
(D) require water cooling

A101. Which of the following items is not affected by a nearby MRI system?

(A) Cardiac pacemaker
(B) Nuclear medicine gamma camera
(C) Credit card
(D) Image intensifier
(E) Optical densitometer

A102. True (T) or False (F). In MR imaging

(A) the RF frequency used is dependent on patient size
(B) T1 for fluids is very long
(C) T2 of bone is longer than T2 of soft tissue
(D) at 1 T, proton signal strength is stronger than ^{31}P
(E) tumors generally have longer relaxation times than normal tissue

A103. MRI reconstruction algorithms commonly use

(A) two-dimensional Fourier transforms
(B) K-space Hankel transforms
(C) patient motion corrections
(D) algebraic reconstruction techniques (ART)
(E) all of the above

A104. The appearance of CSF on a conventional spin echo image with T2 weighting is

(A) isointense with gray matter
(B) darker than white matter
(C) very bright
(D) very dark
(E) cannot be determined

A105. Increasing the main magnetic field will increase all of the following EXCEPT

(A) T1
(B) T2
(C) signal-to-noise ratio
(D) MRI system cost
(E) proton resonance frequency

A106. Match the T1 relaxation time (at 1 tesla) with the tissue type.

(A) 260 ms
(B) 650 ms
(C) 2400 ms

(i) CSF
(ii) Fat
(iii) Kidney

A107. Match the T2 relaxation time with the tissue type.

(A) 45 ms
(B) 90 ms
(C) 180 ms

(i) White matter
(ii) Cerebrospinal fluid
(iii) Liver

A108. All of the following effects give rise to artifacts in MRI EXCEPT

(A) susceptibility changes
(B) motion
(C) chemical shifts
(D) refraction
(E) undersampling

A109. Match the physical density with the tissues found in the breast.

(A) 0.9 g/cm^3
(B) 1.04 g/cm^3
(C) 1.05 g/cm^3
(D) 2.2 g/cm^3

(i) Calcification
(ii) Adipose
(iii) Fibroglandular tissue
(iv) Carcinoma

A110. Mammography examinations use a low kVp primarily to

(A) reduce x-ray tube loading
(B) increase subject contrast
(C) increase the importance of Compton effects
(D) reduce the importance of photoelectric effects
(E) reduce the patient dose

A111. Screen/film mammography uses all the following EXCEPT

(A) half-wave rectification
(B) low kVp (25–35)
(C) molybdenum targets
(D) beryllium windows
(E) molybdenum filtration

A112. Grids in mammography may increase all the following EXCEPT

(A) breast dose
(B) image contrast
(C) x-ray tube loading
(D) object contrast
(E) exposure time

A113. American College of Radiology accreditation of breast imaging centers involves all the following EXCEPT

(A) documentation of a quality control program
(B) assessment of image quality using a phantom
(C) independent evaluation of clinical images
(D) weekly measurement of kVp
(E) annual evaluations by a medical physicist

A114. Match the following mammographic imaging methods with the appropriate technical components and setting.

(A) Screen/film
(B) Xeromammography
(C) Magnification
(D) Two images at ± 15 degrees

(i) 45 kVp, tungsten target, Al filter
(ii) 0.1 mm focal spot
(iii) 28 kVp, Mo target, Mo filter
(iv) Stereotactic localization

A115. Advantages of ultrasound for breast imaging include all of the following EXCEPT

(A) differentiation of cysts from solids
(B) no ionizing radiation
(C) noninvasive
(D) good visualization of micrcocalcifications

A116. All of the following imaging modalities have been used for breast imaging EXCEPT

(A) thermography
(B) magnetic resonance imaging
(C) ultrasound
(D) electron microscopy
(E) diaphanography

A117. If the average number of photons detected in a mm^2 is 10,000, the chance of detecting between 9700 and 10,300 counts in any exposed mm^2 is

(A) 67%
(B) 90%
(C) 95%
(D) 99%
(E) insufficient data to perform calculation

A118. If 100 photons strike each square mm of an imaging system, the corresponding signal-to-noise ratio (SNR) per mm^2 is

(A) > 100:1
(B) 100:1
(C) 10:1
(D) 1:1
(E) cannot be determined

A119. Match the following.

(A) High specificity
(B) High sensitivity
(C) High accuracy

(i) High true-negative fraction (TNF)
(ii) Low false-positive (FPF) and false-negative fractions (FNF)
(iii) High true-positive fraction (TPF)

A120. Adjusting a decision threshold to increase the sensitivity will normally result in an increase in the

(A) area under the ROC curve
(B) false-positive fraction
(C) specificity
(D) accuracy
(E) none of the above

Answers and Explanations

A1–B. Roentgen is the non-SI unit; in SI units, exposures are expressed in C/kg, where $1\ R = 2.58 \times 10^{-4}$ C/kg.

A2. A–iv; B–ii; C–iii; D–i; E–v.

A3. A–iii; B–iv; C–i; D–ii.

A4–D. Binding energy. Inner-shell electrons are tightly bound to the nucleus with binding energies of the order of keV; outer-shell electrons are loosely bound with binding energies of a few eV.

A5. A–iii; B–i; C–iv; D–ii.

A6. A–ii; diagnostic x-rays and 10^{-10} m; **B–iv;** MRI and 7 m radio waves; **C–iii;** ultrasound and 1 mm; **D–i;** visible light and 5×10^{-7} m.

A7–E. Ultrasound is not ionizing radiation. Note that photons and neutrons are indirectly ionizing radiations, whereas charged particles like electrons and alpha particles are directly ionizing.

A8. A–True; emission of an electron results in an increase in the nuclear positive charge of one unit; **B–False;** the mass number A does not change; **C–False;** the emission of a positron reduces the nuclear charge by one; **D–True;** isomeric transition involves the emission of gamma rays; **E–True;** in alpha decay, a helium nucleus is emitted which contains two protons and two neutrons.

A9. A–i; B–ii; neutrinos are emitted in electron capture processes; **C–iii;** in pair production, a photon is transformed into an electron/positron pair; **D–v;** an electric current is a flow of electrons; **E–iv;** ^{222}Rn is an alpha emitter.

A10–D. 1 Ci is 3.7×10^{10} Bq or 37 GBq, and 10 mCi is 1/100 of that, or 3.7×10^8 Bq (370 MBq).

A11–C. The only difference is that half-wave rectification has half the pulses "missing," therefore the output of the full-wave rectified system is twice as large (ripples are the same at 100%).

A12–A. The K-shell binding energy for tungsten is 69 keV, so K-shell vacancies cannot be created using 50 keV electrons.

A13–A. A space charge.

A14–B. The intensity of x-ray production is approximately proportional to the atomic number Z.

A15. A–iv; most of the energy is converted into heat; **B–i;** only about 1% of the incident energy is converted into x-rays; **C–iii;** the incident energy is either converted into x-rays or heat and thus the total must sum to 100%; **D–ii;** only 10% of the photons in this beam will be characteristic x-rays with energies of about 65 keV.

A16–B. Focal-spot ratings are for exposure times of 0.1 s.

A17–A. The total x-ray tube output will primarily determine the film density.

A18–B. The highest x-ray beam intensity is at the cathode edge. At the anode edge, there is significant absorption within the anode itself.

A19–B. Pair production mainly occurs in the strong electric field near the nucleus. The threshold is 1.022 MeV and, therefore, this interaction is not encountered in diagnostic radiology.

A20–B. Scattered photons are generally produced in Compton processes. The incident photon is completely absorbed during the photoelectric effect.

A21. A–False; the photon disappears in photoelectric absorption and produces a photoelectron; **B–False;** Compton scatter has no threshold; 1.022 MeV is the threshold for pair production; **C–False;** the photoelectric effect falls off rapidly as $1/E^3$ above the K-edge; **D–True**.

A22–E. Scattering angle. When the scattering angle is 180 degrees, the backscattered photon has the lowest energy, and the Compton electron the highest energy.

A23. A–photoelectric; Compton is greater than photoelectric at photon energies > 25 keV; the mean energy for 28 kVp beams is < 25 keV; **B–photoelectric;** for calcium with a K-shell binding energy of 4 keV, the Compton effect is greater than the photoelectric effect for energies > 90 keV; **C–Compton effect; D–photoelectric effect; E–photoelectric effect**. Coherent processes are never dominant in diagnostic radiology.

A24–B. The mass attenuation coefficient is equal to the linear attenuation coefficient (μ) divided by the density (ρ) (0.1/2 or 0.05 cm^2/g).

A25–C. Tube loadings must increase since the x-ray tube output is reduced by the added filter. Increased filtration will increase the mean energy of the x-ray beam and therefore decrease subject contrast and skin exposure for a constant film density.

A26–C. Beam quality is the penetrating power measured as the thickness of Al required to attenuate the beam by 50%.

A27–A. kVp affects the subject contrast, which is the difference in x-ray beam intensities emerging from the patient. The other factors determine how subject contrast is transformed into image contrast.

A28–C. Rem is the non-SI unit of dose equivalent.

A29–B. The QF converts dose (rad or Gy) to dose equivalent (rem or Sv). Note that in diagnostic radiology, the QF is generally equal to 1.0.

A30. A–iii; B–i; C–ii.

A31. A–ii; gray and rad are units of absorbed dose; **B–iii;** becquerel and curie are units of activity; **C–i;** sievert and rem are units of dose equivalent; **D–v;** C/kg and roentgen are units of exposure; **E–iv;** joule and erg are units of energy.

A32–A. Increasing the developer temperature will generally increase the film density.

A33. A–iii; mammography requires high contrast; gammas of about 3 are typical; **B–i;** chest radiographs need wide latitudes to visualize both the lung and mediastinum; **C–ii;** penetration through the abdomen is low, and fast screen/film combinations are used to reduce exposure times and patient dose.

A34–C. Wide latitude. Latitude is inversely proportional to contrast, so that a high value of one indicates a low value of the other.

A35. A–i; GM meters are very sensitive and portable, which makes them ideal for detection of contamination; **B–iii;** physicists use ionization chambers to measure the output of x-ray tubes; **C–ii;** thermoluminescent dosimeters are replacing film for personnel monitoring due to their superior energy response and ease of processing without the use of chemicals; **D–iv;** xeroradiography uses charged selenium plates.

A36–B. The intensification factor is typically about 50.

A37–E. None are true. Matching the K-edge with the x-ray photon energy improves the x-ray beam *absorption efficiency*.

A38. A–True; B–True; C–True; D–True; E–False. Note that most films are generally sensitive to blue light.

A39–A. The grid ratio (strip height divided by gap distance) determines how efficiently the scattered radiation is removed.

A40–C. The modulation transfer function (MTF) specifies the resolution properties of an imaging system.

A41–C. Because the HVL for soft tissue is about 3 cm, the nodule will reduce the x-ray intensity by a factor of 2 and change log relative exposure by $\log_{10}2$, which is 0.3; changing log exposure by 0.3 changes film density by 0.6 if the gradient is 2.0.

A42–B. Focal spot blur increases with focal spot size and magnification. Note that there is *no* focal spot blur in contact radiography.

A43–E. All of the listed factors would generally be expected to *increase* image contrast.

A44–C. Thicker screens will increase the efficiency of x-ray absorption but reduce the spatial resolution performance because of increasing screen blur.

A45. A–iv; the air gap introduced in the magnification view causes most of the scatter to miss the film; **B–iii;** a 12:1 grid is necessary because of the large amount of Compton scatter present in abdominal studies due to the large body thickness; **C–i;** because mammography is performed at low (28) kVps, there is less scatter, and a 4:1 grid is usually sufficient; **D–ii;** 6:1 grids are less sensitive to lateral decentering, which is an important consideration in portable examinations.

A46–D. Increasing the screen thickness does not change the total number of x-rays absorbed to give a specified film density, and therefore image noise will not be affected.

A47. A–iv; subject contrast is always reduced as kV increases; **B–i;** a lower mA will require a longer exposure time, which will increase the motion blur; **C–ii;** grids improve image contrast by reducing the amount of scatter reaching the screen/film; **D–iii;** increasing focal spot size will increase focal spot blur.

A48–E. This is a list of the key characteristics of computed radiography.

A49. A–iii; B–ii; C–i.

A50–E. Photocathodes convert light to electrons.

A51–A. The use of CsI crystals limits the spread of light in the input phosphor and therefore improves spatial resolution.

A52–E. All of the statements are true.

A53–D. The dominant source of image noise is quantum mottle, which is reduced by increasing the number of x-ray photons.

A54–A. kVp requirements in fluoroscopy and cine are very similar (70 to 90 kVp) and primarily determined by patient penetration.

A55–B. The distance along one dimension is 250 mm, which is used for 256 pixels, so each has a linear dimension of about 1 mm.

A56–C. The CPU performs all the arithmetic and logical operations in a computer.

A57. A–False; random access memory loses its information when the power is switched off; **B–True; C–False;** floppy disks hold about 1 MByte of information, whereas hard disks can store up to 1000 times more; **D–False;** magnetic tapes are relatively slow devices because the information is stored serially; **E–True;** optical jukeboxes can store over 1 TByte (10^{12} Bytes) of information.

A58–D. PACS are currently very expensive; their justification is in their potential to cut operating costs (e.g., film, clerks).

A59. A–ii; B–iv; C–iii; D–v; E–i.

A60–E. Patient temperature does not significantly affect the attenuation properties of the tissue relative to water.

A61–D. Limiting spatial resolution will increase because the pixel size is reduced when the matrix size is increased.

A62–B. At a higher kVp, attenuation coefficient differences are reduced and subject contrast is decreased.

A63–B. Phase-encoding artifacts only occur on MR images.

A64–C. The mA determines the intensity of the x-ray beam, hence image noise, but has no direct effect on spatial resolution.

A65–A. Displayed contrast is the only factor that will be affected by the display window width.

A66–A. Beam-hardening artifacts occur because the average photon energy of an x-ray beam increases as it passes through the patient. The preferential loss of lower energy x-rays depresses the CT numbers because of an apparent increase in x-ray beam penetration.

A67. A–37 Bq (10^{-9} Ci); **B–370 kBq** (10^{-5} Ci); **C–370 MBq** (10^{-2} Ci); **D–3.7 GBq** (1 Ci); **E–3.7 × 10^{13} Bq** (10^3 Ci); **F–3.7 × 10^{17} Bq** (10^7 Ci).

A68–D. ^{99m}Tc generators can be eluted with saline on a daily basis. The parent ^{99}Mo has a half-life of 67 hours, whereas the daughter ^{99m}Tc has a half-life of 6 hours. The growth of daughter activity reaches its maximum after about 4 daughter half-lives, or 24 hours.

A69–E. All of the statements are true.

A70–A. Spatial resolution decreases with increasing distance from the collimator face.

A71–B. Septal penetration always increases with increasing photon energy.

A72–C. Only MUGA studies absolutely require a computer to place the acquired counts into different parts of the cardiac cycle.

A73–E. Gamma camera imaging time has no effect on organ doses.

A74. A–True; B–False; the Γ factor would be needed to estimate the external radiation exposure level near the patient, but not the thyroid dose; **C–True; D–True; E–True**.

A75–B. Crystal impurities are found in solid crystals such as film grains or semiconductor devices, not radiopharmaceuticals.

A76–D. Multiple views are obtained (typically 64 or 128 as the gamma camera is rotated around the patient).

A77–C. The range of the positrons is only 1 mm in soft tissue. PET makes use of the subsequent 511 keV gammas emitted when the positron annihilates with an electron.

A78–C. Lymphocytes are very radiosensitive.

A79–E. All of the statements are true.

A80. A–iii; B–i; C–ii.

A81–D. The entrance skin dose for a lateral lumbar spine is about 10 mGy (1 rad) so that the dose to the embryo will likely be 0.5 to 1 mGy (50–100 mrad).

A82–E. All of the statements are correct.

A83–C. Most diagnostic radiology lead aprons have a 0.5 mm lead equivalence.

A84–D. None of these are requirements for leaded glasses.

A85. A–True; B–True; C–True; domestic radon may be responsible for 10% of lung cancers in the United States; **D–False;** radon is an alpha emitter; **E–False;** radon's half-life is just under 4 days.

A86–B. Because beam attenuation is proportional to frequency, beam penetration will be markedly reduced.

A87–C. $dB = 10 \times \log_{10}(I/I_o)$.

A88–E. All of the statements are true.

A89–D. Refraction is governed by Snell's law and results in the ultrasound beam changing direction when passing from one medium to another.

A90–C. The Q factor is the bandwidth of the frequencies generated by the ultrasound transducer. A high Q indicates a narrow bandwidth and relatively pure frequency.

A91. A–True; B–False; TGC amplifies returning echoes dependent on depth; **C–True;** prevents an air layer between the transducer and patient that would reflect virtually all the incident beam; **D–False;** stores digital image data which are converted into video signal for display on a TV monitor.

A92–B. TGC increases the echo intensity with increasing echo time to account for increasing signal attenuation with tissue depth.

A93–D. The typical PRF is 1 kHz, not 100 kHz. The penetration depth would be less than 1 cm for a PRF of 100 kHz.

A94–A. Axial resolution is equal to half the pulse length; therefore, increasing the pulse length reduces axial resolution.

A95–C. Doppler provides information about flow from the change in ultrasound frequency produced by a moving object.

A96. A–False; nuclei with even numbers of protons and neutrons (e.g., ^{4}He) have no net magnetic moment; **B–True;** for protons this is 42 MHz/tesla; **C–False;** when aligned parallel, the energy is *lower*; **D–False;** only the excess in the lower energy orientation contribute to the signal (about 3 per million).

A97–D. The Larmor equation ($2\pi f_L = \gamma \times B$) determines the RF frequency, where f_L is the Larmor frequency, B is the applied field, and γ is the gyromagnetic ratio.

A98–B. T2 is the characteristic time that describes loss of phase coherence in the transverse plane in the absence of magnetic field inhomogeneity effects.

A99. A–True; power dissipation in the resistive coils is several tens of kW; **B–False;** maximum fields are about 0.5 T; **C–True;** permanent magnets have poles similar to horseshoe magnets which limit the fringe fields; **D–True;** the large mass of permanent magnets is one of their disadvantages because of siting difficulties; **E–True;** most magnets are shimmed to achieve a uniformity of about 1 ppm; **F–True;** there are a number of whole body 4 T magnets in operation.

A100–D. RF coils do not require water cooling.

A101–E. Optical densitometers are used to measure the density of film and are not affected by magnetic fields.

A102. A–False; RF frequency is determined solely by the type of nucleus and the magnetic field strength; **B–True;** several seconds for water and cerebrospinal fluid; **C–False;** T2 for all solids including bone is very short and is the main reason why bone gives no detectable MR signal; **D–True; E–True;** T1 and T2 generally increase with malignancy, but there are wide ranges for both normal and malignant tissues.

A103–A. Two-dimensional Fourier transforms are generally employed for planar reconstruction on current commercial systems.

A104–C. CSF has a long T2 value and will appear bright on T2 weighted spin echo sequences.

A105–B. For biological tissues, T2 is generally independent of magnetic field strength.

A106. A–ii; B–iii; C–i. Lipids have a short T1 and fluids have a long T1.

A107. A–iii; B–i; C–ii.

A108–D. Refraction gives rise to artifacts in ultrasound, not MRI.

A109. A–ii; B–iii; C–iv; D–i. Fat has the lowest density, and calcifications have the highest. Cancer is only slightly more dense than fibroglandular tissue.

A110–B. The contrast between fibroglandular and malignant tissues increases with reducing kVp because the photoelectric effect predominates at these low kVps.

A111–A. Dedicated mammography units currently use either three-phase or high-frequency generators. Half-wave rectification would reduce the x-ray tube output and significantly increase exposure times.

A112–D. Object contrast, which refers to the physical differences between areas of the imaged breast, is not affected by grids.

A113–D. kV is checked on an annual basis and requires special kVp meters used by physicists.

A114. A–iii; classic requirements for screen/film mammography; **B–i;** classic requirements for xeroradiography; **C–ii;** microfocal spot size is always used in magnification mammography to minimize focal spot blur; **D–iv;** two views are required to localize the lesion stereoscopically.

A115–D. Ultrasound does not visualize microcalcifications.

A116–D. Electron microscopy is used for in vitro tissue analysis.

A117–D. The standard deviation σ is $\sqrt{10,000}$ or 100; 99% of counts will lie between the mean $\pm 3\,\sigma$ or $10,000 \pm 300$.

A118–C. 10:1; signal is 100, the noise is $\sqrt{100}$, or 10, so the SNR is 10:1.

A119. A–i; B–iii; C–ii.

A120–B. When the threshold criterion becomes more lax so that the TPF increases, the FPF also increases, and specificity, which is $(1 - \text{FPF})$, is reduced.

PRACTICE EXAMINATION B

B1. Match the energy source and power level.

(A) 2 W
(B) 50 W
(C) 500 W
(D) 2000 W

(i)   Light bulb
(ii) Flashlight
(iii) Stove burner
(iv) Microwave oven

B2. Match the following.

(A) Radon gas
(B) Magnetic resonance imaging
(C) Radiation therapy
(D) Beta minus decay

(i)   Electrons
(ii) Gamma rays
(iii) Alpha particles
(iv) RF waves

B3. Which of the following have zero rest mass?

(A) X-ray photons
(B) Electrons
(C) Neutrons
(D) Alpha particles
(E) None of the above

B4. Match the K-shell binding energies with the appropriate element.

(A) Iodine (Z = 53)
(B) Oxygen (Z = 8)
(C) Calcium (Z = 20)
(D) Tungsten (Z = 74)

(i)   0.5 keV
(ii) 4 keV
(iii) 33 keV
(iv) 70 keV

B5. Match the following application with the appropriate electromagnetic radiation.

(A) Used in magnetic resonance
(B) Used in diagnostic radiology
(C) Emitted by a CsI scintillator
(D) Emitted by all patients and staff
(E) Used in nuclear medicine

(i)   Visible light
(ii) X-rays
(iii) Radiowaves
(iv) Infrared
(v)   Gamma rays

B6. The process in which a neutral atom is changed into an electrically charged atom is called

(A) fission
(B) fusion
(C) ionization
(D) excitation
(E) scintillation

B7. Match the following nuclides with the appropriate definition.

(A) Isomer
(B) Isobar
(C) Isotone
(D) Isotope

(i)   Same number of nucleons
(ii) Same number of protons
(iii) Same number of neutrons
(iv) Same nucleus

B8. ^{226}Ra

(A) is a naturally occurring radionuclide
(B) emits alpha particles
(C) has a half-life of 1600 years
(D) has a radioactive daughter product ^{222}Rn (radon)
(E) all of the above

B9. A 100 keV x-ray photon and a 100 keV gamma ray differ in their

(A) means of production
(B) position in the electromagnetic spectrum
(C) wavelengths
(D) penetrating power in matter
(E) speed

B10. Compared to an x-ray beam produced by a single-phase generator, an x-ray beam produced by a three-phase generator (6 pulse) will have

(A) lower maximum photon energy
(B) fewer photons
(C) lower HVL
(D) greater heel effect
(E) none of the above

B11. Maximum x-ray energy increases with the

(A) anode angle
(B) atomic number of the target
(C) filament current
(D) tube current
(E) tube kVp

B12. Match the characteristic K x-ray photon energy with the element.

(A) Molybdenum (Z = 42)
(B) Iodine (Z = 53)
(C) Tungsten (Z = 74)
(D) Lead (Z = 82)

(i) 84.9 keV
(ii) 67.2 keV
(iii) 19.6 keV
(iv) 32.3 keV

B13. Which of the following devices CAN-NOT be used to obtain information about the focal spot size?

(A) Pinhole camera
(B) Slit camera
(C) Multiformat camera
(D) Star test pattern
(E) Parallel bar (line pair) phantom

B14. The maximum focus loading will likely increase with

(A) smoother waveform
(B) increasing focal spot size
(C) increasing anode rotation speed
(D) all of the above

B15. How would the exposure time have to be changed to maintain the same film density if the tube current (mA) was tripled?

(A) Kept constant___
(B) Increased by $\sqrt{1/3}$
(C) Reduced to 1/3
(D) Reduced to 1/9
(E) Depends on patient thickness

B16. True (T) or False (F). X-ray tube output (mR) may be increased by increasing the

(A) voltage across the tube (kV)
(B) heat capacity of the target
(C) atomic number (Z) of the target
(D) tube current (mA)
(E) filtration at the x-ray tube window
(F) rotation speed of anode

B17. Radiation that leaves the x-ray tube housing when the collimators are fully closed is known as

(A) primary radiation
(B) secondary radiation
(C) leakage radiation
(D) entrance radiation
(E) backscattered radiation

B18. Coherent scatter is important because it results in

(A) backscatter
(B) increased patient doses
(C) scattered electrons
(D) reduced spatial resolution
(E) none of the above

B19. Following absorption of a single 30 keV photon in a patient

(A) temperature rises significantly (> 1° C)
(B) a large number of ionization events occur
(C) several scatter photons emerge to degrade image quality
(D) internal conversion electrons are produced
(E) "excited" nuclei are produced

B20. True (T) or False (F). When radiation interacts with matter

(A) scattered photons with shorter wavelengths than those of incident photons may be produced
(B) a photon may be totally absorbed by an atom
(C) energy is transferred to electrons
(D) photons may scatter from atoms without losing energy

B21. Backscattered photons in fluoroscopy are most likely due to

(A) Compton scatter
(B) isomeric transitions
(C) coherent interactions
(D) K-shell interactions
(E) photodisintegration interactions

B22. The interaction of diagnostic x-rays in patients involves all of the following EXCEPT

(A) energy transfer from photons to electrons
(B) primarily Compton and photoelectric effects
(C) pair production
(D) coherent scatter
(E) energy deposition in the patient

B23. Approximate values for primary x-ray transmission through a patient are

(A) 10% for chest x-rays
(B) 1% for skulls
(C) 0.5% for abdomens
(D) 5% for mammography
(E) all of the above

B24. In diagnostic radiology, the linear attenuation coefficient (μ) increases with

(A) increasing density (ρ)
(B) increasing atomic number (Z)
(C) reduced photon energy
(D) reduced x-ray tube voltage (kVp)
(E) all of the above

B25. True (T) or False (F). Addition of an Al filter into an x-ray beam (for constant film density) would increase the

(A) patient skin exposure
(B) half-value layer (HVL)
(C) subject contrast
(D) mAs
(E) anode heat loading

B26. Diagnostic x-ray beam quality measured using HVL is

(A) independent of the added filtration
(B) proportional to x-ray tube mAs
(C) independent of kVp
(D) typically 3 mm Al at 80 kVp
(E) not subject to regulations

B27. All the following are related to exposure EXCEPT

(A) linear energy transfer (LET)
(B) ability to ionize air
(C) ionization chambers
(D) Roentgen
(E) output of an x-ray tube

B28. The exposure and absorbed dose is as the

(A) rad and the gray
(B) absorption of ionizing radiation and biological effect
(C) photons and charged particles
(D) ionization in air and absorption in a medium
(E) ionizing and non-ionizing radiation

B29. The f-factor, which converts exposure (R) to absorbed dose, is

(A) independent of photon energy
(B) independent of atomic number (Z)
(C) much greater than 1.0 at high photon energy levels
(D) about 3.0 for bone for diagnostic x-rays
(E) numerically the same in SI and non-SI units

B30. Match the following:

(A) 37 rad
(B) 37 rem
(C) 37 R
(D) 37 Bq

(i) 370 mSv
(ii) 1 nCi
(iii) 370 mGy
(iv) 9.5 mC/kg

B31. Film optical density is all of the following EXCEPT

(A) $\log_{10}$ of the ratio of incident-to-transmitted light
(B) usually measured with a photometer
(C) about 3.0 when most of the silver ions are reduced
(D) about 1.2 at maximum radiographic contrast
(E) best viewed with a hot light when > 2.0

B32. In which film density range will an increase in film fog level most adversely affect image quality?

(A) < 0.5
(B) 0.5 to 1.0
(C) 1.0 to 1.5
(D) > 1.5
(E) Fog does not affect image quality

B33. Increasing the thickness of a scintillation screen will improve

(A) absorption efficiency
(B) conversion efficiency
(C) photocathode efficiency
(D) all of the above

B34. Match the equipment with the associated effect.

(A) X-ray to trapped electrons
(B) Light to electrons
(C) Gamma rays to light
(D) X-ray to light

(i) NaI crystal
(ii) Intensifying screen
(iii) CR imaging plate
(iv) Photomultiplier tube

B35. X-ray photons absorbed by an intensifying screen can produce all of the following EXCEPT

(A) photoelectrons
(B) light photons
(C) characteristic x-rays
(D) auger electrons
(E) Bremsstrahlung

B36. Using a screen/film combination rather than film on its own will reduce

(A) patient dose
(B) x-ray tube loading
(C) patient motion artifacts
(D) exposure times
(E) all of the above

B37. Calcium tungstate screens are

(A) least efficient at photon energies above 70 keV
(B) faster than rare earth screens
(C) able to convert 50% of absorbed x-ray energy to light
(D) commonly rated as 100 speed
(E) popular because they reduce patient blur

B38. Match the following examinations with the most appropriate image receptor.

(A) Mammography
(B) Chest radiography
(C) Computed tomography
(D) Barium enema spot film
(E) Xeroradiography

(i) Double screen and wide latitude, double emulsion film
(ii) Selenium-coated aluminum plate
(iii) Single screen and single emulsion film
(iv) Double screen and fast, double emulsion film
(v) Single emulsion film (no screen)

B39. A Bucky grid will increase all the following EXCEPT

(A) image contrast
(B) exposure times
(C) anode loading
(D) geometric unsharpness
(E) patient dose

B40. A grid will generally _____ image contrast.

(A) improve
(B) keep constant
(C) reduce
(D) eliminate

B41. The limiting spatial resolution in *contact radiography* can be improved by reducing the

(A) focal spot size
(B) kV
(C) filtration
(D) grid ratio
(E) screen speed

B42. In a phototimed diagnostic radiograph, doubling the mA will increase the

(A) x-ray beam output rate
(B) beam HVL
(C) average photon energy
(D) patient penetration
(E) patient entrance skin dose

B43. Match the examination with exposure time.

(A) Digital subtraction angiography (DSA) (1 frame)
(B) Abdominal radiograph
(C) Chest radiograph
(D) Film/screen mammography

(i) 5 ms
(ii) 30 ms
(iii) 100 ms
(iv) 1 second

B44. Choice of screen/film combination affects all the following EXCEPT

(A) subject contrast
(B) patient dose
(C) quantum mottle
(D) low contrast discrimination
(E) high contrast spatial resolution

B45. Match the following imaging systems with the limiting spatial resolution.

(A) 400 speed film/screen
(B) 35 mm cine film
(C) Conventional fluoroscopy
(D) MRI

(i) 0.3 line pair per mm
(ii) 1.0 line pair per mm
(iii) 3.5 line pair per mm
(iv) 7.0 line pair per mm

B46. Entrance skin exposure is generally NOT affected by increasing the

(A) screen thickness
(B) grid ratio
(C) kVp
(D) focal spot size
(E) film speed

B47. Which of the following changes in the radiographic technique would NOT double the screen/film exposure level?

(A) Increase kVp by ~10
(B) Double the kVp
(C) Double the mA
(D) Double the exposure time
(E) Reduce focus-to-film distance by 30%

B48. Subject contrast is increased by decreasing

(A) kVp
(B) mA
(C) screen thickness
(D) film speed
(E) none of the above

B49. The MTF of an image intensifier is primarily affected by the

(A) input grid
(B) input phosphor thickness
(C) lens system
(D) TV camera
(E) all of the above

B50. An image intensifier with a 12" diameter input and a 1" diameter output has a minification gain of

(A) 1/144
(B) 1/12
(C) 12
(D) 13
(E) 144

B51. All of the following are true for fluoroscopy EXCEPT

(A) the conversion gain is typically 100 cd/m^2 per mR/s
(B) a major source of image noise is quantum mottle
(C) the image intensifier input dose is ~2 μR per frame
(D) the image intensifier voltage is 220 V AC
(E) the resolution is about 1 line pair per mm

B52. If the light intensity at the exit phosphor of a typical image intensifier is 100 cd/m^2, then the input exposure rate is most likely about

(A) 10 mR/s
(B) 1 mR/s
(C) 1 mR/minute
(D) 1 mR/hour
(E) none of the above

B53. In cardiac cine filming

(A) spatial resolution is > 8 line pairs per mm
(B) very large IIs are used
(C) patient entrance skin exposures may be 30 μR per frame
(D) images from the II are captured on 35 mm film
(E) typical frame rates are 5/s

B54. True (T) or False (F).

(A) Exact framing utilizes the entire intensifier image
(B) Exact framing provides a magnified image
(C) Overframing records the whole II image
(D) Overframing provides superior spatial resolution

B55. Match the following image receptor exposure per frame and imaging modality.

(A) 2 μR
(B) 25 μR
(C) 150 μR
(D) 300 μR

(i) 400 speed screen/film
(ii) Regular fluoroscopy
(iii) 35 mm cineradiography
(iv) Photospot film

B56. Match the following computer storage medium with access time.

(A) 10 ms
(B) 1 s
(C) > 10 s

(i) Floppy disk
(ii) Magnetic tape
(iii) Hard disk

B57. Match the local area network with the time required to transfer a digital 8 MB chest x-ray image.

(A) < 1 second
(B) 1 minute
(C) 2 hours

(i)   Modem (phone)
(ii) Asynchronous transfer mode (ATM)
(iii) Ethernet

B58. Gamma cameras use 8 bits to code for one pixel; the maximum number of gray levels that can be coded for is

(A) 8
(B) 64
(C) 512
(D) 1028
(E) none of the above

B59. Computers use all the following EXCEPT

(A) COBOL input/output devices
(B) programming languages such as C
(C) magnetic media storage devices
(D) CPUs to perform arithmetic and/or logic functions
(E) array processors for fast computation

B60. Match the digital imaging modality and typical matrix size.

(A) Computed radiography
(B) Nuclear medicine
(C) CT scanner
(D) Magnetic resonance
(E) Digital subtraction angiography

(i) 64×64
(ii) 256×256
(iii) 512×512
(iv) 1024×1024
(v) 2048×2048

B61. CT is better than screen/film for neuroimaging because CT

(A) is quicker
(B) has superior spatial resolution
(C) reduces patient doses (radiation risk)
(D) has excellent contrast discrimination
(E) is less expensive

B62. A material which has an attenuation coefficient 5% greater than water will have a Hounsfield unit value of

(A) – 50
(B) – 5
(C) + 5
(D) + 50
(E) none of the above

B63. Iodine-based contrast results in increased CT numbers in the reconstructed image because of

(A) changes in the image display settings
(B) increased photoelectric absorption
(C) dilation of blood vessels
(D) increased blood flow
(E) none of the above

B64. CT spatial resolution may be expected to increase with increasing

(A) focal spot size
(B) matrix size
(C) field of view
(D) mAs
(E) kVp

B65. Small tumors could be missed on a CT scan because of

(A) large section thickness (10 mm)
(B) incorrect window setting
(C) large table index (20 mm)
(D) use of a bone reconstruction algorithm
(E) all of the above

B66. Detecting large, low-contrast objects by CT is affected by all of the following EXCEPT

(A) focal spot size
(B) mA
(C) slice thickness
(D) scan time
(E) pixel size

B67. The typical dose to the eye lens from a CT scan of the head is approximately

(A) < 1 µGy (< 0.1 mrad)
(B) 1 µGy (0.1 mrad)
(C) 1 mGy (100 mrad)
(D) 1 Gy (100 rad)
(E) none of the above

B68. True (T) or False (F).

(A) The curie is a non-SI unit of activity
(B) 1 curie is 7.3×10^7 disintegrations per second
(C) The curie is based on the activity of 1 g of ^{226}Ra
(D) One becquerel is equal to 1 transformation per second
(E) Specific activity is measured in becquerel per kg (curie per g)

B69. ^{99m}Tc

(A) has a half-life of 67 hours
(B) emits a spectrum of electrons
(C) produces a stable daughter product
(D) emits 140 keV photons
(E) all of the above

B70. Match the radionuclide with the decay mode.

(A) Isomeric transition
(B) Electron capture
(C) Positron emitter
(D) Beta-minus decay

(i) ^{11}C
(ii) ^{131}I
(iii) ^{67}Ga
(iv) ^{99m}Tc

B71. Specify whether the equilibrium for the following generators is considered to be secular or transient.

(A) ^{99}Mo/^{99m}Tc
(B) ^{82}Sr/^{82}Rb
(C) ^{113}Sn/^{113m}In

B72. Match the following radionuclides and primary photopeak energies.

(A) Oxygen-15
(B) Technetium-99m
(C) Iodine-131
(D) Thallium-201

(i) 70 keV
(ii) 140 keV
(iii) 365 keV
(iv) 511 keV

B73. High count rates in nuclear medicine may result in

(A) image distortions
(B) pulse pile-up
(C) poor linearity
(D) long counting times
(E) edge-packing artifacts

B74. The sensitivity of a gamma camera may be improved by increasing the

(A) photomultiplier tube gain
(B) distance to the patient
(C) collimator thickness
(D) collimator hole diameter
(E) none of the above

B75. The biological half-life of a radionuclide depends on the

(A) physical decay mode
(B) administered activity
(C) biological clearance rate
(D) physical half-life
(E) efficiency of detection system

B76. Match the effective dose equivalent (H_E) with the radiographic examination.

(A) 0.03 mSv (3 mrem)
(B) .15 mSv (15 mrem)
(C) 1 mSv (100 mrem)
(D) 10 mSv (1 rem)

(i) Abdominal CT (20 sections)
(ii) PA chest x-ray
(iii) PA + lateral skull examination
(iv) AP + lateral abdominal examination

B77. Iodine-131 administered to a patient for thyroid therapy has

(A) a physical half-life of 8 days
(B) additional biological clearance
(C) an effective half-life shorter than the physical half-life
(D) thyroid dose dependent on the effective half-life
(E) all of the above

B78. A hospital requires all the following before using a radioactive source on a patient EXCEPT

(A) license for the radionuclide in question
(B) a room with 1/16″ lead shielding
(C) designation of a radiation safety officer
(D) the patient's consent
(E) approval of the "radiation safety (isotope) committee"

B79. In PET imaging

(A) scatter is reduced using a thick parallel hole collimator
(B) pulse height analysis is not needed
(C) coincidence detection is employed
(D) off-peak imaging can improve imaging performance
(E) image acquisition is longer than in SPECT

B80. Stochastic effects of radiation exposure include

(A) epilation (hair loss)
(B) cataract induction
(C) leukemia
(D) skin erythema
(E) permanent sterility

B81. The probability of a patient developing a radiation-induced cataract following four head CT examinations is

(A) 0%
(B) 0.1%
(C) 1%
(D) 10%

B82. True (T) or False (F). For low-level occupational exposure to radiation

(A) deterministic radiation effects are likely to occur
(B) cancer and genetic effects are the major concerns
(C) cancer risks are associated with latent periods (years)
(D) quantitative risk estimates are available
(E) radiation risk estimates are about 4% per Sv (100 rem)

B83. All of the following will reduce patient dose EXCEPT

(A) faster screens
(B) higher kVp
(C) higher ratio grids
(D) more beam collimation
(E) photospot film vs screen/film

B84. Which of the following will generally reduce the entrance skin dose during a radiographic examination if the film density is kept constant?

(A) Increase the kVp
(B) Increase the screen/film speed
(C) Reduce the grid ratio
(D) All of the above

B85. During fluoroscopy the

(A) entrance skin exposure (ESE) rate is several mR per minute
(B) legal maximum ESE rate is 10 R/s
(C) ESE rate can never exceed 10 R/min
(D) scattered radiation is reduced by two when distance is doubled
(E) none of the above

B86. Match the following dose equivalents.

(A) Typical annual dose equivalent for a nuclear medicine worker
(B) Current annual dose equivalent limit for workers
(C) ICRP proposed dose equivalent limit for fetus
(D) Minimum detectable dose equivalent for film badge

(i) 0.2 mSv (20 mrem)
(ii) 1 mSv (100 mrem)
(iii) 2.5 mSv (250 mrem)
(iv) 50 mSv (5 rem)

B87. A technologist standing 1 meter from a patient during fluoroscopy receives a significant radiation dose from

(A) Compton electrons
(B) photoelectrons
(C) Compton scattered photons
(D) characteristic x-rays generated in the patient

B88. The effective dose equivalent would exceed 4 mSv in which of the following?

(A) Ten transcontinental high altitude air flights
(B) A secretary working in a radiology department for one year
(C) The annual fallout from nuclear weapons exploded in the atmosphere
(D) X-rays for the average US citizen per year
(E) Someone living in Leadville, CO (3000 m elevation) for a year

B89. Indoor radon involves all the following risks EXCEPT

(A) lung cancer
(B) lung irradiation by alpha emission
(C) deposition of radioactive aerosols in lung
(D) skin irradiation by beta particles

B90. Ultrasound acoustic impedance is

(A) measured in ohms
(B) independent of density
(C) inversely proportional to the speed of sound
(D) very low for air
(E) very low for bone

B91. Match the following energy reflection values for normal incidence with the type of interface.

(A) 0.1%
(B) 1%
(C) 40%

(i) Bone/muscle
(ii) Blood/muscle
(iii) Fat/muscle

B92. Which of the following does NOT apply to ultrasound echos?

(A) Usually detected by the emitting transducer
(B) Occur after 13 μs for tissue interfaces at depths of 1 cm
(C) Strong for interfaces with large acoustic impedance differences
(D) Increase in intensity with ultrasound frequency
(E) Require the interface to be almost perpendicular (< 3 degrees) to the beam

B93. The angle of reflection of an ultrasound beam at an interface is equal to the

(A) ratio of velocities in the two media
(B) ratio of the impedances of the two media
(C) angle of incidence
(D) angle of refraction
(E) sine of the angle of incidence

B94. The frequency of an ultrasound transducer is most affected by the

(A) applied voltage intensity
(B) crystal thickness
(C) thickness of backing material
(D) crystal density
(E) crystal atomic number

B95. Low Q ultrasound transducers are likely to have

(A) a large Fraunhofer zone dispersion angle
(B) a short focal zone
(C) no focussing
(D) a narrow band of ultrasound frequencies
(E) a wide band of ultrasound frequencies

B96. Real-time images may be obtained with all of the following transducers EXCEPT

(A) linear arrays
(B) rotating single element
(C) rotating multiple element
(D) continuous wave Doppler
(E) annular phased array

B97. How long will it take to receive the echo from an ultrasound beam transmitted through soft tissue to an object 10 cm away?

(A) 1.3 μs
(B) 130 μs
(C) 13 ms
(D) 1.3 s
(E) Cannot be determined from information provided

B98. Match the following ultrasound display modes with the most appropriate clinical application.

(A) A mode
(B) M mode
(C) B mode
(D) Continuous wave Doppler

(i) Detection of stenosis
(ii) Measurements in ophthalmology
(iii) Assessment of the mitral valve
(iv) Liver scanning

B99. Cavitation is most likely to occur at

(A) frequencies above 10 MHz
(B) depths beyond the fresnel zone
(C) low pulse repetition frequencies
(D) interfaces with large acoustic impedance differences
(E) high ultrasound intensities

B100. Continuous wave Doppler uses

(A) the same transducers for pulse generation/detection
(B) high frequencies for better axial resolution
(C) frequency shifts to determine blood flow velocity
(D) transducers with a low Q factor
(E) blood vessels flowing perpendicular to the beam

B101. Match the relative MR sensitivity with the nucleus.

(A) 1.0
(B) 0.83
(C) 0.066

(i) ^{31}P
(ii) ^{19}F
(iii) ^{1}H

B102. True (T) or False (F). The following tissue parameters are likely to affect the image intensity in MR.

(A) Physical density
(B) Proton density
(C) Electron density
(D) Atomic number
(E) T1 relaxation time
(F) T2 relaxation time

B103. Match the tissue with the approximate T1 relaxation time (at 0.5 tesla).

(A) 200 ms
(B) 320 ms
(C) 650 ms
(D) 2000 ms

(i) Gray matter
(ii) Cerebrospinal fluid (CSF)
(iii) Fat
(iv) Liver

B104. The magnetic field strength of resistive magnets used in MR imaging is normally limited by the

(A) poor field inhomogeneities
(B) RF power deposition in coils
(C) weight of the magnet
(D) large fringe fields
(E) large heating in magnet coils

B105. The gradient coils used in MR

(A) cause radiowave emission from the total sample
(B) provide spatial localization
(C) measure the spin coupling
(D) impose the main field along the patient axis
(E) none of the above

B106. True (T) or False (F). The bio-effects of static magnetic fields used in MRI include

(A) magnetophosphes
(B) switching of pacemakers
(C) displacement of aneurysm clips
(D) significant tissue heating
(E) induction of amnesia

B107. All the following signals are associated with MRI, EXCEPT

(A) reverberation echo
(B) free induction decay
(C) gradient echo
(D) spin echo
(E) frequency encoded

B108. A Fourier transform is used in MRI to convert the free induction decay signal into what components?

(A) T1
(B) T2
(C) T2*
(D) Proton spin density
(E) None of the above

B109. Which of the following is NOT true of MRI pulse sequences?

(A) Inversion recovery commences with a 180-degree RF pulse
(B) T2 weighted spin echo sequences have long TE times
(C) FLASH sequences use gradient recalled echos
(D) Echo planar imaging (EPI) uses long TR times
(E) EPI needs very rapid gradient switching

B110. The MRI signal-to-noise ratio depends on all of the following EXCEPT the

(A) strength of the magnetic field
(B) number of excitations (acquisitions)
(C) image reconstruction algorithm
(D) voxel size
(E) nucleus being imaged

B111. The total examination time in MRI is affected by all of the following EXCEPT the

(A) number of frequency encoding steps
(B) number of phase encoding steps
(C) TR time
(D) number of acquisitions

B112. To perform MR spectroscopy with current scanners generally requires all of the following EXCEPT

(A) strong magnetic fields
(B) good magnetic field uniformity
(C) signal from a volume of tissue of at least 1 cm^3
(D) administration of a spectroscopy contrast agent
(E) frequency analysis of acquired FID signals

B113. Match the following breast tissues and linear mass attenuation coefficients.

(A) Adipose
(B) Fibroglandular
(C) Carcinoma
(D) Calcification

(i) 12.5 cm^{-1}
(ii) 0.85 cm^{-1}
(iii) 0.8 cm^{-1}
(iv) 0.45 cm^{-1}

B114. Compression is used in mammography to

(A) make the breast more uniform
(B) allow a lower kVp to be used
(C) reduce focal spot blur
(D) reduce the radiation dose
(E) all of the above

B115. The mean glandular dose in mammography could be reduced by increasing all of the following EXCEPT the

(A) kVp
(B) half-value layer
(C) screen/film speed
(D) exposure time
(E) processing temperature

B116. Advantages of xeromammography over screen/film include

(A) lower doses
(B) wider latitude
(C) increased large area contrast
(D) reduced scatter
(E) all of the above

B117. Advantages of MRI for breast imaging include all of the following EXCEPT

(A) no ionizing radiation
(B) three-dimensional imaging
(C) fat suppression
(D) spatial resolution comparable to screen/film

B118. Light diaphonography for breast imaging

(A) involves detection of light
(B) has been associated with poor clinical results
(C) has a problem with too much light scatter
(D) primarily detects increases in vascularity
(E) all of the above

B119. Match the following mean counts and corresponding standard deviations.

(A) 100
(B) 1000
(C) 10,000
(D) 100,000

(i) 316
(ii) 1%
(iii) 32
(iv) 10%

B120. True (T) or False (F). Concerning the area under a receiver operating characteristic (ROC) curve

(A) it is a measure of imaging performance
(B) smaller values indicate better performance
(C) an area of 0.5 (50%) is obtained by guessing
(D) an area equal to 0.95 corresponds to an ideal performance
(E) it is normally expressed by the parameter A_z

Answers and Explanations

B1. A–ii; B–i; C–iv; D–iii.

B2. A–iii; ^{222}Rn and its daughters emit alpha particles; **B–iv;** MR uses RF pulses for imaging; **C–ii;** radiation therapy uses gamma emitting radioactive sources such as ^{60}Co; **D–i;** electrons with a spectrum of energy levels are emitted during beta minus decay.

B3–A. X-rays, like all photons, are not particles and have no rest mass.

B4. A–iii; I and 33 keV; **B–i;** O and 0.5 keV; **C–ii;** Ca and 4 keV; **D–iv;** W and 70 keV. Note that the K-shell binding energy always increases with atomic number Z.

B5. A–iii; the resonance frequency for protons at 1 T is 42 MHz, which corresponds to a wavelength of 7 m, which is in the radiofrequency region of the electromagnetic spectrum; **B–ii;** diagnostic x-rays are high frequency electromagnetic radiation with energy in the range of 20 to 150 keV; **C–i;** light photons have an energy in the range 1 eV (red) to 3 eV (blue); **D–iv;** this is in the form of heat; as bodies get hotter, the photon energy increases; **E–v;** gamma rays are used in nuclear medicine.

B6–C. Ionization occurs when electrons are ejected from a neutral atom leaving behind a positively charged atom.

B7. A–iv; isomers refer to excited energy levels of the given nucleus; **B–i;** isobars have the same mass number; **C–iii;** isotones have the same number of neutrons; **D–ii;** isotopes have the same number of protons.

B8–E. All of the statements are true.

B9–A. X-rays are generally produced by electrons, whereas gamma rays are generated in nuclear processes. All of the physical properties of x-rays and gamma rays are *identical*.

B10–E. None are correct. For the same kVp, the three-phase generator has the same maximum energy, more photons, and a higher HVL.

B11–E. Tube kVp determines the maximum energy of electrons striking the anode and therefore the maximum x-ray photon energy that can be produced in a bremsstrahlung process.

B12. A–iii; Mo and 19.6 keV; **B–iv;** I and 32.3 keV; **C–ii;** W and 67.2 keV; **D–i;** Pb and 84.9 keV. The characteristic x-ray energy increases with Z and is a little less than the corresponding atomic K-shell binding energy.

B13–C. Multiformat cameras are used to produce film images of video displays. Pinhole and slit cameras measure focal spot dimensions directly. Star and parallel bar phantoms measure the loss of spatial resolution due to the finite size of the focal spot.

B14–D. All are generally true.

B15–C. Reduced to 1/3. The mAs should be kept constant to maintain the same film density.

B16. A–True; output increases approximately as kV^2; **B–False;** output depends on anode Z, but not heat capacity per se; **C–True;** output is approximately proportional to Z; **D–True;** output is directly proportional to tube current; **E–False;** filters increase the average photon energy but reduce the tube output; **F–False;** x-ray production is independent of anode rotation speed whose purpose is to spread anode heat loading.

B17–C. Leakage radiation.

B18–E. None of the statements are true. Coherent scatter is the result of x-rays that have changed direction but deposit energy in the patient.

B19–B. Energy will be deposited and produce a large number of ionizations as the photoelectron loses energy.

B20. A–False; scattered photons have less energy and therefore lower frequencies and longer wavelengths; **B–True;** photoelectric effect; **C–True; D–True;** coherent scatter.

B21–A. Compton scatter is the major interaction in fluoroscopy which results in backscattered x-rays.

B22–C. Pair production has a threshold energy of 1.022 MeV, which is much greater than that used in diagnostic radiology.

B23–E. All of the given values are reasonable for the transmission of primary x-ray beams for an average patient (there will also be scattered radiation).

B24–E. All of these statements are generally true.

B25. A–False; patient entrance skin exposure is reduced as the effective energy is increased; **B–True; C–False;** higher effective energy levels reduce subject contrast; **D–True;** requires a higher mAs because the filter reduces the beam intensity; **E–True;** because the tube output must be increased, the anode loading must increase.

B26–D. The regulatory minimum HVL is 2.5 mm Al at 80 kVp and 3 mm would be a typical value. The HVL should not be confused with the filtration, which is the actual amount of Al added at the x-ray tube to increase the HVL.

B27–A. The LET determines the radiation quality.

B28–D. Exposure is ionization by photons per unit mass in air, whereas absorbed dose is the energy absorbed per unit mass.

B29–D. The f-factor (rad/R) is about 3 for bones and about 1.0 for soft tissues at diagnostic x-ray energies.

B30. A–iii; B–i; C–iv; D–ii; 1 gray = 100 rad; 1 sievert = 100 rem; 1 R = 2.58×10^{-4} C/kg; 1 C = 3.7×10^{10} Bq.

B31–B. Photometers are used to measure the illuminance level (lux) in a room or brightness levels (cd/m^2) of a viewbox or display screen. Densitometers are used to measure the optical density of film.

B32–A. Fog will reduce image contrast, and this will be most marked at low film densities.

B33–A. A thicker crystal will stop more photons and thereby increase the absorption efficiency.

B34. A–iii; CR imaging plates use photostimulable phosphors that store x-ray energy as trapped electrons and release light when stimulated with a laser scanner; **B–iv;** photomultiplier tubes absorb light and emit electrons; **C–i;** scintillation crystals such as NaI absorb gamma rays and emit light; **D–ii;** screens absorb x-rays and convert between 5% and 20% of this energy into light.

B35–E. Bremsstrahlung is produced when electrons interact with matter.

B36–E. Because less radiation is required, all the items listed will be reduced.

B37–D. Modern rare earth screens are normally much faster (commonly rated as 400 speed) than calcium tungstate (commonly rated as 100 speed).

B38. A–iii; single screens and emulsions are used to achieve high spatial resolution by minimizing blur; **B–i;** chest radiographs require wide latitude; **C–v;** in CT, films are printed using lasers that only use single emulsions; **D–iv;** the limited penetration requires the use of relatively fast systems with no special requirements for spatial resolution; **E–ii;** xeroradiography uses selenium photoconductors as the detection medium, which require a special powder development process to visualize the latent image.

B39–D. Geometric unsharpness will not be affected by the introduction of a Bucky grid.

B40–A. Grids remove scatter and therefore improve image contrast.

B41–E. Reducing screen speed (use of thinner screens) will reduce screen blur. Note that there is no focal spot blur in *contact* radiography because there is no magnification.

B42–A. Doubling the mA will double the exposure rate and require only half the exposure time to give the required film density.

B43. A–i; DSA exposure times are very short; **B–iii;** a typical abdomen is 23 cm thick and longer exposures are required to adequately expose the film; **C–ii;** the exposure time should be short enough to minimize heart motion; **D–iv;** mammography exposure times are generally longer because of the low photon energy levels used and the low x-ray tube outputs for Mo targets operated at 28 kVp.

B44–A. Subject contrast is determined by the x-ray beam (kVp and filtration) and the tissue characteristic (atomic number, density, and thickness), and is independent of the choice of screen/film combination.

B45. A–iv; B–iii; C–ii; D–i.

B46–D. Focal spot size normally does not affect the entrance skin exposure.

B47–B. Doubling the kVp would increase the screen/film exposure by much more than a factor of two.

B48–A. Decreasing kVp always increases subject contrast. Changes in screen/film combination and film processing affect *image* contrast but do not affect the *subject* contrast.

B49–B. Input phosphor thickness is the primary determinant of the blur associated with the image intensifier. The TV camera will affect fluoroscopic performance, but not the II itself.

B50–E. The minification gain is the ratio of the input area to the output area, or $(12:1)^2$.

B51–D. The II potential is in the range of 25,000 to 30,000 volts and is direct current, not alternating current.

B52–B. 1 mR/s. A typical II conversion factor is 100 cd/m^2 per mR/s.

B53–D. 35 mm film is used at about 30 frames per second using small II sizes to improve resolution to about 3 line pairs per mm in the cardiac region. The *typical II exposure rate* is about 30 µR per frame, which corresponds to a patient dose over 100 times higher.

B54. A–True; B–False; C–False; D–True. In exact framing, the entire circular II image is recorded and only 80% of the film is used. In overframing, the II image is magnified so that the entire film is used, but only 64% of the image is recorded.

B55. A–ii; B–iii; C–iv; D–i.

B56. A–iii; B–i; C–ii.

B57. A–ii; B–iii; C–i.

B58–E. None of the answers are correct; with 8 bits per pixel, the maximum number of gray levels is 2^8 or 256.

B59–A. COBOL is a programming language, not an input/output device.

B60. A–v; CR is 2 k^2; **B–i;** nuclear medicine is usually 64^2 or 128^2; **C–iii;** CT is generally 512^2; **D–ii;** 128 × 256 to 256^2 are common MR matrix sizes; **E–iv;** most current DSA is 1 k^2.

B61–D. CT can differentiate between two adjacent tissues that differ in attenuation properties by as little as 5 HU (i.e., 0.5% difference), and thus has excellent contrast discrimination.

B62–D. +50. HU is $1000 \times (\mu - \mu_w)/\mu_w$, where μ is the attenuation coefficient of the material and μ_w is that of water.

B63–B. Iodinated contrast has a high atomic number (Z = 53 for iodine), which increases x-ray absorption and the attenuation coefficient and, therefore, the computed HU value.

B64–B. Increasing the matrix size will reduce the pixel size and thereby improve spatial resolution.

B65–E. All are possible reasons for missing a small (low contrast) tumor. Thick sections contribute to volume averaging; window settings affect displayed contrast; a large table index may result in the lesion falling between sections; and a bone reconstruction algorithm will increase image noise.

B66–A. Focal spot size affects spatial resolution, but all the other parameters affect image noise, which impacts the ability to detect low contrast objects.

B67–E. None of the doses listed are correct. Typical eye lens dose is approximately 40 mGy (4 rad).

B68. A–True; B–False; 1 curie = 3.7×10^{10} disintegrations per second; **C–True;** 1 g of ^{226}Ra produces 3.7×10^{10} disintegrations per second; **D–True; E–True**.

B69–D. ^{99m}Tc emits 140 keV photons. The daughter product (^{99}Tc) is radioactive, with a half-life of 210,000 years.

B70. A–iv; B–iii; C–i; D–ii.

B71. A–Transient; ^{99}Mo half-life is 67 hours, and ^{99m}Tc half-life is 6 hours; **B–Secular;** ^{82}Sr has a 25-day half-life, and ^{82}Rb has a half-life of 1.3 minutes; **C–Secular;** ^{113}Sn has a half-life of 120 days, and ^{113m}In has a half-life of 100 minutes.

B72. A–iv; ^{15}O is a positron emitter; **B–ii;** ^{99m}Tc at 140 keV; **C–iii;** ^{131}I at 365 keV; **D–i;** ^{201}Tl at 70 keV.

B73–B. Pulse pile-up occurs when two absorption events occur simultaneously and the total energy deposited in the crystal is summed as one event.

B74–D. Larger collimator holes allow more primary photons to pass through to the NaI crystal.

B75–C. The biological half-life is determined by biological clearance (i.e., no biological clearance corresponds to an infinite biological half-life).

B76. A–ii; B–iii; C–iv; D–i.

B77–E. All of the statements are true.

B78–B. The issue of room shielding for dispensing radiopharmaceuticals is irrelevant.

B79–C. Coincidence detection of two 511 keV annihilation photons is used in PET, which results in high count rates and short imaging times.

B80–C. Leukemia is a stochastic effect. All the other effects listed are deterministic and have a threshold dose below which the effect does not occur.

B81–A. Zero. The eye lens dose will be about 160 mGy (16 rad), which is below the threshold dose of 2 Gy (200 rad) for cataract induction.

B82. A–False; dose limits are set to prevent deterministic effects such as skin erythema; **B–True;** in the 1930s, genetic effects were considered the main risk, but in the last 30 years, the estimated cancer risks have increased and the genetic risks decreased; **C–True;** the latent period is shorter for leukemia (a few years) than for solid cancers (5- to 20-year latent period); **D–True;** ICRP, UNSCEAR, and BEIR all publish radiation risk estimates, but uncertainties in these risk estimates at low occupational exposure levels are very large and much debated; **E–True;** this is the best estimate of the radiation risk currently available from groups such as the ICRP, UNSCEAR, and BEIR.

B83–C. Higher grid ratios *increase* the patient dose. The other factors listed reduce patient doses.

B84–E. All will reduce the patient skin dose.

B85–E. None of the statements are true. ESE values are a few R per minute. The legal maximum is 10 R/min, but may be exceeded if a high dose option is used, or if the image is being recorded. Doubling the distance from the patient will reduce the scatter exposure rate by a factor of four.

B86. A–iii; B–iv; C–ii; D–i.

B87–C. It is only Compton scattered photons that have a significant probability of reaching the operator.

B88–E. The average US citizen receives an average annual exposure, including medical exposures, of about 3.6 mSv (360 mrem) per year. The additional dose to a person living in Leadville, as a result of both the elevation (higher cosmic background) and living in the Colorado plateau (higher external background), would result in an average annual dose > 4 mSv (400 mrem) per year.

B89–D. There is no significant risk of skin irradiation by beta particles.

B90–D. Acoustic impedance is the product of the velocity of sound and the density. For air, both velocity of sound and density are low; therefore, the acoustic impedance of air is very low.

B91. A–ii; B–iii; C–i.

B92–D. The echo strengh is not determined by the frequency per se, and the echo intensity will be lower at higher frequencies due to increased tissue attenuation.

B93–C. As in the case of light, the angle of reflection is equal to the angle of incidence.

B94–B. The crystal thickness (t) is generally one half the wavelength (λ) and thus determines the resultant transducer frequency ($f = v/\lambda = v/(2 \times t)$, where v is the speed of sound in the crystal.

B95–E. Low Q transducers have a wide band of ultrasound frequencies, and they also have short pulses, a characteristic that improves axial resolution.

B96–D. Continuous wave Doppler does not provide spatial information, only frequency shifts, which are related to movement such as blood flow.

B97–B. 130 μs. The total distance travelled is 20 cm, and speed of travel is 1540 m/s; therefore, time is 0.2 m/1540 m/s, or 130 μs.

B98. A–ii; B–iii; C–iv; D–i.

B99–E. Cavitation is the creation and collapse of tiny bubbles, and only occurs at high ultrasound intensities.

B100–C. For any fixed angle, the ultrasound frequency shift is directly proportional to blood flow.

B101. A–iii; B–ii; C–i.

B102. A–False; B–True; C–False; D–False; E–True; F–True.

B103. A–iii; B–iv; C–i; D–ii.

B104–E. Resistive magnets dissipate large amounts of power in the coils and generally require water cooling. The practical upper magnetic field strength is about 0.5 T.

B105–B. Gradient coils permit the origin of the MR signal to be determined by superimposing small gradients (mT/m) on the large fixed field.

B106. A–False; these are light flashes induced by time-varying magnetic fields; **B–True; C–True; D–False;** applied RF can result in tissue heating; **E–False.**

B107–A. Reverberation echoes occur in ultrasound imaging, not in MRI.

B108–E. None of the answers are correct. A Fourier analysis decomposes the signal into its *frequency* components.

B109–D. EPI obtains the image from a single "excitation" by rapidly switching the gradients, and there is no repetition of a basic pulse sequence separated by a repetition time TR, as in SE or IR imaging sequences.

B110–C. The image reconstruction technique does not affect the signal-to-noise ratio.

B111–A. The frequency encoding gradient does not affect the image acquisiton time, but determines matrix size.

B112–D. Spectroscopy is commonly performed on the naturally occurring metabolites of ^{31}P.

B113. A–iv; adipose tissue has a low density; **B–iii; C–ii;** carcinoma is slightly more attenuating than fibroglandular tissue; **D–i;** the high atomic number of calcium results in a high attenuation coefficient.

B114–E. All of the listed statements are true.

B115–D. Increasing exposure time may result in film reciprocity law breakdown and hence require an increase in exposure to maintain film density. All other factors reduce the mean glandular breast dose.

B116–B. Xeroradiography has a wide latitude.

B117–D. The spatial resolution of MR (< 1 line pair/mm) is markedly inferior to that of screen/film (15 to 20 line pairs/mm).

B118–E. All of the listed statements are correct.

B119. A–iv; B–iii; C–ii; D–i; note that if the count is N, the standard deviation is given by $\sqrt{N}$ and the percentage standard deviation is $100/\sqrt{N}$.

B120. A–True; B–False; increasing the area under the ROC curve corresponds to improved imaging performance; **C–True; D–False;** an ideal performance would correspond to an area of 1.0; **E–True**.

Appendix—Units

I. Summary of SI and Non-SI Units for General Quantities

Quantity	SI Unit	Non-SI Unit
Length	meter (m)	centimeter (cm), foot
Mass	kilogram (kg)	gram (g), pound (lb), ton
Time	second (s)	minute (min), hour (h)
Electrical current	ampere (A)	electrostatic unit (ESU) per second (s)
Amount of substance	mole (mol)	-
Frequency	hertz (Hz)	revolutions per minute (rpm)
Force	newton (N)	dyne, poundal
Energy, work, heat	joule (J)	erg, dyne-cm, electron volt (eV), British thermal unit (BTU)
Power	watt (W)	erg/s, BTU/h
Electrical charge	coulomb (C)	ESU
Electrical potential	volt (V)	-
Magnetic field	tesla (T)	gauss (G)

II. Summary of Units for Radiologic Quantities

Quantity	SI Unit Equation	Non-SI Unit	SI to Non-SI Conversions	Non-SI to SI Conversions
Exposure $X = Q/M$	C/kg	roentgen ($1\ R = 2.58 \times 10^{-4}$ C/kg)	1 C/kg = 3876 R	$1\ R = 2.58 \times 10^{-4}$ C/kg
Absorbed dose $D = E/M$	gray (1 Gy = 1 J/kg)	rad (1 rad = 100 erg/g)	1 Gy = 100 rad 1 mGy = 100 mrad	1 rad = 10 mGy 1 mrad = 10 µGy
Dose equivalent $H = D \times QF$	sievert (1 Sv = 1 J/kg)	rem (1 rem = 100 ergs/g)	1 Sv = 100 rem 1 mSv = 100 mrem	1 rem = 10 mSv 1 mrem = 10 µSv
Effective dose equivalent $H_E = \Sigma_i H_i \times w_i$ (*ICRP 26 w_i* values)	sievert	rem	1 Sv = 100 rem 1 mSv = 100 mrem	1 rem = 10 mSv 1 mrem = 10 µSv
Effective dose $H_E = \Sigma_i H_i \times w_i$ (*ICRP 60 w_i* values)	sievert	rem	1 Sv = 100 rem 1 mSv = 100 mrem	1 rem = 10 mSv 1 mrem = 10 µSv
Activity	becquerel (1 Bq = 1/s)	curie ($1\ Ci = 3.7 \times 10^{10}$/s)	1 MBq = 27 µCi 1 GBq = 27 mCi	1 mCi = 37 MBq

III. Summary of Units for Photometric* Quantities

Quantity	SI Unit	Non-SI Unit	To Convert Non-SI Units to SI Units
Luminance[†] (light scattered or emitted by a surface)	cd/m^2 (nit)	foot-lamberts	1 cd/m^2 = foot-lamberts × 3.426
Illuminance[†] (light falling on a surface)	$lumen/m^2$ (lux)	foot-candles	1 $lumen/m^2$ = foot-candles × 10.76

*Photometric units take into account the spectral sensitivity of the eye; radiometric units, however, do not and may, therefore, be used outside the "visible" part of the electromagnetic spectrum.

[†]One lux falling on a perfectly diffusing surface with no absorption produces a luminance of $1/\pi$ cd/m^2.

IV. Approximate Luminance Values

Luminance (cd/m^2)	Viewing Conditions
> 10^7	Causes retinal damage
~3000	Average mammography viewbox
~1500	Standard viewbox
~600	Brightest commercial monitor display for use in radiology
60–200	Typical commercial monitor display brightness

V. Approximate Illuminance Values

Illuminance (lux)	Conditions
5000	Full daylight
500	Overcast day
100–500	Office illumination for reading text
20	X-ray reading room illumination
5	Twilight
0.1	Moonlight
0.001	Starlight

VI. Summary of Prefix Names and Magnitudes

Prefix Name	Symbol	Magnitude
exa	E	10^{18}
peta	P	10^{15}
tera	T	10^{12}
giga	G	10^{9}
mega	M	10^{6}
kilo	k	10^{3}
hecto	h	10^{2}
deca	da	10
deci	d	10^{-1}
centi	c	10^{-2}
milli	m	10^{-3}
micro	μ	10^{-6}
nano	n	10^{-9}
pico	p	10^{-12}
femto	f	10^{-15}
atto	a	10^{-18}

Glossary

90-degree pulse - in magnetic resonance, radio frequency pulse that rotates the equilibrium magnetization vector through 90 degrees

180-degree pulse - in magnetic resonance, radio frequency pulse that rotates the equilibrium magnetization vector through 180 degrees

A-mode ultrasound - displays echo strength versus time

absolute risk model - theory of cancer induction in which radiation induces a given number of cancers

absorbed dose - radiation energy absorbed per unit mass of a medium measured in gray or rad

acceleration - rate of change in velocity measured in meters per second per second (m/s^2)

acoustic impedance - product of density and the velocity of sound in a medium measured in Rayls

activity - number of nuclear transformations per unit of time measured in becquerels or curies

air gap - gap between a patient and imaging receptor used in magnification examinations that reduces scattered radiation that reaches the film

ALARA - **a**s **l**ow **a**s **r**easonably **a**chievable is the principle for minimizing all radiation exposures

algorithms - step by step computer protocols

aliasing - artifacts in imaging modalities (e.g., magnetic resonance and ultrasound) caused by under-sampling

alpha decay - emission of an alpha particle by a radionuclide

alpha particle - particle consisting of two neutrons and two protons emitted from the nucleus of a radioisotope

analog-to-digital convertor (ADC) - converts analog signals into digital values for subsequent use in a computer

anode - positive side of an electric circuit such as the x-ray tube anode that includes the target

antineutrino - particle with no rest mass and no electric charge emitted in beta minus decay

array processor - hard-wired computer component used for performing rapid calculations

atom - constituent of all matter consisting of a positively charged nucleus surrounded by a cloud of electrons

atomic mass unit (AMU) - one-twelfth of the mass of a carbon atom

atomic number (Z) - number of protons in the nucleus of an atom

attenuation coefficient (μ) - measure of the x-ray attenuating property of a material measured in cm^{-1}

Auger electron - electron (rather than characteristic x-ray) emitted by an excited (energetic) atom

automatic brightness control (ABC) - regulates x-ray tube output to maintain a constant brightness at image intensifier output

autotransformer - allows the number of windings included in the circuit to be increased or decreased to produce the output voltage needed

axial resolution - ability to separate two objects lying along the axis of the ultrasound beam

B-mode ultrasound - brightness mode that displays a cross-sectional image

background radiation - radiation exposures from naturally occurring radioactivity and extraterrestrial cosmic radiation

bandwidth - range of frequencies that can be satisfactorily processed by a system

beam hardening - increase in mean energy of a polychromatic x-ray beam as lower energy photons are preferentially absorbed

beam quality - penetrating ability of an x-ray beam, usually expressed as the aluminum thickness, which reduces beam intensity by 50%

becquerel - the SI unit of radioactivity (1 Bq = 1 disintegration per second)

BEIR - the United States National Academy of Sciences Committee on the **B**iological **E**ffects of **I**onizing **R**adiation

beta minus decay - nuclear process in which a neutron is converted to a proton with emission of an electron and antineutrino

beta particle - electron or positron emitted from a nucleus during beta decay

beta plus decay - nuclear process in which a proton is converted to a neutron with emission of a positron and neutrino

biological half-life - time required to biologically clear one-half of the amount of a stable material in an organ or tissue

bit - smallest unit of computer memory that holds one of two possible values, 0 or 1

blur - the "smeared out" image of an object produced by an imaging system

bremsstrahlung radiation - general or "braking radiation" x-rays produced when electrons lose energy

brightness gain - ratio of image brightness on an image intensifier output to brightness produced on the input phosphor

Bucky - moving grid

Bucky factor - ratio of incident to transmitted radiation for a given grid

byte - unit of computer memory equal to 8 bits

cathode - negative side of an x-ray tube containing the filament

characteristic curve - plot of film density against the logarithm of relative exposure, also known as a Hurter and Driffield (H and D) curve

characteristic radiation - x-ray photon of characteristic energy emitted from an atom when an inner shell vacancy is filled by an outer shell electron

chi-square test - nonparametric statistical test used to determine if the categorical information from two groups is equivalent or independent

coherent scatter - photon scattered by an atom without suffering any energy loss, also known as Raleigh scatter

collimation - restriction of an x-ray beam or gamma rays by use of attenuators

Compton interaction - photon interaction with an outer shell electron resulting in a scattered electron and photon of lower energy

contrast - difference in signal intensity between an object and the surrounding background

contrast improvement factor - ratio of image contrast levels obtained with, and without, the use of scatter reduction systems such as grids or air gaps

controlled area - area with potentially high exposure rates that must be supervised by a radiation safety officer

converging collimator - a collimator used to image small organs, resulting in a magnified image

conversion efficiency - the percentage of energy deposited into a screen that is converted into light photon energy

conversion factor - in image intensifiers, the light output (Cd/m^2) per input exposure rate (mR/s); usually about 100

computed radiography (CR) - digital radiography that uses photostimulable phosphor plates rather than screen/film systems

coulomb (C) - unit of electric charge

count density - used in nuclear medicine to specify the number of counts per unit area

coupling gel - material used to couple sodium iodine crystals to the photomultiplier tube in a gamma camera

cumulative activity - a measure of the total number of radioactive disintegrations obtained by integrating the activity over time (area under the curve of activity versus time)

curie (Ci) - the non-SI unit of activity ($1\ Ci = 3.7 \times 10^{10}$ disintegrations per second)

current - rate of flow of electric charge measured in amperes

cyclotron - charged particle accelerator used to make radioisotopes

decay constant (λ) - the rate of decay of radionuclides ($\lambda = 0.693/T_{1/2}$, where $T_{1/2}$ is the half-life)

densitometer - device used to measure optical density on film

deterministic effect - nonstochastic biological effect of radiation that has a threshold dose

digital - quantity specified by discrete numbers as opposed to being continuous (analog)

digital subtraction angiography (DSA) - imaging modality in which digital images made before and after the introduction of iodine contrast are digitally subtracted from each other

directly ionizing radiations - charged particles, such as electrons, protons, and alpha particles, which can directly ionize atoms

diverging collimator - collimator used to image large organs (e.g., lungs), resulting in a minified image

Doppler shift - change in ultrasound frequency with motion

dose - absorbed energy per unit mass, expressed in grays or rads

dose area product - product of the entrance skin dose and cross-sectional area of the x-ray beam

dose calibrator - ionization chamber used in nuclear medicine to measure the amount of radioactivity in a syringe before injection into the patient

dose equivalent - product of the absorbed dose and radiation quality factor expressed in sieverts (Sv) or rem

echo planar imaging (EPI) - fast MR imaging mode that can create images in as little as 50 ms

edge enhancement - enhancement of tissue margins achieved in xeroradiography or by using digital processing techniques

effective atomic number - average atomic number obtained from a weighted summation of the atomic constituents of a compound

effective dose (*E*) - conceptually similar to the effective dose equivalent but obtained using the *International Commission on Radiological Protection Publication 60* organ weighting factors

effective dose equivalent (*H*$_E$) - uniform whole-body dose that has the same radiation risk as a given dose distribution and obtained using the *International Commission on Radiological Protection Publication 26* organ weighting factors

effective half-life - half-life of a radioactive material in an organ that is also being cleared biologically

effective voltage - constant voltage that produces the equivalent x-ray spectrum as an applied waveform

electromagnetic force - force that results from stationary or moving charges and that holds atoms together

electromagnetic radiation - transverse wave in which electric and magnetic fields oscillate perpendicular to wave motion

electron - fundamental constituent of matter with 1/1836 of the mass of a proton and a negative charge

electron binding energy - energy that must be supplied to extract a bound atomic electron

electron capture - nuclear process in which a proton is converted to a neutron by capturing an electron and emitting a neutrino

electron traps - in solid-state devices, energy levels that may temporarily trap an electron

emulsion - layer of film that contains silver halide grains

energy - ability to do work measured in joules (J)

entrance skin exposure - x-ray exposure measured at the skin surface

ethernet - wiring or fiberoptic cable used to transmit digital data to distant computers, stores, or displays

exact framing - the entire circular image of an image intensifier is recorded on the film

excited state - any energy level above the lowest energy ground state in an atom or nucleus

exposure - measure of the ability of a source of x-rays to ionize air measured in coulombs per kilogram (C/kg) or roentgens (R)

extrinsic flood - gamma camera image obtained using a collimator of a uniform source of activity

f-factor - photon energy dependent factor used to convert exposures into absorbed dose for a specified absorbing medium

faraday cage - radio frequency shielding that normally consists of copper sheets built into the wall structures around a magnetic resonance scanner

fast spin echo - magnetic resonance imaging technique that uses multiple spin echoes to reduce imaging times in comparison to spin-echo imaging

ferromagnetic - material (e.g., iron and nickel) with large intrinsic magnetic fields produced by a regular array of unpaired atomic electrons in a domain

field uniformity - a measure of the uniformity of a nuclear medicine image obtained using a uniform (flood) source of activity

filament - wire on the cathode of an x-ray tube that emits electrons

film dosimetry (film badge) - film used to estimate the radiation dose obtained from a measure of film blackening

film gamma - the maximum gradient of a film characteristic curve

film latitude - the range of exposure levels over which the film may be used without being under- or overexposed

film mottle - random fluctuations in film density due to the granular nature of the emulsion

filter - thin plate, usually made of aluminum, placed in an x-ray beam to absorb unwanted low-energy x-rays

filtered back projection - computed tomography image reconstruction technique

flip angle - the angle through which the net magnetization vector is rotated by an applied radio frequency pulse

flux gain - number of light photons at the output phosphor of an image intensifier per light photon produced at the input phosphor

focal spot - area of anode where x-ray beam is produced

focusing cup - directs electrons leaving the x-ray tube filament

focused transducer - ultrasound transducer that can focus the beam using acoustical lenses

fog level - film blackening in the absence of radiation exposure

force - directed energy that can change the motion of a mass

Fourier analysis - analysis of time signals which identifies the individual frequencies and intensities of the signal

Fraunhofer zone - the far zone of an ultrasound beam where it diverges

free induction decay (FID) - decreasing magnetic resonance signal following a 90-degree frequency pulse caused by the dephasing of nuclear spins

frequency - the number of oscillations per second measured in hertz (1 Hz = 1 oscillation per second)

frequency encode gradient - magnetic field gradient applied during the acquisition (readout) of a free induction decay signal

Fresnel zone - near zone of an ultrasound beam used for imaging

fringe field - magnetic field at a distance from a magnet

full width half maximum (FWHM) - a measure of spatial resolution equal to the width of an image of a line source, defined at points where the intensity is reduced to one-half the maximum intensity

gamma camera - nuclear medicine imaging system that uses a scintillation crystal to detect gamma rays

gamma rays - high-frequency electromagnetic radiation produced by nuclear processes

Gaussian distribution - a bell-shaped statistical distribution that is symmetrical about the mean value and whose spread is characterized by the standard deviation σ

Geiger counter - ionization chamber with a high voltage resulting in amplified output following the detection of an ionizing particle (x-ray photon)

generator - produces radionuclides such as ^{99m}Tc in nuclear medicine

genetically significant dose (GSD) - a population dose indicator that estimates the genetic significance of radiation exposures by taking into account the child expectancy of exposed individuals

gradient - the average slope of a film characteristic curve, normally obtained between the film densities of 0.5 and 2.0

gradient coils - current-carrying coils in magnetic resonance that create small magnetic field gradients superimposed on the large stationary magnetic field

gradient recalled echo (GRE) - magnetic resonance spin-echo created using gradients rather than 180-degree rephasing radio frequency pulses

gravity - force responsible for attraction between all matter

gray (Gy) - the SI unit of absorbed dose (1 Gy = 1 J/kg)

grid - strips of lead in a radiolucent matrix used to reduce scattered radiation

grid line density - the number of grid lines per centimeter

grid ratio - ratio of height to separation gap of lead strips in a grid

ground state - lowest energy level of an atom or nucleus

gyromagnetic ratio (γ) - a value characteristic of any magnetic nucleus that determines the Larmor precession frequency, f_L, in a given magnetic field B ($\omega = 2\pi \times f_L = \gamma \times B$)

H and D (Hurter and Driffield) curve - characteristic curve of a film showing the relationship between exposure and optical film density

half-life (physical) - time for the activity of a radioisotope to decrease by a factor of 2

half-value layer (HVL) - thickness of specified material (e.g., aluminum) needed to reduce the x-ray beam intensity by 50%

heat unit (HU) - for single-phase x-ray units, the product of exposure time, peak voltage, and amperage (1 J = 1.35 HU)

heel effect - the x-ray intensity is greater at the cathode side and is lower at the anode side because of anode absorption

Helmholtz coils - coaxial coils used to generate a magnetic field gradient along the main axis of a cylindrical magnetic resonance scanner

Hounsfield unit (HU) - the attenuation coefficient of a material relative to that of water as used in computed tomography

ICRP (International Commission on Radiological Protection) - international radiation protection agency founded in 1928 that issues recommendations regarding radiation safety

image intensifier (II) - converts incident x-ray pattern to a light image that can be viewed, recorded, or photographed

incidence - the number of new cases of a disease each year

indirectly ionizing radiation - uncharged radiation that produces ionization by way of intermediate charged particles such as photoelectrons (for x-rays) and recoil protons (for neutrons)

integral dose - a measure of the total amount of energy imparted to a patient during a radiological examination

intensification factor - ratio of x-ray exposure without, and with, an intensifying screen to produce a given film density

intensifying screen - converts x-rays to light, producing many light photons for each absorbed x-ray photon

internal conversion - electron emitted from an atom in lieu of a gamma ray

intrinsic flood - gamma camera (without collimator) image obtained of a uniform source of activity

inverse square law - exposure decreases in proportion to the square of the distance from the source

inversion recovery (IR) - magnetic resonance pulse sequence designed to emphasize T1 differences

ionization - production of electrons and positive ions following the absorption of radiation energy

ionization chamber - gas chamber used to accurately determine radiation levels based on measurements of charge liberated in a given mass of gas (air)

ionizing radiation - radiation that can result in the ejection of electrons from atoms

isobar - nuclides with the same total number of neutrons and protons (mass number)

isomer - nuclides with an excited nuclear state

isometric state - metastable state that exists for more than 10^{-12} seconds

isotone - nuclides with the same number of neutrons

isotope - nuclides with the same number of protons

joule (J) - SI unit of energy

K-edge - binding energy of K-shell electrons

Kell factor - correction factor of about .7 used to calculate the actual vertical resolution on a television system based on the theoretical resolution

KERMA - (*k*inetic *e*nergy *r*eleased in the *m*edium) refers to the transfer of energy from uncharged to charged particles

kinetic energy - energy associated with motion

lag - afterglow of an image on a screen or television camera

Larmor frequency - precession frequency of a magnetic nucleus in an applied magnetic field

lateral resolution - ability to resolve two laterally adjacent objects with ultrasound

latitude - the range of exposures over which an image recording system can operate

law of transformers - the ratio of voltages in two linked coils is proportional to the number of turns in each coil

LD$_{50/60}$ - radiation dose that will kill 50% of the exposed population within 60 days

leakage radiation - the radiation emerging from an x-ray unit when the collimators are fully closed

limiting resolution - the highest spatial frequency resolved by an imaging system measured in line pairs per millimeter

line focus principle - result of viewing a sloped surface (x-ray tube anode) at an angle, thus reducing its apparent size

line spread function - image of a narrow line used as a measure of the blurring associated with any imaging system

line density - in ultrasound, the number of lines used to generate an image

linear attenuation coefficient - the fraction of photons lost from an x-ray beam in traveling a unit of distance measured in cm^{-1}

linear energy transfer (LET) - energy absorbed by the medium per unit of length traveled, measured in keV per μm

longitudinal magnetization - component of magnetization that is oriented parallel to the main magnetic field in a magnetic resonance scanner

luminance - the brightness of a light-emitting source such as a lightbox or computer monitor

M-mode ultrasound - displays depth versus time and permits motion to be observed

magnetic moment - strength of nuclear or electronic magnetism

magnetic susceptibility - the inherent property of a substance that modifies the local magnetic field when placed in a strong applied (external) field

mass - resistance to acceleration (inertia) of matter measured in kilograms (kg)

mass attenuation coefficient - linear attenuation coefficient divided by the physical density, measured in square centimeters per gram (cm^2/g)

mass number (A) - total number of nucleons (protons and neutrons) in the nucleus of an atom

matching layer - layer of material placed in front of an ultrasound transducer to improve the efficiency of energy transfer into a patient

matrix size - the number of pixels allocated to each linear dimension in a digital image

mean - the average value of any distribution of values

mean glandular dose (MGD) - the average dose to the glandular breast tissue from an x-ray procedure

median - value of a statistical distribution where half the distribution is higher and half is lower

metastable state - transient unstable energy state of an atom with a half-life exceeding 10^{-12} seconds

minification gain - ratio of the area of the image intensifier input to output

mode - the value of a distribution with the highest frequency

modulation transfer function (MTF) - ratio of output to input contrast amplitude plotted as a function of spatial frequency

mole - measure of the amount of substance (number of atoms), where 1 gram mole is about 6×10^{23} atoms

monochromatic radiation - radiation in which all photons have the same energy

negative predictive value - probability of not having a disease given a negative diagnostic test result

neutrino - particle with no rest mass and no charge that is emitted during beta plus decay and in electron capture processes

neutrons - uncharged particles found in the atomic nucleus

noise - random fluctuations in image intensity for the same nominal input exposure

nonoccupational exposure - exposure of members of the public as opposed to radiation workers

nonspecular reflection - diffuse ultrasound reflections (scatter) that occur at irregular (rough) surfaces

nonstochastic effects - radiation effects such as epilation that do not occur below a threshold (also called deterministic effects)

NRC (Nuclear Regulatory Commission) - United States federal agency ultimately responsible for regulating nuclear materials

nucleon - neutron or proton

nuclides - nuclei with differing numbers of protons or neutrons

occupational dose limit - regulatory dose limits applied to radiation workers

OID - object to image distance

operating system - software program used by computers for housekeeping functions such as copying files

optical density - measure of the degree of film blackening using a logarithmic scale

optical disk - large capacity digital data storage device used to store digital radiographic images

overframing - capturing a circular image intensifier image with a square film frame with the square circumscribed by the circle

***p* value** - a number representing the probability that a given result occurred by chance

PACS (picture archiving and communications system) - system in which a radiology department replaces film with digital images

pair production - an electron and positron pair produced in an atomic nucleus by a high-energy photon (> 1.022 MeV)

paramagnetism - substance with a positive susceptibility, which enhances the local magnetic field due to the presence of unpaired atomic electrons (e.g., gadolinium chelates)

parametric test - statistical test, such as the t-test, which makes assumptions regarding how the results are distributed

partial volume artifact - an artifact caused by a mixture of tissues with two different attenuation coefficients within any given voxel

penumbra - geometric unsharpness caused by focal spot size

phase encode gradient - magnetic resonance gradient applied perpendicular to the frequency encode gradient and before the free induction decay readout gradient and applied in the perpendicular direction within the excited section

photodisintegration - disintegration of a nucleus after absorbing a high-energy photon (greater than 15 MeV)

photoelectric effect - a photon is absorbed by an atom and a photoelectron is emitted

photomultiplier tube - converts light into an electric signal

photons - bundle of electromagnetic radiation that can behave like a particle and has an energy proportional to frequency

photopeak - signal produced in a gamma camera crystal as a result of a photoelectric interaction in which all the incident gamma ray energy is absorbed by the crystal

photospot film - small film produced by photographing the image intensifier output

photostimulable phosphor - barium fluorohalide material used to capture radiographic images in computed radiography systems

piezoelectric effect - conversion of electric energy into mechanical motion (and vice versa)

pin cushion distortion - linear distortion due to increased magnification of the periphery associated with all image intensifiers

pinhole collimator - collimator used in nuclear medicine for high-resolution images of small structures

pixel - picture element comprising the smallest component of a digital image

Poisson distribution - random distribution in which the variance is equal to the mean value

positive predictive value - probability of having a disease given a positive diagnostic test result

positron emission tomography (PET) - nuclear medicine imaging modality that detects the annihilation radiation (511 keV gamma) of positron emitters such as ^{15}O

positrons - particles identical to electrons but with a positive electric charge

potential energy - energy associated with the location of a particle at a high-energy potential, such as an electron at a cathode

power - rate of doing work measured in watts (W)

prevalence - the total number of existing disease cases in a population

primary transmission - the fraction of the primary x-ray beam, excluding scatter, that penetrates a patient or a grid

protons - positively charged particle found in the nucleus

pulse repetition frequency (PRF) - the number of ultrasound pulses generated by the transducer each second

pulse sequence - sequence of radio frequency pulses and magnetic gradients used to generate a magnetic resonance image

Q-factor - determines the purity of an ultrasound pulse; high Q values correspond to pure frequencies and vice versa

quality factor (QF) - determined from the linear energy transfer (LET) value of each type of radiation and used to convert absorbed dose into dose equivalent

quantum mottle - image noise caused by the discrete nature of x-ray photons

quenching gases - gases added to Gieger counters and ionization chambers to minimize electronic discharges

rad - stands for "radiation absorbed dose," which is a non-SI unit of absorbed dose (1 rad = 100 erg/g)

radiographic mottle - random density fluctuations (noise) observed in an image after a uniform exposure

radiochemical purity - a measure of chemical impurity; usually checked using thin layer chromatography

radioisotopes - atoms with unstable nuclei

radionuclide - an unstable nuclide that decays exponentially

radionuclide purity - a measure of radioactive contaminants (other radionuclides)

radiopharmaceutical - chemical or pharmaceutical that is labelled with a radionuclide

radon (^{222}Ra) - radioactive gas produced when naturally occurring radium (^{226}Ra) decays; found at high levels in some home basements

random access memory (RAM) - volatile computer memory that loses information when the computer power supply is switched off

range - distance traveled by an energetic charged particle, such as an electron, before losing all of its energy

rare earth screen - radiographic screen containing rare earth elements

read only memory (ROM) - permanent memory in computers

real time ultrasound imaging - cross-sectional image updated 20 to 40 times per second, allowing motion to be followed

receiver operating characterisitic (ROC) curve - plot of the true-positive fraction versus false-positive fraction used to evaluate imaging performance

reciprocating grid - a grid that moves during a radiographic exposure and smears out the grid lines in the resultant image; also known as a Bucky

reconstruction algorithm - a set of mathematical rules for reconstructing an image from projection data

rectification - changing an alternating voltage into one that retains a selected polarity (AC to DC)

refraction - change of direction of any wave when moving from one medium to another

relative risk model - theory of cancer induction in which radiation exposure increases the natural incidence by a fixed percentage

rem - stands for "radiation equivalent man;" non-SI unit of dose equivalent

reverberation - artifact in ultrasound caused by multiple echoes from parallel tissue interfaces

ring artifact - artifact resembling a ring produced by a defective detector in third-generation computed tomography and single photon emission computed tomography

ring down time - the time an ultrasound transducer requires for a generated pulse intensity to be reduced to a negligible value

roentgen (R) - unit of exposure that measures charge liberated in air

SID - source-to-image distance

scatter - radiation deflected from its initial direction

scintillator - material that emits light after absorption of radiation

screen mottle - random fluctuations in image density produced because of imperfections and variations in screen thickness

screen unsharpness - blur caused by light diffusion within the intensifying screens

secondary radiation - radiation such as characteristic x-rays produced as a result of the absorption of primary radiation

self-rectification - a reference to the fact that electrons cannot flow from the anode to the cathode in an x-ray tube

sensitivity - the ability of a test to detect disease

septal penetration - gamma rays that penetrate the collimator septa

shim coils - current-carrying coils used in magnetic resonance magnets to improve the magnetic field homogeneity

signal-to-noise ratio (SNR) - used in imaging to measure the ratio of signal intensity to the image noise level

solid-state material - one of the three states of atomic matter, with the other two being liquid and gas

space charge - result of an electron cloud around the filament in an x-ray tube

spatial frequency - alternate physical regions of oscillating signal intensity expressed in line pairs or cycles per millimeter

spatial peak pulse average (SPPA) - ultrasound intensity obtained at a single point and averaged over a single ultrasound pulse

spatial peak temporal average (SPTA) - ultrasound intensity obtained at a single point and averaged over many pulses

spatial resolution - ability to discriminate between two adjacent high-contrast objects

specificity - the ability to identify the absence of disease

SPECT (single photon emission computed tomography) - nuclear medicine tomographic imaging technique achieved by rotating a gamma camera around a patient

spectroscopy - magnetic resonance mode that yields an analysis of the chemical species present in a given volume such as ^{31}P, which may be present as adenosine triphosphate, inorganic phosphor, and so on

specular reflection - ultrasound reflections from large smooth surfaces

spin echo (SE) imaging - magnetic resonance imaging pulse sequence in which echoes are generated by rephasing spins in the transverse plane using radio frequency pulses or magnetic field gradients

standard deviation - a measure of the spread of a statistical distribution

stochastic effect - radiation effect, including carcinogenesis and genetic effects, that occurs at a rate proportional to dose

streak artifacts - artifacts seen in computed tomography that may be caused by patient motion or metallic implants

strong force - holds the nucleus of an atom together

subject contrast - difference in x-ray beam intensities emerging from an object

superconducting - property of certain conductors of having zero electrical resistance when cooled to very low temperatures

superparamagnetism - magnetic property similar to ferromagnetism but occurring in small aggregates of atoms (single domains)

T1 - spin lattice or longitudinal relaxation time

T2 - spin–spin or transverse relaxation time

T2* - rapid reduction of free induction decay signals due to spin dephasing as a result of magnetic field inhomogeneities

t-test - parametric statistical test to evaluate whether a given experimental result could have occurred by chance

TE (echo time) - time from the initial 90-degree radio frequency pulse to the echo signal in magnetic resonance spin-echo sequences

tenth-value layer (TVL) - thickness of material needed to reduce an x-ray beam intensity to 10% of its initial value

thermoluminescent dosimeter (TLD) - solid-state device that, after x-ray exposure, emits light when heated

threshold dose - dose below which deterministic effects do not occur

TI - time to inversion or the time interval between the initial 180-degree pulse and subsequent 90-degree radio frequency pulse in an inversion recovery pulse sequence

time gain compensation (TGC) - used in ultrasound to correct for increased attenuation of sound with tissue depth

TR - repetion time in magnetic resonance pulse sequences, corresponding to the time interval before the basic pulse sequence is repeated

transducer - device that converts mechanical energy into electric current and vice versa

transformer - device used to increase or decrease voltages

transient equilibrium - equilibrium between the parent and daughter radionuclides in which the parent half-life is relatively short

transmittance - the fraction of light transmitted by an exposed radiographic film

transverse magnetization - magnetization vector oriented in a plane perpendicular to the main external magnetic field in magnetic resonance

velocity - rate of change of position in a specified direction

vignetting - peripheral reduction of light intensity in image intensifiers

voltage - electrical potential difference

voxel - volume element obtained from the product of pixel size and the image section thickness

wavelength - the distance between two consecutive crests of a wave

weak forces - account for beta decay processes

weight - gravitational attractive force due to gravity

window width and center - method for displaying digital images; determines the allocation of stored image data to shades of white, black, and gray in the displayed image

word - unit of computer memory equal to 2 bytes (or 16 bits)

work - product of force and distance, measured in joules

x-rays - high-frequency (energetic) electromagnetic radiation produced using electrons

xeroradiography - imaging modality based on selenium photoconducting detectors

Bibliography

General Radiologic Imaging (Residents)

Bushberg JT, Seibert AJ, Leidhodt EM Jr, Boone JM: *The Essential Physics of Medical Imaging*. Baltimore, Williams & Wilkins, 1994.

Curry TS, Dowdey JE, Murray RC Jr: *Christensen's Physics of Diagnostic Radiology*, 4th ed. Philadelphia, Lea & Febiger, 1990.

Hendee WR, Ritenour R: *Medical Imaging Physics*, 3rd ed. St. Louis, Year Book, 1992.

Sprawls P Jr: *Physical Principles of Medical Imaging*, 2nd ed. Gaithersburg, MD, Aspen, 1993.

Wolbarst AB: *Physics of Radiology*. Norwalk, CT, Appleton & Lange, 1993.

General Radiologic Imaging (Technologists)

Bushong SC: *Radiologic Science for Technologists*, 5th ed. St. Louis, CV Mosby, 1993.

Graham BJ, Thomas WN: *An Introduction to Physics for Radiologic Technologists*. Philadelphia, WB Saunders, 1975.

Kelsey CA: *Essentials of Radiology Physics*. Warren Green Inc. St. Louis, Warren Green, 1985.

Malott JC, Fodor J III: *The Art and Science of Medical Radiography*. St. Louis, CV Mosby, 1993.

Selman J: *The Fundamentals of X-ray and Radium Physics*, 7th ed. Springfield, IL, Charles C. Thomas, 1985.

Nuclear Medicine

Chandra R: *Introductory Physics of Nuclear Medicine,* 4th ed. Philadelphia, Lea & Febiger, 1992.

Mettler FA, Guibertean MJ: *Essentials of Nuclear Medicine Imaging*, 3rd ed. Philadelphia, WB Saunders, 1991.

Sorensen JA, Phelps ME: *Physics in Nuclear Medicine*, 2nd ed. Orlando, Grune and Stratton, 1987.

Radiobiology and Radiation Protection

Hall EJ: *Radiobiology for the Radiologist*, 4th ed. Philadelphia, JB Lippincott, 1993.

National Council on Radiation Protection and Measurements (NCRP) Report No. 91: *Recommendations on Limits for Exposure to Ionizing Radiation*. Washington, DC, National Council on Radiation Protection and Measurements, 1987.

National Council on Radiation Protection and Measurements (NCRP) Report No. 100: *Exposure of the US Population from Diagnostic Medical Radiation.* Washington, DC, National Council on Radiation Protection and Measurements, 1989.

Pizarello DJ, Witcofski RL: *Medical Radiation Biology*, 2nd ed. Philadelphia, Lea & Febiger, 1982.

Ultrasound

Fish P: *Physics and Instrumentation of Diagnostic Medical Ultrasound.* Chichester, John Wiley, 1990.

Smith H, Zagzebski J: *Basic Doppler Physics.* Madison, Medical Physics Publishing, 1991.

Wells PNT: *Biomedical Ultrasonics.* London, Academic Press, 1977.

Magnetic Resonance

Andrew ER, Bydder G, Griffiths J, et al: *Clinical Magnetic Resonance Imaging and Spectroscopy.* Chichester, John Wiley, 1990.

Lufkin RB: *The MRI Manual.* Chicago, Year Book, 1990.

Smith HJ, Ranallo FN: *A Non-Mathematical Approach to Basic MRI.* Madison, Medical Physics Publishing Corporation, 1989.

Breast Imaging

Haus AG, Yaffe MJ (eds): *Syllabus: A Categorical Course in Physics, Technical Aspects of Breast Imaging.* Presented at the 78th Radiological Society of North America (RSNA), Oak Brook, IL, 1993.

National Council of Radiation Protection and Measurements (NCRP) Report No. 85: *Mammography - A User's Guide.* Bethesda, MD, National Council of Radiation Protection and Measurements, 1986.

Examination Review Books

Carlton RR: *Radiography Exam Review.* Philadelphia, JB Lippincott, 1993.

Cummings GR, Meixner E: *Corectec's Comprehensive Set of Review Questions for Radiography*, 3rd ed. Corectec, 1993.

Leonard WL: *Examination Review: Radiography.* Norwalk, CT, Appleton & Lange, 1991.

Saia DA: *Appleton and Lange's Review for the Radiography Examination*, 2nd ed. Norwalk, CT, Appleton & Lange, 1993.

Odwin CS, Bubinsky T, Fleischer AC: *Appleton and Lange's Review for the Ultrasonography Examination*, 2nd ed. Norwalk, CT, Appleton & Lange, 1993.

Phlipot D, Carlton RR, McLaughlin MJ, et al: *Mammography Exam Review.* Philadelphia, JB Lippincott, 1992.

Index